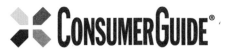

1,001
Amazing
Home
Remedies
& Cures

Linnea Lundgren

Michele Mann

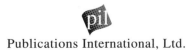

Publications International, Ltd.

Linnea Lundgren has ten years' experience researching, writing, and editing for newspapers and magazines. She is the author of four books, including *Living Well with Allergies.*

Michele Mann has written numerous magazine articles and books on health- and fitness-related topics. Her favorite way to stay healthy is enjoying the country life with her husband and four children.

Cover illustration by **Kurt Pfaff**.
Interior illustrations by **Jeff Moores**.

Facts verified by Alice Lesch Kelly and Timothy Gower.

Acknowledgments:
Page 16 (sage), 54 (lemon juice, cumin, ginger), 55 (peppermint), 118 (orange juice), 173 (basil), 183 (lemon), 201 (cumin), 230 (papaya): Adapted with permission from *The Complete Book of Ayurvedic Home Remedies* by Vasant D. Lad, 1998, Harmony Books, New York. Page 416 (tooth eruption chart): ©American Dental Association. Used with permission. All rights reserved.

Louis Weber, CEO
Publications International, Ltd.
7373 North Cicero Avenue
Lincolnwood, Illinois 60712

Permission is never granted for commercial purposes.

ISBN-13: 978-1-4127-3881-1
ISBN-10: 1-4127-3881-4

Manufactured in Canada.

8 7 6 5 4 3 2 1

Library of Congress Control Number: 2009932727

Contents

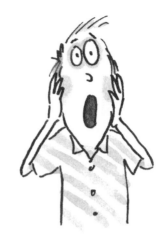

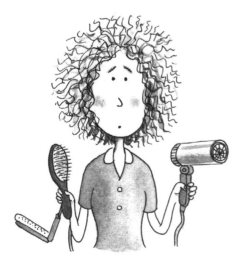

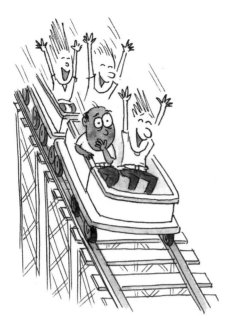

Introduction

These days, we're bombarded by advertisements for prescription and over-the-counter medications. There's a drug for every symptom and every condition—and then some! The constant promotion would have you believe that medications are our only treatment options.

But there are simple solutions to everyday problems, using common products that are sitting on your shelves, in your cabinets, and even in your refrigerator. Many of these are time-tested remedies that your great-grandparents used often. Others are more recent discoveries, based on the latest scientific information.

1,001 Amazing Home Remedies & Cures is your antidote to the skyrocketing costs of medications and doctor visits. It's always on call, ready to help with more than 90 health issues. You'll find a wealth of inexpensive ways to ease discomfort, treat ailments, and even prevent problems.

Each profile gives a short explanation of the causes and symptoms of the condition, then provides remedies categorized by type. There are dietary remedies, herbal remedies, lifestyle remedies, and more. The profiles also tell you when to forgo home remedies and seek professional medical intervention. As an extra bonus, *1,001 Amazing Home Remedies & Cures* is also brimming with fascinating facts, enlightening statistics, and unusual stories.

With *1,001 Amazing Home Remedies & Cures* on your bookshelf, you'll have both Great-Grandma and the doctor in residence. Consult their wisdom for all your health-related concerns.

Allergies
BREATHING EASIER

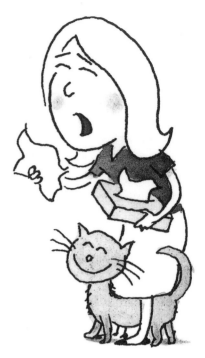

Every March, like clockwork, Mark O'Connor's nose begins to run. He sniffles and wipes, and his nasal passages become stuffy. Miserable, he's certain he has a cold. But his symptoms don't follow the usual trajectory of an illness—they don't get worse, and they don't get better…for weeks.

Mark's son Jason gets red-eyed every June. When the trees bloom green, the whites of his eyes turn the color of an autumnal maple. His eyes itch, and he can't help rubbing them, which further inflames them and sometimes causes an infection.

Mark and Jason, along with approximately 40 million Americans, have seasonal allergies. But there are many other types of allergies, including animal allergy, food allergy, dust-mite allergy, and insect-sting allergy. Allergies can be called a haywire response of the immune system, which guards against intruders it considers harmful to the body, such as certain viruses and bacteria. In allergic people, however, the immune system goes a bit bonkers. It overreacts when you breathe, ingest, or touch a harmless substance. The benign culprits that trigger the overreaction, such as dust, pet dander, and pollen, are called allergens.

The body's first line of defense against invaders includes the nose, mouth, eyes, lungs, and stomach. When the immune system reacts to an allergen, it causes an inflammatory response in these battleground body parts. It releases chemicals that cause runny nose; sneezing; watery, swollen, or red eyes; nasal congestion; wheezing; shortness of breath; a tight feeling in the chest; difficulty breathing; coughing; diarrhea; nausea; headache; fatigue; and a general feeling of misery. Symptoms can occur alone or in combination and can range from mild to severe.

What Causes Allergies?

Blame your genes. The tendency to become allergic is inherited, and allergies typically develop before age 30. Children with two allergic parents have a 70 percent chance of developing allergies, while children with one allergic parent have a 33 percent chance, according to the Asthma and Allergy Foundation of America. The inherited predisposition doesn't mean you'll develop the same kind of allergy as your predecessors, however. What you become allergic to is based on the substances you are exposed to and how often you are exposed to them. Generally, the more often you encounter the allergen, the more likely it is to trigger a reaction and the greater your reaction will be.

Although allergies cannot be cured, there are plenty of ways to diminish symptoms. Allergies should be properly diagnosed by a medical doctor, particularly an allergy specialist, to avoid the inappropriate use of medications or other remedies. Many mild allergies, however, can be eased without drugs—or by a combination of self care and pharmaceutical treatments.

Dietary Remedies

Wasabi. If you're a hay fever sufferer and sushi lover, this remedy will please. Wasabi, that pale-green, fiery condiment served alongside California rolls, is a member of the horseradish family. Anyone who has taken too big a dollop of wasabi or plain old horseradish knows how it makes sinuses and tear ducts spring into action. That's because allyl isothiocyanate, a constituent in wasabi, promotes phlegm flow and has anti-asthmatic properties. The tastiest way to get in

Ach-Choo! God Bless You!

Pope Gregory the Great gets bragging rights on coining the phrase "God bless you" after a sneeze. During his reign in the 6th century, a plague ravaged the region. He insisted on a quick prayer as a response to the very contagious sneeze.

Sneeze and the World Sneezes with You

When it comes to allergies, take comfort in the fact that you aren't alone in your misery. An estimated 50 million Americans— that's one out of every five people—suffers from all types of allergies, including indoor/outdoor (seasonal), food and drug, latex, insect, skin, and eye allergies. It's the fifth leading chronic disease in the United States, among all age groups.

SPEEDY SNEEZES

Blink and you just might miss that sneeze. Sneezing, a reflex beyond your control, is caused by the irritation of nerve endings in the nose and mucous membranes. A sneeze can whip out at 100 miles per hour—quicker than you can grab a tissue to catch it. Also, your eyes naturally close when one approaches, so yes, you will blink and miss it.

those allyl isothiocyanates is by slathering horseradish on your sandwich or plopping wasabi onto your favorite sushi. A harder-to-swallow option is to purchase grated horseradish and take ¼ teaspoon during an allergy attack.

HERBAL REMEDIES

Basil. To help ease a topical allergic reaction or hives, try dousing the skin with basil tea, a traditional Chinese folk remedy. Basil contains high amounts of an antiallergic compound called caffeic acid. Place 1 ounce dried basil leaves into 1 quart boiling water. Cover and let cool to room temperature. Use the tea as a rinse as often as needed.

Mint tea. Allergy sufferers throughout the centuries have turned to hot tea to relieve clogged noses and irritated mucous membranes. Mint tea is one of the best for symptom relief. It's been used by the Chinese to treat allergies since the seventh century. Mint smells delicious, and its essential oils have decongestant properties. Substances in mint also contain anti-inflammatory and mild antibacterial constituents. To make mint tea, place ½ ounce dried mint leaves in a 1-quart jar. Fill two-thirds of the jar with boiling water and steep for five minutes (inhale the steam). Let cool, strain, sweeten if desired, and drink.

TOPICAL REMEDIES

Baking soda. One-half cup baking soda poured into a warm bath is an old New England folk remedy for soothing hives. Soak for 20 to 30 minutes.

Ice. Wrap a washcloth around ice cubes and apply them to your sinuses for instant relief and refreshment.

Milk. Milk does the body good, especially when it comes to hives. Wet a cloth with cold milk and lay it on the affected area for 10 to 15 minutes.

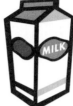

Salt. Nasal irrigation, an effective allergy-management tool that's done right at the sink every morning, uses a mixture of salt water to rid the nasal passages of mucus, bacteria, dust, and other gunk, as well as to soothe irritated passageways. All you need is 1 to 1½ cups lukewarm water (do not use softened water), a bulb (ear) syringe, ¼ to ½ teaspoon salt, and ¼ to ½ teaspoon baking soda. Mix the salt and baking soda into the water and test the temperature. To administer, suck the water into the bulb and squirt the saline solution into one nostril while holding the other closed. Lower your head over the sink and gently blow out the water. Repeat this, alternating nostrils until the water is gone. Nasal irrigation isn't a pretty sight, yet it works wonders on sore noses and rids the passages of unwanted matter.

Steam. Breathing steam refreshes and soothes sore sinuses, and it helps rid the nasal passages of mucus. It takes some time, but you will feel wonderful! Boil several cups of water and pour into a big bowl (or a plugged sink). Place your head carefully over the bowl and drape a towel over your head. Breathe gently for 5 to 10 minutes. When you're finished breathing steam, use the hot water for a second purpose. Let the water

BOOST THAT IMMUNE SYSTEM

If you suffer from allergies, your immune system needs more of certain nutrients to protect your body and to help rebuild defenses. Make sure to get sufficient amounts of

- Vitamin A. If you eat a well-balanced diet, you should have an ample supply. If you don't, eat more of the following: milk, liver, fortified foods, and bright orange and yellow vegetables, such as carrots and cantaloupe.
- Vitamin B complex. B vitamins are found in almost every food, but the best sources are from fresh vegetables and meats.
- Vitamin C. Citrus fruits are high in vitamin C.
- Vitamin E. Vegetable oils, nuts, and seeds have high amounts. Moderate amounts are in avocados, asparagus, mangoes, apples, and sweet potatoes.
- Iron. The best sources are meats, oysters, whole grains and cereals, beans, and green vegetables.
- Selenium. Find this mineral in meats, seafood, and whole grains.
- Zinc. Find good amounts in meats, oysters, dairy products, and some beans.

WHEN TO CALL THE DOCTOR

Allergies can be difficult to self diagnose. How you treat your symptoms depends, however, on an accurate appraisal. What you have might be an infection, an intolerance, or a specific disease rather than an allergy. Check with your doctor if you experience any of the following:

- Nasal problems that cause secondary symptoms, such as chronic sinus infections, nasal congestion, or difficulty breathing
- Symptoms that last for several months
- Inability to get relief from over-the-counter medications or unacceptable side effects, such as drowsiness, from them
- Symptoms that interfere with your ability to carry out daily activities or decrease your quality of life
- Any of these symptoms, which can be warning signs of asthma or more serious conditions: struggling to catch your breath; wheezing and coughing, especially at night or after exercise; shortness of breath; tightness in your chest

cool until warm, saturate a washcloth, and hold it on the sinuses (to the sides of your nose, below the eyes and above the eyebrows).

LIFESTYLE REMEDIES

Dehumidify. Dust mites are champion procreators, so deprive them of the moist environment that encourages them to breed. Run a dehumidifier or an air conditioner to keep the air dry and to prevent mold growth, another allergy culprit. You can also keep humidity lower when you're showering or cooking by running an exhaust fan. Keep the windows shut. Sure, fresh air fills your home with the fragrance of a beautiful day, but it also can fill it with pollen. Allergy sufferers should keep their windows shut tight.

Shampoo before bedtime. During pollen prime time, the hair acts as one gigantic magnet, attracting flying pollen and stray mold spores. The more hair you have, and the oilier and more elaborately styled it is, the better its collection capabilities. When you lie down, these hair hitchhikers drop onto the pillow and are quickly inhaled, causing allergy symptoms that night or the next morning. To avoid being a walking collection agency, cover your hair when out for a walk or wash it before bedtime.

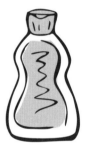

More Do's and Don'ts

- Pass up the milk. When allergies act up, skip that extra-large, whole-milk latte since dairy products thicken mucus. Try herbal tea instead.

Alzheimer's Disease

ALLEVIATING SYMPTOMS

Alzheimer's disease (AD) is many people's worst nightmare. Most diseases destroy either a physical or a mental function. Alzheimer's seizes both, slowly and steadily destroying memory, logical thought, and language. Simple tasks—how to eat or comb hair—are forgotten, and once AD sets in, there's no turning back the clock.

The disease is named for Dr. Alois Alzheimer, a German doctor who, during an autopsy in 1906, discovered physical changes in the brain of a woman who had died of a strange mental illness. He found plaques and tangles in her brain, signs that are now considered hallmarks of AD.

A Progressive Disease

AD is one of a group of brain disorders called dementia, which are progressive degenerative brain syndromes that affect memory, thinking, behavior, and emotion. Alzheimer's is the most common cause of dementia: Between 50 and 70 percent of all cases of dementia can be attributed to Alzheimer's.

Early symptoms include difficulty remembering names, places, or faces

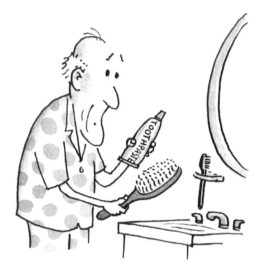

and trouble recalling things that just happened. Personality changes and confusion when driving a car or handling money are also early symptoms. Eventually mild forgetfulness progresses to problems in comprehension, speaking, reading, and writing. And physical breakdown occurs, too, partly because tasks such as eating and drinking are forgotten or too difficult to accomplish.

We don't know the cause of AD yet, but we do know that there are genetic, dietary, and environmental factors. The greatest risk factor is simply advancing age. One out of every eight people older than age 65 has Alzheimer's, while half of those older than 85 have it. Those who have a parent, brother, or sister with AD have a two to three times greater risk of developing the disease, and one gene has been identified as increasing the risk. For several decades, aluminum was considered a possible cause, and there was concern about the everyday use of items that contain aluminum, such as pots and pans, foils, beverage cans, and even deodorant. Scientific studies have failed to confirm that aluminum is a factor, however, and most researchers don't believe that it plays a role in the development of AD. They've turned their attention to other areas of investigation.

Scientists have found a strong link between serious head injury and the development of AD. And there is some evidence that a healthy lifestyle, including eating a balanced diet; exercising regularly; controlling weight, blood pressure, and cholesterol; mental stimulation; and social interaction, helps guard against developing AD.

Since we don't know what causes AD, we also do not yet have a cure for it. However, research is turning up some remedies that can help alleviate symptoms as well as slow the advancement of the disease.

DIETARY REMEDIES

Almonds. Evidence suggests that vitamin E deficiency raises Alzheimer's risk, and almonds are a good source. One ounce of almonds supplies 35 percent of your daily vitamin E requirement.

Blueberries. Some evidence suggests they contain an antioxidant that may slow down age-related motor changes, such as those seen in Alzheimer's.

Other studies have found that eating blueberries, and other fruits that are high in antioxidants, three times a week or more may help prevent AD and may improve memory.

Carrots. These are loaded with beta-carotene, which is a memory booster. Carrot and beet juices are good for the memory, too. So are okra and spinach.

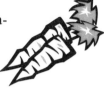

Citrus fruits. These fruits are loaded with vitamin C, which is believed to help protect brain nerves. Berries and some vegetables, including peppers, sweet potatoes, and green leafy vegetables, are also rich sources of vitamin C.

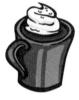

Cocoa. The flavonoids in cocoa are particularly powerful antioxidants that reduce inflammation and free-radical damage in the brain, which have been cited as potential contributors to the memory problems and cognitive decline that are characteristic of dementias. Constituents in cocoa also improve the health and function of blood vessels and increase circulation, which may be beneficial to those with dementia.

Curry. New research suggests that curcumin, an antioxidant and anti-inflammatory compound in turmeric, a spice used in yellow curry, might prevent AD. This could explain why India has one of the lowest rates of AD in the world.

Fish. Eating fish three times a week may prevent AD and other types of dementia. Omega-3 fatty acids, which AD sufferers often lack, are important in keeping those brain nerves healthy. Fish are high in fatty acids (that's why

---

ACCIDENT REMEDIES FROM THE PANTRY

People with Alzheimer's will eventually begin to have embarrassing bathroom accidents. Here are some simple, straight-from-the-pantry cleaners that will take care of those situations.

- For cleaning urine accidents, rinse the carpet, bedding, or upholstery immediately with warm water. Then mix 3 tablespoons white vinegar and 1 teaspoon liquid soap. Apply solution to stained area and leave on 15 minutes. Rinse and rub dry.
- For carpet and upholstery shampoo, use an eggbeater to combine 1 quart water, ¼ cup mild powdered detergent, and 1 tablespoon white vinegar. Whip until a stiff foam forms. Gently rub solution into fabric or carpeting, then remove soiled foam with a dull knife. Follow with a rinse of clean water.

EASY EATING

Using utensils can become difficult for people with Alzheimer's, so solve the problem by offering finger foods. Keep them simple, handy, and nutritious. Some suggestions:

- Fortified breads
- Peanut butter sandwich
- Easy to grab fruits, such as bananas, apricots (especially dried apricots, which are high in potassium), peeled apple wedges (apple peels can cause choking), carrots, and celery sticks
- Chocolate-covered almonds or almond M&Ms. Almonds are rich in vitamin E, which may delay the progression of AD. Two ounces of almonds per day supplies the recommended amount of vitamin E.

EXERCISE EATING RESTRAINT

Recent studies indicate that the less you eat, the slower you age. "Old-age genes" may actually stop functioning when daily calories are cut back by as little as 25 percent. Some of these genes that switch off may be linked to AD.

they're often called "brain food"). Good choices include salmon, mackerel, sardines, and anchovies.

 Green leafy vegetables. These are high in B vitamins such as folic acid, which may stimulate cognitive function. Other good sources of folic acid include beets, black-eyed peas and other legumes, brussels sprouts, and whole-grain foods.

Green tea. A Japanese study of 1,000 people older than age 70 found that those who drank two or more cups of green tea per 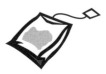 day were half as likely to develop dementia and memory loss as those who drank fewer than two cups per week. This effect was much weaker for black and oolong teas. And laboratory experiments on mice and rat brain cells show that the antioxidants in green tea seem to prevent the formation of beta-amyloid, a protein that accumulates in the brain as plaque and has been associated with memory loss and Alzheimer's disease.

Meal supplements. These meal-in-a-can beverages are easy to drink, and they're fortified with vitamins and minerals. They don't replace healthy eating, but they're a good resource for people who are having trouble keeping their weight up.

Nuts. The Alzheimer's Association includes almonds, pecans, and walnuts as part of its "Brain-Healthy Diet." These nuts are a good source of the most active form of vitamin E, alpha-tocopherol. Walnuts are also rich in melatonin, which research shows helps slow the progression of AD.

Orange juice. This is another way to up your vitamin C intake, but don't combine it with buffered aspirin. The two, taken together, form aluminum citrate, which is absorbed into the body five times faster than normal aluminum.

Red vegetables. Research from the Netherlands suggests that people who eat large amounts of dark red, yellow, and green vegetables may reduce their risk of dementia by 25 percent.

Seeds. Pumpkin, sesame, and sunflower seeds are packed with essential fatty acids necessary for brain function.

Soy products. Animal studies suggest that isoflavones found in soy protein may reduce AD risk. Try these: soy milk over cereal, soy meat substitutes, tofu frozen treats. And substitute tofu for ricotta or cream cheese in recipes. Dietary guidelines suggest 20 to 25 grams soy protein a day.

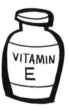

Vitamin E. According to one large federal study, vitamin E may help delay the loss of ability to carry out daily activities. Check with your doctor about vitamin E supplements but do not self-treat, as vitamin E can cause negative interactions and interfere with medications. Including vitamin E-rich foods in your diet, however, will enhance your health and may be protective.

Wheat germ or powdered milk. Add to foods for extra protein.

HERBAL REMEDIES

Many people with AD experience a decrease in taste, so spice up that food to tempt the taste

BANANA BASICS

It's one of nature's true miracles, and for those with Alzheimer's, it's a nutritional miracle. 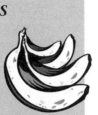 One of the most common problems plaguing people with AD is low fluid intake. Those with the disease simply forget to drink, or they choose not to in order to avoid bathroom emergencies and accidents. The result is dehydration, which can cause a loss of potassium, contributing to confusion. The simple solution for restoring essential potassium to the body is to force fluids—water or sports drinks with potassium—but that's often easier said than done. So the next best solution grows in bunches, is easy to eat, and tastes great.

Here are the banana facts you need to know:

- One ripe, medium-size banana supplies about 13 percent of the body's daily need for potassium.
- Bananas are a great source of fast energy. Very ripe bananas are loaded with sugar, about 23 grams, which is digested quickly and easily, then converted into energy. Ripe bananas are not recommended for people with diabetes.
- Bananas are easy to chew and swallow, which can be very important in AD since these functions may become impaired.

buds and appetite. Chili powder, pepper, sage, oregano—anything that tastes good and makes food interesting will work. Don't overload on salt, though.

Ginger. This spice can stimulate a poor appetite. Try some ginger tea or gingersnaps, or chop up some fresh 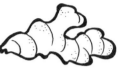 ginger and mix it with a little lime juice and a pinch of rock salt, then chew. It will not only increase appetite but thirst, too.

Sage. For depression associated with AD, drink a tea made with ½ teaspoon sage and ¼ teaspoon basil steeped in 1 cup hot water twice per day.

TOPICAL REMEDIES

Lemon oil. Steep a few drops of lemon or peppermint oil in hot water, then inhale. These are aromatherapy stimulants; they can perk up those suffering typical AD symptoms such as lethargy or depression.

Salt. For dry skin that occurs with age: After a shower or bath, and while the skin is still wet, sprinkle salt onto your hands and rub it all over the skin. Then rinse. This salt massage will remove dry skin and make skin more smooth to the touch. It will also invigorate the skin and get circulation moving. Try this first thing in the morning to help you wake up. If the skin is itchy, soak in a tub of saltwater. Just add 1 cup table salt or sea salt to bathwater. This solution will also soften skin and encourage relaxation.

Sesame oil. Depression associated with AD may be relieved with nose drops of warmed sesame oil. Use about 3 drops per nostril, twice per day. Some say you can also help relieve depression by rubbing a little of that warmed sesame oil on the top of the head and bottoms of the feet.

Vinegar. To prevent the itching that can come with incontinence, clean the genital area thoroughly with equal parts vinegar and water. Cider vinegar can help relieve itchy skin. Add 8 ounces apple cider vinegar to a bathtub of warm water. Soak for at least 15 minutes.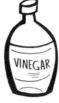

LIFESTYLE REMEDIES

Mental activity. Stimulate your brain every day by doing puzzles or playing games, reading, and working on hobbies. Mental workouts keep your brain vital, helping to create important connections between brain cells and even to generate new brain cells.

Physical activity. Being physically active helps keep the blood flowing to the brain and encourages development of new brain cells. Aerobic exercise, such as walking and dancing, helps deliver more oxygen to your brain and reduces the loss of brain cells in older adults.

Social activity. Research shows that people who continue to be socially engaged are less likely to develop AD and other forms of dementia.

Weight control. Obesity in middle age doubles your risk of developing dementia during your senior years, according to one long-term study. And those who had high cholesterol and high blood pressure were six times more likely to suffer from dementia. Make sure your calorie consumption is moderate and eat a balanced, low-fat, low-cholesterol diet.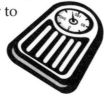

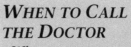

WHEN TO CALL THE DOCTOR

- When memory becomes a problem
- When normal reasoning and decision-making turns difficult
- When the ability to recall simple, everyday tasks is a struggle
- When friends or family mention that there's a noticeable change in personality or memory
- When there is disorientation about time and place

Anemia
BUILDING YOUR BLOOD

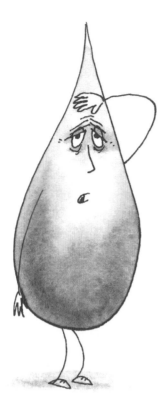

Anemia is a condition in which your red blood cell count is so low that it can't carry enough oxygen to all parts of your body. Not having enough oxygen in the blood is like trying to drive a car with no oil. Your car may run for a while, but you'll soon end up with a burned-out engine. In the same way that oil nourishes your car's engine, oxygen provides needed nourishment for your body's tissues (organs, muscles, etc.), and if they aren't getting enough of that vital sustenance, you'll start feeling weak and tired. A short climb up the stairs will leave you breathless, and even a couple days of rest won't perk you up. If that describes how you feel, check with your doctor. If you do have anemia, you should take action as soon as possible. And you need to be sure you don't have a more serious condition.

Anatomy of Anemia

Your red blood cells are the delivery trucks of the body. They carry oxygen throughout your blood vessels and capillaries to feed tissues. Hemoglobin, the primary component of red blood cells, is a complex molecule and is the oxygen carrier of the red blood cell.

The body works very hard to ensure that it produces enough red blood cells to successfully carry oxygen but not too many, since that can cause the blood to get too thick. Red blood cells live only 90 to 120 days. The liver and spleen get rid of the old cells, though the iron in the cells is

FASCINATING FACT

Blood travels 60,000 miles per day through the body. That's equivalent to traveling around the world two-and-a-half times.

recycled and sent back to the marrow to produce new cells.

When you're diagnosed with anemia, it usually means your red blood cell count is abnormally low, so it can't carry enough oxygen to all parts of your body, or that there is a reduction in the hemoglobin content of your red blood cells. Anemia's not a disease in itself but instead is considered a condition. However, this condition can be a symptom of a more serious illness. That's why it's always important to check with your doctor if you think you may be anemic.

The Most Common Causes of Anemia

There are many types of anemia. Some rare types are the result of a malfunction in the body, such as early destruction of red blood cells (hemolytic anemia), a hereditary structural defect of red blood cells (sickle cell anemia), or an inability to make or use hemoglobin (sideroblastic anemia). The most common forms of anemia are the result of some type of nutritional deficiency and can often be treated easily with some help from the kitchen. These common types are:

- **Iron deficiency anemia.** Iron deficiency anemia happens when the body doesn't have enough iron to produce hemoglobin, causing the red blood cells to shrink. And if there's not enough hemoglobin produced, the body's tissues don't get the nourishing oxygen they need. Children younger than three years of age and premenopausal women are at highest risk for developing iron deficiency anemia. Most young children simply don't get enough iron in their diet, and heavy menstrual periods are the most common cause of iron deficiency anemia in

ANEMIA: FOR WOMEN ONLY? Is anemia a gender-biased condition? The answer is yes. Men are not immune from the condition, but the group at highest risk for nutritional deficiency anemias are premenopausal women and adolescent girls. So why are women so lucky?

The Magic of Menstruation. Blood loss is a major cause of iron deficiency anemia, and because women lose blood through their menstrual cycle every month, they are more at risk for becoming anemic.

The Power of Pregnancy. Women's blood volume increases so much during pregnancy, they literally carry around almost three pints of extra blood. The body needs more iron to adequately supply the red blood cells.

The Downside of Dieting. You'll be hard pressed to meet a woman who hasn't dieted at least once in her life. Most women end up sacrificing iron-rich foods, such as meats, to make the numbers on the scale go down.

BAD BLOOD

For centuries before bad blood took on quite a different meaning, folk medicine experts used it in a more literal sense. Even current folk medicine wisdom believes that if you're feeling run-down, you might be suffering from "bad blood." Folk healers use "blood builders" to help restore needed nutrients to the body and the blood to good standing. Two of the most common "blood builders": beets and molasses.

women who are premenopausal. In addition, during pregnancy a woman's blood volume increases by 50 percent, boosting iron needs. Contrary to popular belief, men and older women aren't at greater risk for iron deficiency anemia. If they do end up developing the condition, it's most often the result of an ulcer.

- **Vitamin B12 deficiency anemia.** While iron deficiency anemia produces smaller than usual red blood cells, a vitamin B12 deficiency anemia produces oversized red blood cells. This makes it harder for the body to squeeze the red blood cells through vessels and veins. It's like trying to squeeze a marble through a straw. Vitamin B12-deficient red blood cells also tend to die off more quickly than normal cells. Most people get at least the minimum amount of B12 that they need by eating a varied diet. If you are a vegetarian or have greatly limited your intake of meat, milk, and eggs for other health reasons, however, you may not get enough of the vitamin. Older people are more at risk for vitamin B12 deficiency; in fact, 1 out of 100 people older than age 60 are diagnosed with pernicious anemia, a vitamin B12 deficiency that is caused by a lack of intrinsic factor. This age group is at increased risk because they are more likely to have conditions that affect the body's ability to absorb vitamin B12. Surgical removal of portions of the stomach or small intestine; atrophic gastritis, a thinning of the stomach lining; and diseases such as Crohn's disease can all interfere with the body's ability to absorb vitamin B12, as can drugs such as metformin. But the most common cause of B$_{12}$ deficiency anemia is a lack of a protein called intrinsic factor. Intrinsic factor is normally secreted by the stomach; its job is to help vitamin B$_{12}$. Without intrinsic factor, the vitamin B$_{12}$ that you consume just floats out as waste. In some people, a genetic defect causes the body to stop producing intrinsic factor. In others, an autoimmune reaction, in which the body mistakenly attacks stomach cells that produce the protein, results in a lack of intrinsic factor. Called pernicious anemia, this condition can be particularly dangerous because it causes neurological problems, such as difficulty walking, poor concentration, depression, memory loss, and irritability. These can usually be reversed if the condition is treated in time. Unfortunately, if you have pernicious anemia, the stomach cannot absorb the vitamin no matter how much B$_{12}$-rich food you eat. Treatment requires injections of B$_{12}$, usually once a month, that deposits the vitamin directly into the bloodstream.

- **Folic acid deficiency anemia.** A deficiency of folic acid produces the same oversized red blood cells as a vitamin B$_{12}$ deficiency. One

IRON'S ABSORPTION EQUATION

You may not be absorbing as much iron from your foods as you think. How much you absorb is dependent on two primary factors: what kind of iron is in the food and what other nutrients the food contains. There are two types of iron: heme and non-heme. Heme, found primarily in foods of animal origin, is much more easily absorbed than non-heme iron, which is found primarily in plant products. But if you eat a vitamin C–rich food or a food rich in heme iron with your non-heme iron food, your body will take in more iron.

Here's a guide to top iron sources:

- Sources of mostly heme iron: beef liver, lean sirloin, lean ground beef, skinless chicken, pork
- Sources of non-heme iron: fortified breakfast cereal, pumpkin seeds, bran, spinach
- Sources of vitamin B$_{12}$: salmon (3 ounces) 2.6 mcg, beef tenderloin (3 ounces) 2.5 mcg, yogurt (1 cup) 1.4 mcg, shrimp (3 ounces) 1.3 mcg,
- Sources of folic acid: spinach (½ cup) 130 mcg, navy beans (½ cup) 125 mcg, wheat germ (¼ cup) 80 mcg, avocado (½ cup) 55 mcg, orange (1 medium) 45 mcg

of the most common causes of this condition is simply not getting enough in the diet. The body doesn't store folic acid for long periods, so if you aren't getting enough in your diet, you will quickly become deficient. Pregnant women are most at risk because the need for folic acid increases by two-thirds during pregnancy. Adequate folic acid intake is essential from the start of pregnancy because it protects against spinal defects in the fetus.

Symptoms of Anemia

Symptoms of more severe anemia include rapid heartbeat, dizziness, headache, ringing in the ears, irritability, pale skin, restless legs syndrome, and confusion. A vitamin B_{12} or folic acid deficiency may even cause your mouth and tongue to swell. These symptoms may sound scary, but the most common forms of anemia are easily treated, especially if caught early.

Symptoms of mild to moderate anemia:
- weakness
- fatigue
- shortness of breath

Symptoms of moderate to severe anemia:
- rapid heartbeat
- dizziness
- headache
- ringing in the ears
- pale skin (especially the palms of your hands), pale or bluish fingernails
- hair loss
- restless legs syndrome
- confusion

Symptom specific to severe vitamin B_{12} or folic acid deficiency anemia:

• swelling of the mouth or tongue

Symptoms specific to pernicious anemia:

• numbness, tingling
• depression and/or irritability
• memory loss

Because all but pernicious anemia are the result of a nutritional deficiency, the best ways to treat them is with dietary changes.

DIETARY REMEDIES

Beef liver. Beef liver is rich in iron and all the B vitamins (including B_{12} and folic acid). In fact, beef liver contains more iron per serving—5.8 mg per 3 ounces—than any other food. Other animal sources of iron include eggs, cheese, fish, lean sirloin, lean ground beef, and chicken. However, sometimes older people have trouble absorbing B_{12} from animal products, and doctors may recommend supplements.

Beets. Beets are rich in folic acid, as well as fiber and potassium. The best way to cook beets is in the microwave. Keep the skin on, but peel before eating. The most nutrient-dense part of the beet is right under the skin.

Blackstrap molasses. Long known as a nutritional powerhouse, blackstrap molasses contains 3.5 mg of iron per tablespoon.

SUPER SUPPLEMENTS

Though most people can get adequate amounts of iron, vitamin B_{12}, and folic acid through their diet, experts believe that people who are at highest risk for nutrient deficiency anemias can benefit from taking supplements. If you are at higher-than-usual risk for a deficiency of iron, vitamin B_{12}, or folic acid, discuss it with your doctor, take a good look at your diet, and follow these recommendations.

• Take it on empty. The iron you absorb from supplements can be decreased by as much as 50 percent if you eat food with your supplement. Absorption is best when iron is taken on an empty stomach and washed down with juice or water.

• Don't overload. The government has done extensive testing on how much of a nutrient is adequate for a healthy diet. Overdoing the amounts can be harmful instead of beneficial. For example, taking too much folic acid may mask symptoms of pernicious anemia. Follow the Recommended Daily Allowances (RDAs) guideline and to avoid nutrient overload.

• Be a label reader. Be cautious when choosing a supplement, and be sure that it meets your unique needs. Some vitamin supplements don't contain any folic acid at all. And some may contain large amounts of nutrients that you don't need, which can be not only a waste of money but, depending on the nutrients, also harmful to your health. In addition, be sure to check the expiration date on the bottle; you don't want to buy a 500-count bottle of a once-a-day supplement that expires in six months!

Dry cereal. Fix yourself a bowl of your favorite fortified cereal (go for one without the sugar and the cartoon characters on the box), and you'll be waging a battle against anemia. These days many cereals are fortified with a nutrient punch of iron, vitamin B12, and folic acid. Check the label for amounts per serving, pour some milk over your flakes, and dig in.

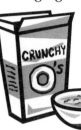

Spinach. Green leafy vegetables contain loads of iron and folic acid. We're talking dark and green, so choose your leaves carefully. Iceberg lettuce is mostly water and is of little nutritive value. Spinach, on the other hand, has 3.2 mg of iron and 130 mcg of folic acid per ½ cup.

Vitamin C. Eat foods rich in vitamin C at the same time that you eat whole grains, spinach, and legumes, in order to increase absorption of the iron they contain. Also, ask your doctor if you should take a vitamin C supplement.

MORE DO'S AND DON'TS

- If you're a vegetarian or have cut way down on your intake of meats, milk, and eggs, be sure that you're getting adequate amounts of iron and vitamin B12 in your diet. Vegetarians are at greater risk for nutritional deficiency anemias because iron from plant sources isn't absorbed as well as iron from animal sources and because vitamin B12 is found almost exclusively in animal foods. Consider taking a multivitamin with B12.

- If you drink coffee or tea, do so between meals rather than with meals. The caffeine in these beverages reduces iron absorption.

Anxiety

QUASHING THE QUIVERS

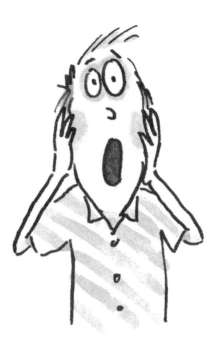

Anxiety is a feeling everyone experiences sooner or later. Perhaps you're sitting in the waiting room, anticipating the horse-size needle your doctor has waiting for you on the other side of the door. Or you've spent all day cooking but the look on your mother-in-law's face says your best efforts were wasted. Or you really hate your job.

These very different experiences can bring on anxiety and its typical symptoms:

- heart palpitations
- sense of impending doom
- inability to concentrate
- muscle tension
- dry mouth
- sweating
- queasy, jittery feeling in the pit of the stomach
- hyperventilation

Anxiety can be short- or long-lived, depending on its source. The more long lasting the anxiety, the more additional symptoms you will experience.

If your anxiety is a reaction to a single, isolated event—the shot the doctor is about to give you—your anxiety level will decrease and your symptoms will disappear after the event. If your anxiety is from friction between you and your mother-in-law, you're likely to experience anxiety for a period of time before and after you see her. In this case, the symptom list probably has grown to include diarrhea or constipation and irritability.

Then there's that job, a source of anxiety that never leaves you. You dread getting up in the morning because you have to go to work, dread going to bed at night because when you wake up you have to go to work, dread the weekend because when it's over you'll have to go to work. When the source of your anxiety is ever-present,

TIPS ON CUTTING THE CAFFEINE

Because caffeine can cause anxiety, and caffeine addiction symptoms mimic anxiety, this morning pick-me-up is at the head of the no-no list. But cutting it out all at once can cause withdrawal symptoms, including anxiety, irritability, headache, and fatigue.

To stop, cut back gradually until you are caffeine free and have no withdrawal symptoms. If you do experience withdrawal symptoms, especially as you near the end of all caffeine consumption, continue drinking 1 cup of a caffeinated beverage daily, then gradually cut back on that.

FASCINATING FACT

Generalized anxiety disorder affects twice as many women as men.

you can probably add the following to the list of symptoms: chest pain, over- or under-eating, insomnia, loss of sex drive.

All three situations described above are types of everyday anxiety, or as some would put it, the cost of living. But the cost can be huge, taking its toll on you physically, mentally, and emotionally.

What Causes Anxiety?

Essentially, anxiety is part of the "fight or flight" mechanism, a carryover from our ancient ancestors. They were hunters as well as the hunted; ready either to attack or flee. Their anxiety kept them alive, kicking in when adrenaline was released into the bloodstream. That big ol' bear was breathing down our ancestor's neck, and his adrenaline surged as a warning, causing his liver to release energy-stimulating sugars into his system to ready him for the fight. That was definitely an anxiety-filled situation, but that warning system was, and still is, necessary for today's emergencies.

Trouble is, we experience the physical manifestations of the "fight or flight" mechanism even when it's not really necessary. Certainly, your mother-in-law's visit may not be pleasant, but it's not life threatening, either. You feel your muscles knot up at the very mention of her name. That, in itself, isn't a problem. But when anxiety is severe or prolonged, the powerful "fight or flight" chemicals can damage your body's organs. Eventually, anxiety can cause a full-fledged illness, such as headaches and high blood pressure.

Although emotion is most often at the root of anxiety symptoms, they can be caused by physical problems as well. Rule out the following before assuming your symptoms are stress-related:

- Hyperthyroidism, which may produce symptoms that resemble those of anxiety
- Heart disorders, which can cause rapid heartbeat, often associated with anxiety
- Caffeine, which can produce nervous symptoms even in moderate amounts
- Premenstrual syndrome (PMS)
- Diet pills
- Anemia
- Diabetes
- Hypoglycemia

So now that you know what anxiety can do, it's time to learn what you can do to control it. Mild anxiety can be treated successfully at home with a little calming music, a little quiet time, and some soothing remedies from the kitchen.

DIETARY REMEDIES

Almonds. Soak 10 raw almonds overnight in water to soften, then peel off the skins. Put almonds in blender with 1 cup warm milk, a pinch of ginger, and a pinch of nutmeg. Drink at night to relax you before going to bed.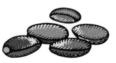

 Orange. The aroma of an orange is known to reduce anxiety. All you have to do to get the benefits is peel an orange and inhale. You can also drop the peel into a small pan or potpourri burner. Cover with water and simmer. When heated, the orange peel will release its fragrant and calming oil.

HERBAL REMEDIES

Chamomile. Sipping chamomile tea calms the nerves and aids in getting to sleep. Simply steep

---

AMISH ANXIETY ANTIDOTES

Because lifestyle has such a huge impact on anxiety, the Amish simply trust their lifestyle to alleviate the problem. Here are some Amish ways that can help.

- Avoid chocolate and caffeinated coffee, tea, and soda.
- Be physically active outside every day.
- Get at least 8 hours sleep every night.
- Avoid nonprescription drugs.
- Use alcohol only in moderation.
- Do something every day to help others.
- Replace negative thoughts with positive thoughts.
- Turn to your religious faith to sustain you.

Don't Ignore Chest Pains!

Symptoms of hyperventilation may actually be the signs of other more serious health problems such as diabetes, heart disease, or thyroid disease. If you experience chest pains, numbness, shortness of breath, or dizziness, call your doctor or 9-1-1 immediately. Remember: a heart attack is a life-threatening medical emergency!

Fascinating Fact

Charles Darwin suffered such severe panic attacks that he isolated himself from society. His symptoms were overwhelming feelings of impending death and bouts of hysterical crying.

1 tablespoon chamomile flowers in 1 cup water for 15 minutes, then strain and drink as needed. Breathe in its aroma, too, for a soothing effect. Use chamomile in an aroma lamp, sachet, or potpourri. However, since chamomile contains pollen, be careful if you have allergies.

Rosemary. Rosemary has a calming effect on the nerves. Make a tea by adding 1 to 2 teaspoons of the dried herb to 1 cup boiling water; steep for 10 minutes, then drink. Inhaling rosemary can be relaxing, too. Burn a sprig, or use rosemary incense to ease anxiety.

Topical Remedies

Baking soda. Add ⅓ cup baking soda and ⅓ cup ginger to a nice warm bath. Soak in the tub for 15 minutes to relieve tension and anxiety.

Ice. This is for muscle tension associated with anxiety. Wrap ice or a bag of frozen vegetables in a kitchen towel and apply it to tight muscles. Some people react better to heat applications. Try each to see which works best for you.

Oil. Sesame oil is great, but sunflower, coconut, or corn oil will work, too. For a wonderful, anxiety-busting massage, heat 6 ounces oil until warm, not hot. Rub over entire body, including your scalp and the bottoms of your feet. A small rolling pin feels marvelous! Use 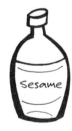 the oil as a massage before the morning bath to calm you down for the day's activities. If anxiety is keeping you awake, try using it before you go to bed, too.

LIFESTYLE REMEDIES

Breathe. Slowly inhaling and exhaling is a well-known antidote to anxiety. It counteracts the "fight or flight" mechanism and prevents hyperventilating.

Chat it away. Talk with a friend, a psychotherapist, or a clergyman. Talking about your anxiety can help relieve it.

Exercise. Noncompetitive exercising, such as walking, bicycling, or swimming, is a boon to your mental health as well as your physical well-being.

Meditate. Or pray or indulge in a mental flight of fantasy. Do whatever it takes to give your mind a break.

WHEN TO CALL THE DOCTOR

- If you're chronically experiencing severe symptoms: chest pain, shortness of breath or hyperventilation, dizziness, headache
- If your anxiety has progressed to panic attacks
- If you begin to alter your life in order to avoid situations that make you feel anxious

FOLK REMEDY HERBAL CURES

If you experience frequent anxiety, it might be wise to keep these herbs on hand.

Warning! If you are taking any medication, whether it's over-the-counter or prescription, do not use any herbal remedy without first consulting your doctor. These cures can have bad side effects when mixed with other drugs!

Catnip. You may keep this one around for Fluffy, but it can help alleviate human anxiety. Make a tea by steeping 3 teaspoons catnip in 1 cup boiling water for 10 minutes. Sweeten to taste and drink three times per day.

Valerian. Ancient Greeks used valerian as a sedative, and it was a folk cure used in Tibet, India, and Japan. Today, valerian is used in the Appalachian regions as a cure for the jitters, and in Louisiana the root is tucked into the pillowcase to be inhaled as you sleep. Place 2 to 3 teaspoons dried valerian root in 1 cup boiling water. Cover and steep for 15 minutes. Drink 2 to 3 cups per day for up to three weeks. Using this any longer may cause lethargy and hangover effects.

Warning! Valerian has a disagreeable odor.

Arthritis
PROTECTING YOUR JOINTS

Arthritis means inflammation of the joints. To the 46 million Americans afflicted with arthritis, every day can be painful. The two most prevalent forms of arthritis are osteoarthritis and rheumatoid arthritis.

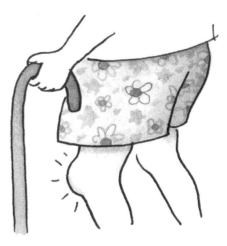

Osteoarthritis (OA), the most common form, is the result of joint cartilage wearing down over time. When the durable, elastic tissue is gone, bones rub directly against one another. This causes stiffness and dull pain in the weight-bearing joints (hips, knees, and spine) and in the hands. The elderly are most susceptible to OA, but athletes and those in jobs requiring repetitive movements are also vulnerable.

Rheumatoid arthritis (RA) is the inflammation of the joint lining. The cause is unknown, but it is thought that the symptoms are the result of the body turning against itself. Symptoms of RA vary from individual to individual. In its mildest form, it causes minor joint discomfort. More often, however, the inflammation causes painful, stiff, swollen joints, and in prolonged cases, severe joint damage. Unlike OA, whose symptoms are joint-specific, RA tends to cause body-wide symptoms such as fatigue, fever, and weight loss.

Old age puts one at risk for osteoarthritis, but this isn't the case with RA. RA usually develops between the ages of 30 and 50 and is more common in women than in men.

Waking up with a stiff back or swollen finger joint doesn't necessarily indicate arthritis; however, should pain, stiffness, or swelling last more than two weeks, you may have arthritis. Other symptoms include:

- Swelling in one or more joints
- Early morning stiffness
- Recurring pain or tenderness in a joint

- Inability to move a joint in a normal fashion
- Redness or warmth in a joint
- Unexplained weight loss, fever, or weakness accompanied by joint pain

There is no cure for arthritis, but many kitchen-crafted remedies can help ease the pain.

DIETARY REMEDIES

Dairy products. Some medicines used to treat arthritis can lead to a loss of calcium from the bones, resulting in osteoporosis. To counteract this effect, make sure you get enough calcium in your diet. A cup of low-fat yogurt, for instance, supplies 300 to 400 mg calcium—about one-third of your daily requirement. Calcium-fortified orange juice will also help you meet your daily calcium needs. The Recommended Daily Allowance is 1,000 mg calcium per day for adults younger than 50 and 1,200 per day for adults older than 50. If you don't get enough calcium in your diet, be sure to supplement to protect your bones.

Food. Decreasing arthritis pain and stiffness may be as easy as eliminating certain foods from your diet. However, the deduction process requires time and observation. There are no set guidelines for this remedy. Rather, it is intuitive. Do you ache more after eating a certain food? Keep a food diary, record what you've eliminated from your diet that week, and rate your discomfort level. There are no guarantees, but you may discover that certain foods contribute to stiffness.

Gamma linolenic acid. Recent research suggests that high doses of an omega-6 essential fatty acid, known as gamma linolenic acid (GLA), can help

DUCKS AREN'T THE ONLY ONES WHO QUACK

Millions of people suffer from ar- 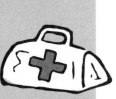 thritic pain, and many will do just about anything to stop the suffering. Such desperation brings out the quacks who equate vulnerability with profit and promote miracle cures for a high price. Be careful when seeking arthritis treatment outside the established medical realm or you may suffer both physically and financially.

- Remember, there is no cure for arthritis. Beware any person, food, drug, liquid, therapy, or retreat that promises a cure.
- Watch for words such as "Secret Formula," "Special Product," or "Quick, Simple Cures." All are sure signs of quackery.
- Be a critical reader. Is the article you're reading an "advertorial," written and paid for by the product's manufacturer, or was it written by an objective source?
- Beware testimonials, especially when the person "testifying" only uses a first name and last initial.

reduce joint inflammation. You'll find GLA in some plant seed oils, such as evening primrose and borage, and in black currants. Research also indicates that the benefits of GLA may be enhanced by supplementation with omega-3 fatty acids, which are plentiful in cold-water fish. You can also take GLA supplements—1,800 mg per day is recommended for rheumatoid arthritis. There is no evidence that applying GLA oils to the skin is effective.

Glucosamine. Glucosamine supplements, often found in products that contain a combination with chondroitin, help relieve the pain and may slow the joint degeneration associated with osteoarthritis. The recommended dosage is 500 mg of glucosamine three times per day. It usually takes two to three months of supplementation for maximum benefit.

TOPICAL REMEDIES

Epsom salts. Magnesium sulfate, otherwise known as Epsom salts, is commonly used to relieve aching joints and reduce swelling. Mix a few heaping tablespoons into the bathwater and soak. More localized soaks are sometimes necessary, especially for the feet. Rest painful feet in a tub of warm water combined with 2 tablespoons Epsom salts. Relax for 15 minutes, pat your tootsies dry, and massage them with your favorite lotion.

Heat and cold treatments. Heat relieves pain primarily by relaxing muscles and joints and decreasing stiffness. However, it may aggravate a joint that's already "hot" from inflammation, as is sometimes the case with rheumatoid arthritis. Osteoarthritis may respond better to heat treatments. Cold is used to reduce pain in specific joints and can be helpful if you have gout. Heat can be applied in the form of a hot, moist towel, with a heating pad, or by taking a warm bath or shower. Cold can be applied with a compress or with a plastic bag filled with crushed ice or a frozen package of vegetables (peas are perfect). If you use ice, wrap the cold pack in a towel to prevent burning your skin.

LIFESTYLE REMEDIES

Exercise. Movement will keep joints functioning better for longer. Range-of-motion exercises are the simplest and easiest, and they help reduce the risk of joint injury and maintain and improve flexibility. Aerobic exercise, such as walking or swimming, increases endurance of muscles that support the joints, and weight-bearing exercises like playing tennis also strengthen bones. Resistance exercises, such as lifting weights or isometrics, strengthen muscles, too.

Don't overuse over-the-counter creams. These arthritis rubs may provide temporary relief by heating up the joints. However, using them too often may activate enzymes that can break down the cartilage in the joints.

Give your hands a workout. Try doing hand exercises in a sink full of warm water for added ease and comfort.

Watch your weight. Being overweight puts more stress on joints. In fact, a weight gain of 10 pounds can mean an equivalent increase in stress of 40 pounds on the knees. If you're carrying excess pounds, losing weight can help improve joint function.

WHEN TO CALL THE DOCTOR

- When stiffness and pain last more than a few weeks
- If joint pain is accompanied by unexplained weight loss, fever, or weakness
- If the pain is severe enough to disrupt your daily routines and well-being

Asthma
WEATHERING THE WHEEZE

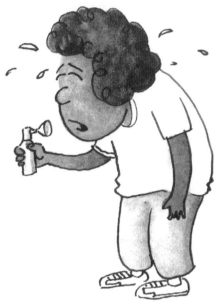

Recent statistics about asthma don't paint a pretty picture. The National Center for Health Statistics estimates that 34 million Americans have been diagnosed with asthma in their lifetime. Almost 30 million Americans reported currently having asthma in 2007. Asthma is the number one cause of chronic illness in kids, affecting more than 6.7 million children. Despite this discouraging news, there is reason to be hopeful if you are one of the millions of asthmatics across the country. As the numbers of asthma cases continue to climb, researchers are even more determined to find asthma's causes and develop more effective treatments.

Breathing Basics

When you take a breath, the air goes from your mouth or nose to the windpipe (or trachea). It then travels to the lungs. It enters the lungs through the bronchi, a group of tubes that branch off from the windpipe. The bronchi then branch off into bronchioles. Imagine a car driving from the interstate to a state highway to a country road and you get the picture.

Asthma happens when the bronchi and bronchioles come in contact with a foreign invader, or asthma "trigger." There are many different triggers, and each person has their own set. Once a foreign material enters the body, the airways quickly become inflamed, causing the muscles that rest on the outside of the airways to tighten and narrow. This allows a thick mucus to enter the airways. The mucus causes swelling and makes it very difficult to breathe. The classic symptoms of an asthma attack include wheezing, tightening in the chest, dry coughing, and increased heart rate. These are frightening symptoms to experience, and they're also quite alarming for someone to observe.

Asthma Instigators

About half of all asthma attacks are caused by allergies. The most common allergens are dust mites, cockroaches, chemicals, pollen, mold, and animal dander.

There are quite a few additional asthma triggers aside from allergens. Other triggers include:

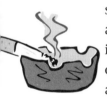

- Tobacco smoke. There is a direct relationship between secondhand smoke and asthma. Secondhand smoke is a lung irritant, and it contains an abundance of harmful chemicals such as formaldehyde, arsenic, and benzene. It's especially bad for children and teenagers to be around tobacco smoke.
- Exercise. Working out, especially outside in the cold, can cause exercise-induced asthma. This is not an excuse for people with asthma to shy away from exercise; they just need to consult the doctor about how to control the attacks.
- Weather. Cold air can act as an asthma trigger. Other weather conditions, such as rain, wind, or a sudden change in the weather, can also cause an attack.

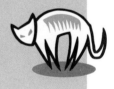

STAY AWAY FROM SULFITES

Some asthma sufferers are particularly sensitive to the chemical preservatives sulfites, which are found in many kinds of foods and beverages. If you have a question about a food, check out the label. Sulfites will probably be listed among the ingredients.

Here are some common foods with high concentrations of sulfites:
• Wine
• Lemon juice
• Dried fruits
• Fresh shrimp
• Instant potatoes
• Canned veggies
• Fruit topping
• Molasses
• Wine vinegar
• Corn syrup
• Pizza dough
• Grapes
• Beer
• Instant tea

• Chemicals. This includes chemical fumes, such as from paint or perfume, and chemical additives, such as the sulfites that are used as preservatives in food. Any of these can trigger an asthma attack in susceptible people.
• Respiratory infections. Colds, sinus infections, and even the flu can predispose one for or aggravate asthma. It's a good idea for asthmatics to get a flu shot each year.
• Stomach acid. Excess stomach acid can irritate the esophagus lining and create a reaction in the lungs that may cause an attack.
• Pregnancy. One-third of pregnant women with asthma get worse, but one-third of pregnant women with asthma get better, too. And one-third remain the same.
• Emotional stress. Though a stressful day at work won't cause an asthma attack, it can aggravate the condition.
• Drugs. Some people with asthma are sensitive to certain drugs. The most common culprits are aspirin and nonsteroidal anti-inflammatory drugs (NSAIDs).

Though there are many natural ways to help asthma sufferers breathe easier, experts recommend that combining certain natural remedies with prescription anti-inflammatories and bronchodilators are your best bet to attack your asthma. Here are some helpful remedies.

DIETARY REMEDIES

Chili peppers. Hot foods such as chili peppers open up airways. Experts believe this is because peppers stimulate fluids in the mouth, throat, and lungs. The increase in fluids thins out the mucus formed during an asthma attack so it can be coughed up, making breathing easier. Capsaicin, the stuff that makes hot peppers hot, acts as an anti-inflammatory when eaten and a bronchodilator when inhaled in small doses.

Coffee. The caffeine in regular coffee can help prevent and treat asthma attacks. Researchers have found that caffeinated coffee drinkers have one-third fewer asthma symptoms than 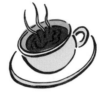 those who don't drink it. And caffeine has bronchodilating effects. In fact, caffeine was one of the main anti-asthmatic drugs during the 19th century. Don't load up on java, though. Three cups per day will provide the maximum benefit.

 Onions. Onions are loaded with anti-inflammatory properties. Studies have shown that these properties can reduce the constriction of the airways in an asthma attack. Use cooked onions, as raw onions are generally too irritating.

Orange juice. Vitamin C is the main antioxidant in the lining of the bronchi and bronchioles. Research discovered that people with asthma had low levels of vitamin C and that eating foods that had at least 300 mg of vitamin C per day—equivalent to about 3 glasses of orange juice—cut wheezing by 30 percent. Other foods high in vitamin C include red bell pepper, papaya, broccoli, blueberries, and strawberries.

Salmon. Fatty fish such as sardines, salmon, mackerel, and tuna contain omega-3 fatty acids. These fatty acids seem to help the lungs react better to irritants in people who have asthma and may even help

IT'S IN THE GENES
Heredity is a major factor in whether or not you have asthma. If you have one parent with asthma, you have a 50 percent chance of developing asthma, too. And if both parents are allergic, you have a 75 to 80 percent chance of being allergic.

WHEN TO CALL THE DOCTOR

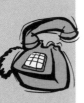

Asthma attacks can be deadly. In 2005, asthma was responsible for 3,384 deaths in the United States. Those deaths are preventable, but you need to know when to take quick action. If you have any of these symptoms, get to an emergency room fast.

- If breathing gets difficult, especially if your neck, chest, or ribs pull in every time you take a breath, or if you have a feeling of suffocation
- If nostrils begin to flare
- If walking or talking is a chore
- If fingernails or lips turn blue
- If you are dizzy
- If ears, palms, genitals, or soles of feet begin itching
- If you have hives
- If you have a feeling of imminent doom

prevent asthma in people who have never had an attack. Studies have found that kids who eat fish more than once a week have one-third the chance of getting asthma as children who don't eat fish. And researchers discovered that people who took fish oil supplements, equivalent to eating 8 ounces of mackerel per day, increased their body's ability to avoid a severe asthma attack by 50 percent.

HERBAL REMEDIES

Peppermint extract. This is a folk remedy for a homemade vaporizer. Put 1 quart nonchlorinated water in a stainless steel, glass, or enamel pan, and put it on the stove. Add 10 drops peppermint extract or peppermint oil and bring to a boil. Let it simmer for about 1 hour until all the water is gone. The volatile oil will saturate the room air.

LIFESTYLE REMEDIES

Cheesecloth. Put a fine cheesecloth over each room's heat outlet for a homemade dust filter. Stick-on commercial fine filters are also available.

Consider a vegan diet. Eliminating animal products from the diet gets rid of many food allergens (cow's milk, for example) and, if you add asthma-aiding nutrients such as vitamin C to your diet, you can greatly improve asthma symptoms.

Exercise your options. Research has shown that getting regular aerobic exercise increases exercise tolerance in people with asthma. At first, keep your bronchodilator with you. If you feel tightness in your chest and can't work through it, use the device. If one type of exercise induces an

attack, try another type. You may not be able to tolerate running, for instance, but you may be able to swim regularly.

Athlete's Foot
FIGHTING THE FUNGUS

Athlete's foot itches, burns, and is downright ugly to look at. But it's not a condition unique to athletes. Blame the misnomer on the ad man who gave it its name in the 1930s. In fact, athlete's foot, or *tinea pedis,* is the most common fungal infection of the skin. This fungus loves moist places, especially the soft, warm, damp skin between the toes. Certainly the athlete's locker room environment, with its steamy showers, is a good place for the fungus to thrive. But *tinea pedis* is actually present on most people's skin all the time, just waiting for the right opportunity to develop into an infection.

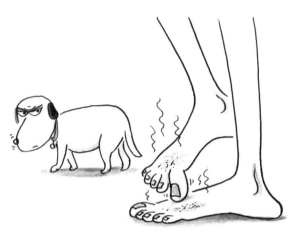

Who Gets It?
So what causes athlete's foot to rear its ugly little fungal head? Skin that's irritated, weakened, or continuously moist is primed for an athlete's foot infection. And certain medications, including antibiotics, corticosteroids, birth control pills, and drugs that suppress immune function, can make you more susceptible. People who are obese and those who have diabetes mellitus or a weakened immune system, such as those with AIDS, also are at increased risk. And some people may be genetically predisposed to developing athlete's foot.

Anyone can get athlete's foot—and most people will at some time in their lives. Teenage and adult males, though, are at the top of the fungus-footed list. Who's at the bottom? The following are those who are least likely to succumb:

- People who spend a lot of time barefoot
- Women
- Children under the age of 12

Signs and Symptoms
Just because you're not in the high risk category doesn't mean you're safe. Here's how you can tell whether you have an athlete's foot infection:

- Itching, scaling, red skin
- Red, cracking, peeling skin between the toes

FUNGUS TOENAIL

Yep, the creeping athlete's foot fungus can spread right on up to your toenail if your infection goes untreated long enough. Called *tinea unguium*, toenail fungus turns the nail yellowish or brown and makes it thicken and crack. As the fungus grows, the nail will give off a foul odor. Eventually the toe under and around the nail can start to throb as the infection takes a firm hold and pus builds up in the irritated areas.

Athlete's foot is easily treated but fungus toe is not. It may respond to any of the remedies in this profile or to an over-the-counter or prescription antifungal treatment, but occasionally the nail must be surgically removed. The simplest solution is to treat the initial athlete's foot infection as soon as it appears to keep it from spreading.

- Dry, flaking skin
- Blisters
- Unpleasant and unusual foot odor

Keep It From Spreading

In extreme cases, the fungus that causes athlete's foot can spread to other moist areas of the body, such as the groin and even the armpits. So take precautions when coming into contact with that athlete's foot. Be sure to wash your hands with soap and water. Keep your linens and towels clean, and never wear the same pair of socks twice without first washing them. You can also spread athlete's foot with contaminated sheets, towels, and clothing.

There are any number of antifungal creams on the market that can rid you of your foot fungus. They're costly, and you may have to buy several tubes or cans before the problem is cleared. So before you trudge off to the pharmacy on those poor, itchy feet, try some of the following kitchen concoctions.

DIETARY REMEDIES

Garlic. Eat some garlic, as it has antifungal properties.

Immune-boosting foods. Because low immunity can make you more susceptible to a fungal infection, diets rich in immune-boosting foods might make it possible for you to tiptoe through the shower without getting infected. These foods might help: broccoli, garlic, onions, red meats, sweet potatoes, rice, scallions, sunflower seeds, and whole-grain breads,

Yogurt. One of the greatest of all fungus-fighting foods in your fridge is yogurt that contains acidophilus. It doesn't matter what the flavor is as long as the yogurt contains the active bacteria (check the label; it will tell you). Acidophilus helps control vaginal and oral yeast, but it may give other fungi a pretty good fight too. And if nothing else, it tastes good and is good for you as well.

TOPICAL REMEDIES

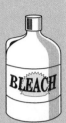

Baking soda. Sprinkle baking soda directly into your shoes to absorb moisture.

Cornstarch. Rub cornstarch, which absorbs moisture, on your feet. Very lightly browned cornstarch is even better because any moisture content already contained in the cornstarch is removed, allowing for better absorption. To brown, sprinkle cornstarch on a pie plate and bake at 325 degrees Fahrenheit for just a few minutes, until it looks brownish. Then dab some on your feet and toes.

Cinnamon. A good soak in a cinnamon-tea foot bath will help slow down the fungus. Boil 8 to 10 broken cinnamon sticks in 4 cups water, then simmer for five minutes. Let steep for another 45 minutes. Soak your feet for 15 to 30 minutes. Repeat daily as needed.

Garlic. You can also swab the affected area with garlic juice or oregano oil twice a day. If your toenail appears to have the fungus, use this recipe, which is usually effective:

Crush 1 clove garlic and mix with a few drops of olive oil to make a paste. Apply to the nail and leave on for 15 to 30 minutes, then clean off in warm, soapy water. Dry feet thoroughly. Repeat daily. Because the fungus can return, you may wish to continue this treatment for several weeks after it has disappeared to ward off another fungal visit.

Lemon. This remedy will help you in the sweaty feet–odor department. Squeeze the juice from a lemon and mix it with 2 ounces water. Rinse your feet with the lemon water.

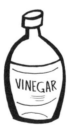 **Salt.** Soak your infected foot in warm salt water, using 1 teaspoon salt for each cup of water, for ten minutes. Dry your foot thoroughly, then dab some baking soda between your toes.

Tea. The tannic acid in tea is soothing, helps to dry the foot, and helps kill the fungus. Make a foot soak by putting 6 black tea bags in 1 quart warm water.

Vinegar. Soak your feet in a solution of 1 cup vinegar mixed with 2 quarts water for 15 to 30 minutes every night. Or make a solution of 1 cup vinegar to 1 cup water, and apply it directly to the affected areas with a cotton ball. If the infection is severe and the skin is raw, the solution will sting. Make sure your feet are completely dry before putting on your socks or slippers.

Cider vinegar can also be used as a remedy. Mix equal parts apple cider (or regular) vinegar and ethyl alcohol. Dab on the affected areas.

LIFESTYLE REMEDIES

Don't wear tight-fitting or watertight shoes. Skip shoes made of plastic and rubber, too. The best shoe choices are those made of natural materials that "breathe," such as leather.

Don't share or swap shoes with anybody. If you find yourself with a pair of someone else's vintage shoes, treat them with antifungal powder before you put them on.

Wear sandals or thongs on your feet in fungus-harboring public places such as beach showers and locker rooms; don't go barefoot.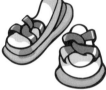

Set your shoes outside to air on a warm, sunny day. This will help dry them out and kill the fungus. Alternate shoes every day. Wear one pair while you dry out the other. When selecting socks, try both natural and synthetic fabrics to see which keep your sweaty feet the driest. You may wish to try synthetic sock liners to absorb the moisture and keep it away from your skin.

Give your socks a double washing in extra hot water to kill the fungal spores.

Make sure to dry thoroughly between your toes after bathing. That's where athlete's foot usually starts.

When you're not in a wet environment, go barefooted as often as you can. This will get your foot outside the moist shoe environment where fungus loves to lurk. This is best done indoors, however, where you are less likely to cut, scrape, or otherwise injure your feet.

WHEN TO CALL THE DOCTOR

- If the infection gets worse no matter what you do
- If one or both feet swell
- If you see pus in the cracks
- If the fungus spreads to your hands or elsewhere
- If you see an obvious change in color in your toenails, especially the nail of your big toe
- If you develop pain in the feet along with angry-looking inflammation, general malaise, fever, or chills. Your athlete's foot could be turning into a much more serious condition called cellulitis, which MUST be treated by a physician immediately.

Back Pain
ANSWERING THE ACHE

People are bad to their backs, crouching over keyboards for eight hours, struggling to lift heavy objects, or quickly transforming themselves from sedentary office workers to weekend warriors. Whatever the action, the back often can't handle such stress, and it reacts with pain.

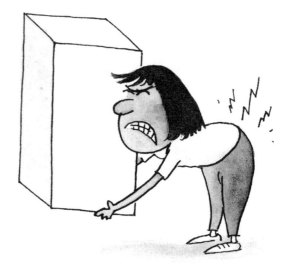

Almost everyone will experience back pain at some point in their life. Lower back pain has many causes, including common muscle strain and more serious problems with the bones in the spine (vertebrae) and the disks of shock-absorbing material that separate them. Why is the lower back such a glutton for punishment? Unlike the upper back, it isn't supported by the rib cage, and many people don't exercise the back and the supporting abdominal muscles as they should.

Back pain remedies rely primarily on rest, strengthening and stretching exercises, and modification of daily routine. However, your shelves do hold a few ingredients that can help get that back back into shape.

DIETARY REMEDIES
Milk. Bone up on milk. Women should be sure to include plenty of calcium in their diets. (Older women are at greater risk for developing osteoporosis, the disease of eroding bones.) Calcium helps build strong bones and protect the spine from osteoporosis.

HERBAL REMEDIES
Chamomile tea. This calms and soothes tense muscle tissue. Steep 1 tablespoon chamomile flowers in 1 cup boiling water for 15 minutes. Or, you can use a prepackaged chamomile tea. Drink 1 to 3 cups per day.

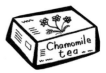

Warning! Chamomile contains allergy-inducing proteins related to ragweed pollen. Ask your doctor about drinking chamomile if you are allergic to ragweed. Packaged tea may be safer to drink than tea made from the flowers. Your doctor can advise you.

Gingerroot. Fragrant ginger-root has long been known to help ease nausea, but back pain, too? Ginger does contain anti-inflammatory 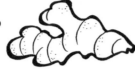 compounds, including some with mild aspirinlike effects. When your back aches, cut a 1- to 2-inch fresh gingerroot into slices and place in 1 quart boiling water. Simmer, covered, for 30 minutes on low heat. Cool for 30 minutes. Strain, sweeten with honey (if desired), and drink.

Rosemary. Its leaves are packed with these anti-inflammatory substances: carnosol, oleanolic acid, rosmarinic acid, and ursolic acid—all of which work to ease swollen tissues. To make a pain-relieving tea: Place ½ ounce dried rosemary leaves into 1 quart boiling water. Cover and steep for 30 minutes. Drink 1 cup tea at bedtime and another cup before eating breakfast.

TOPICAL REMEDIES

Cayenne Pepper. The hot stuff contains capsaicin, the source of its heat. Capsaicin causes nerve endings to release substance P, a chemical that transmits pain signals from the body to the brain. When the nerve endings have lost all their substance P, no pain 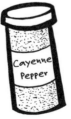 signals can be transmitted back to the brain. Make a cayenne back rub by placing 1 ounce cayenne pepper into 1 pint boiling water. Simmer for 30 minutes, remove from heat, and add a pint

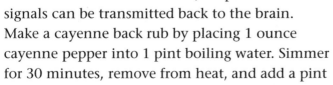

FASCINATING FACT
Eight out of ten Americans have back pain at some point in their lives. No age is immune, but it is most common in middle age. Low back pain is the most common type of chronic pain, reported by 27 percent of respondents in a recent national survey.

LEARN TO LIFT

Working in the home requires more lifting, bending, and standing than you may think. You lug in the groceries, reach to put them away, lift a heavy saucepan from the cabinet, stand over the stove for an hour. Here are some back-saving tips to use when in the home.

- Always stand with your feet shoulder-width apart. This gives you a solid base of support. If you'll be peeling potatoes for hours, place one leg on a stool to relieve back strain.
- Keep knees slightly bent. Never lock your knees.
- Suck that stomach in! Abdominal muscles help support your back.
- When lifting, position the person or object close to your body, and lift using your leg muscles. Squat; don't bend at the waist.
- Try not to twist and turn when lifting. To move, point your toes in the direction you want to move and pivot in that direction.
- Push, don't pull, grocery carts, baby buggies, or anything else with wheels.
- Wear flat shoes or heels no higher than one inch.
- Ask for assistance if an item is too heavy to lift.

of rubbing alcohol. Cool and use when needed. A pepper poultice, made with a mixture of flour and water, can also bring relief. Simply make a paste of the two ingredients, then spread it onto cotton, muslin, or gauze, and fold over. Apply to the back.

Warning! Never apply cayenne pepper directly to the skin or you may suffer a burn or blisters. Do not touch your eyes while handling cayenne, and always wash your hands well after handling peppers of any sort. Better yet, wear disposable rubber gloves. Capsaicin ointment, 0.025 percent, is also available over the counter.

Cold compresses. Cold compresses or ice packs should be applied immediately after back strain or injury. When the back suffers injury, blood rushes to the damaged area. Even though the resulting swelling is normal, too much inflammation can increase pain and lengthen your recovery period. An icy application reduces inflammation and helps numb pain. (Hot compresses can be used 48 hours after the injury.) To make a cold compress, pack a few crushed cubes of ice into a plastic, reclosable bag, cover with a washcloth or towel, and apply to the back for 15 minutes. Take it off for 30 minutes and then replace it for 15 more minutes. (A bag of frozen vegetables also works well. Wrap in a towel, too.)

Epsom salts. Epsom salts ease back pain by reducing swelling. Fill your bathtub as usual and add 2 cups salts. Soak for 30 minutes.

Hot compresses. You can begin to apply heat to your back 48 hours after an injury. Warmth relaxes tight muscles, increases blood flow, and feels terrific. Soak a washcloth in water that you've heated on the stove, use a heating pad, or take a hot shower or bath.

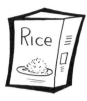

Rice. Fill a clean, thick sock with 1 cup uncooked rice and place in the microwave for 30 to 60 seconds on medium-low. Check the temperature and apply to the back as a compress.

LIFESTYLE REMEDIES

Get some zzzz's. Back muscles work all day to hold you erect; lying down takes the stress off. Lie flat on your back with two pillows underneath your knees. Don't overdo it, though. More than a day or two of rest may actually prolong your recovery. If you are still in too much pain to walk after two days, call your doctor.

Relax! When you're tense, so are those back muscles. Try some relaxation exercises.

Sit in comfort. Are your kitchen chairs padded? Does your car seat support the small of your back? Comfort should always come first wherever you park yourself. Buy inexpensive cushions for wooden or metal chairs and a small cushion for the car seat. Watch how you sit, too. It is better to lean back at an angle of 110 degrees than to sit straighter than an arrow.

Less is more. Maintaining your ideal weight helps take pressure off back muscles. The less you have to carry, the less burden to the supporting muscles and bones. Beer bellies and pendulous abdomens can make you sway-backed, which only accentuates back pain.

Invest in a new mattress. A soft, sagging mattress may contribute to the development of back problems or worsen an existing one. If you can't afford a new mattress, place a three-quarter-inch-thick piece of plywood between the mattress and the box spring.

WHEN TO CALL THE DOCTOR
- When the pain radiates from your lower back to the buttocks or down your legs
- If you experience numbness in the leg, foot, groin, or rectal area
- If the back pain is accompanied by fever, nausea, vomiting, stomachache, weakness, or excessive sweating
- If you lose control of your bowel and/or bladder functions
- When the pain is intense
- When a back injury is cramping your lifestyle

Bad Breath
HALTING HALITOSIS

Most people are worried about having bad breath—they don't want their breath to walk into a room before they do. That's why Americans spend a billion dollars per year on mints, mouthwash, and minty-fresh toothpastes.

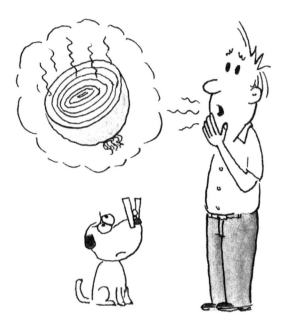

Having a concern and awareness about the possibility of bad breath is certainly normal, and even desirable, but the truth is there is no absolutely reliable way to assess the odiferousness of your breath. And some people take the concern over halitosis, as bad breath is technically called, to an obsessive extreme. A study, published in the *Journal of the American Dental Association*, found that some people think their breath smells bad even if the smell isn't all that offensive. And they go to great lengths to ensure their breath is fresh. Researchers called this a "negative breath odor self image" and found that people who tend to have a poor self-image in general think they have a breath odor problem.

Harboring Halitosis?

Only about 25 percent of the population deal with chronically bad breath. Are you one of them? You can try breathing into a handkerchief, running floss through your mouth, or licking the back of your hand, waiting a few minutes, and then sniffing. The Japanese have even tried to develop an electronic breath-sniffing device. But the truth is, people are immune to their own odors, offensive or not. So have a spouse or a (really) close, honest friend sniff your breath (use the same friend who always tells you when you have green stuff in your teeth) and give you the verdict.

More than likely, your fears of halitosis are all in your head. But if you discover your breath does have an unpleasant odor, there is usually a very treatable reason. Ninety percent of bad breath is a result of bacteria from something you ate setting up house in your mouth. Even when you brush and floss regularly, you can still miss some food particles. This can cause smelly breath. Other reasons for bad breath include:

- Potent foods. Garlic and onions, among other foods, contain sulfur compounds that move on to the lungs after they are absorbed in the bloodstream. Unfortunately, the chemicals that make these foods so tasty and pungent stick around. And they don't smell so great as you whisper sweet nothings into your sweetheart's ear. In some cultures, however, garlic and onion are so common in the food that they're considered desirable aromas, even on the breath.
- Periodontal (gum) disease. Caused by a buildup of plaque on the teeth, periodontal disease can result in chronically bad breath.
- Dry mouth. Saliva is the mop of the mouth. It cleanses and removes potentially smelly particles. When you don't produce enough saliva, you end up with bad breath. That's why when you wake up in the morning you go running for the nearest toothbrush. You produce less saliva while you sleep, and that causes you to wake up with icky breath.
- High-protein diet. Eating a high-protein diet such as the Atkins diet causes the body to produce ketones, which are eliminated in the urine and the breath. Ketones have an unpleasant odor.
- Hunger. If you haven't eaten in a while, you develop a very distinctive breath smell.

FIVE STEPS TO FRESH BREATH

- Brush teeth twice a day and floss regularly.
- Use your tooth-brush to brush your tongue after you've brushed your teeth.
- Chew sugarless gum or candy to keep your mouth moist.
- Rinse your mouth with water after you eat.
- Chew on parsley after eating.

FASCINATING FACT

Believe it or not, most people can tell, within 95 percent accuracy, if a person is a man or woman by the way their breath smells.

Is Mouthwash Worth It?

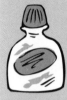

As much as most people would like to think mouthwash gets rid of offending odors, it only covers odors temporarily (from 20 minutes to 2 hours). Look for mouthwashes that contain cetylpyridinium chloride (CPC); essential oils of lime, cinnamon, or cloves; zinc chloride; or chlorhexidine. These compounds neutralize odors and/or inhibit bacterial growth.

Top Ten Breath Offenders:

Garlic
Raw onions
Cabbage
Horseradish
Eggs
Broccoli
Brussels sprouts
Fish
Red meat
Coffee

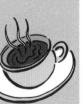

Some scientists believe this happens because pancreatic juices pass into the stomach when a person doesn't eat for some time. This is another factor in morning breath.

- Smoking. Tobacco is a major factor in bad breath. Ever heard the saying, "Kissing a smoker is like licking an ashtray"? Tobacco causes bad breath, stains the teeth, and interferes with your ability to taste food. Tobacco also irritates gum tissue, making smokers more likely to suffer periodontal disease.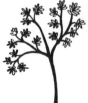
- Sinus infections and stuffy noses can cause smelly breath.
- Other, more serious illnesses can cause distinctive breath odors. People with kidney failure may have breath that smells like urine. Liver failure can cause a "fishy" breath smell. And fruity breath can signal diabetes.
- Some prescription drugs can cause bad breath.
- Certain fish, such as anchovies, and seaweed are high in "fishy" amine odors.

Dietary Remedies

Fresh vegetables. Fresh vegetables, such as carrots and celery, fight plaque and keep your breath smelling nice.

Parsley. Parsley has long been used as a breath neutralizer. It won't get rid of bad breath, but it may help mask the garlic shrimp you had for dinner.

Sugarless gum or candy. To keep your mouth moist and increase saliva flow, the American Dental Association suggests chewing sugarless gum or sucking on sugarless candy.

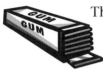

These are made with sorbitol, mannitol, or xylitol (sugar alcohols), which do not support oral bacterial growth.

Water. Water is essential for fresher breath. Swish water around your mouth for at least 20 seconds to loosen food particles and clean your mouth. Water may even work as well as mouthwash in removing trapped food particles and keeping your breath fresh.

HERBAL REMEDIES

Aromatic spices. Chewing on the seeds of spices such as clove, cardamom, or fennel after meals is a common practice in South Asia and the Middle East. The seeds of these spices contain antimicrobial properties that can help halt bad breath.

TOPICAL REMEDIES

Baking soda. Baking soda is a great way to clean your teeth and get fresh breath. For fresher breath, sprinkle some baking soda into your palm, dip a damp toothbrush into the baking soda, and brush.

If brushing with plain baking soda sounds icky, try adding a little artificial sugar, such as saccharine or aspartame. Or you can make your own toothpaste: Mix 3 parts baking soda with 1 part salt; add 3 teaspoons glycerin and 10 to 20 drops of your favorite flavoring (peppermint, wintergreen, anise, cinnamon); add enough water to make a paste.

To create a tooth powder, mix 3 parts baking soda with 1 part salt. Add a few drops of peppermint or wintergreen oil.

WHEN TO CALL THE DOCTOR

If you have chronic bad breath and your dentist gives your mouth a clean bill of health. Make an appointment with your doctor to rule out any other conditions that might be causing your bout with foul breath. Some specialists now treat chronic halitosis.

ANCIENT REMEDIES FOR BAD BREATH

Yes, bad breath has been a bane of existence for centuries. According to the Academy of General Dentistry, ancient Greeks rinsed with white wine, aniseed, and myrrh. Italians created a mouthwash of sage, cinnamon, juniper seeds, root of cypress, and rosemary leaves.

FASCINATING FACT

The average person produces more than two quarts of saliva per day.

Belching
ELIMINATING ERUPTIONS

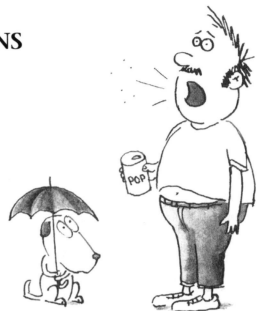

It's not a big deal, not even a medical condition most of the time. It's simply the result of swallowing air. But the air that goes down has to go somewhere, so most of the time it leaves the same way it came in—through the mouth. We all belch. Even the most prim of the proper is not exempt from this oftentimes untimely eruption.

Belching does serve a purpose other than embarrassment, however. It removes gas from the stomach by forcing it up into the esophagus and then on out your mouth. Without this escape device, we'd blow up like one of those big balloons in the Macy's Thanksgiving Day Parade, not to mention the sharp cramps we'd feel running all the way from our stomach to our throats. So belching is a good thing. And no matter how many good ones we let out during the course of a day, the swallowed air that turns into a burp is only a tiny fraction of the intestinal gas that we all have. (For more on gas, see Flatulence, page 180.)

The Cause
Swallowing air, which is called aerophagia, is the primary offender when it comes to producing a belch. We swallow air all the time, especially when we:
- Eat and drink
- Talk
- Yawn and sigh
- Breathe through the mouth
- Smoke
- Chew gum or suck on hard candy

Here are some other reasons we belch:
- Belching occurs when we eat because food in the belly displaces the air that was already swallowed and is sitting in the stomach.
- Anxiety is a cause of belching, too. We get nervous, we swallow more air. The more nervous we are, the more air we swallow, and

the more we belch. Anxiety belching is usually habitual and subconscious. We swallow air into the esophagus and expel it before it hits the stomach.

- An improper denture fit can cause you to swallow air.
- Drinking carbonated beverages.
- Excessive swallowing due to postnasal drip.
- Although belching is not normally a symptom of illness, some gastrointestinal disorders are accompanied by belching, including infections, gastrointestinal blockage, gallstones, hiatal hernia, ulcer, irritable bowel syndrome, celiac disease, and gastritis.

Even with all the conditions belching could potentially indicate, most often belching is simply belching for the sake of letting out unneeded gasses.

Medically, belching is called eructation, and the definition from *Taber's Encyclopedic Medical Dictionary* is, "Producing gas from the stomach, usually with a characteristic sound."

In many Eastern cultures, that characteristic sound is accepted as an appreciative expression of a good meal. In Western society, however, no matter how good that meal was, eructation is not acceptable. Bottom line—we try not to belch in public. Of course, that occasional and inadvertent little burp may slip out, and often at the most embarrassing moment. If its escape is indeed occasional, there's nothing to worry about. If it happens more often than you'd like, or if your life is just plain plagued by belching, you can either relocate to a country where your eructation routine is looked upon favorably, or you can use some home-remedy help.

DIETARY REMEDIES

Ginger. Ginger tea can help relieve the need to belch. Pour 1 cup boiling water over 1 teaspoon freshly grated gingerroot. Steep for 5 minutes, then drink.

Lemon juice. This works whether it's fresh or from the bottle. Mix 1 teaspoon lemon juice with ½ teaspoon baking soda in 1 cup cool water. Drink it quickly after meals.

Papaya. Most cures for belching aren't found in the fridge. But there is one surefire belch begone in the fruit drawer: papaya! It's full of an enzyme called papain that can get rid of whatever's causing that burp.

Yogurt. Eat some yogurt with live cultures (check the label) every day. It aids digestion.

HERBAL REMEDIES

Most of the belching cures are found right here, if you know what to mix. Here are a few remedies that might just squelch that belch.

Caraway. Try some caraway seeds, either straight or sprinkled on a salad. They help calm the digestive tract.

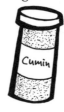

Cumin. Roast equal amounts of cumin, fennel, and celery seed. Combine. After you eat, chew well about ½ to 1 teaspoon of the mixture, then chase it down with ⅓ cup of warm water.

Ginger. Mix 1 teaspoon fresh ginger pulp with 1 teaspoon lime juice, and take after eating.

Peppermint. Pour 1 cup boiling water over 1 teaspoon dried mint. Steep for five minutes.

LIFESTYLE REMEDIES

Avoid carbonated drinks when you can. Or, pour them out into a glass and let them defizz for a few minutes before you drink. This includes beer too!

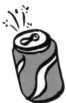

Don't chew gum or suck on hard candy. You may enjoy them, but they cause air-swallowing.

Don't drink through straws or narrow-mouthed bottles.

Don't gulp your food. Gulping makes you swallow air. Instead, eat slowly.

Don't lie down after you eat. Activity will force the belches out instead of letting them build up.

Keep a belching diary. Note foods and beverages consumed, as well as specific incidents prior to the start of belching. You may discover that you are more burp-prone immediately after you eat dairy foods (see Lactose Intolerance, page 289) or when you're stressed.

Exercise. Lie on your back and pull your knees up to your chest. Count to ten. Release, and repeat if necessary.

Quit smoking. That can cure the burps as well as many other problems.

WHEN TO CALL THE DOCTOR

- If your belching is accompanied by symptoms such as nausea, vomiting, jaundice, gastric juices backing up into the mouth, upper abdominal pain, loss of appetite, sweating, or dark or bloody stools
- If belching is persistent and without apparent cause

Bites and Stings
REDUCING THE REACTION

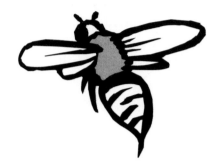

With billions of bugs out there, you're bound to be bitten or stung sometime in your life. Typically, the worst reactions are to bees, yellow jackets, hornets, wasps, and fire ants. Other nasty creatures, such as blackflies, horseflies, black or red (not fire) ants, and mosquitoes, also bite and sting, but their venom usually does not cause as intense a reaction. No matter what attacks, once you're zapped, the body reacts with redness, itching, pain, and swelling at the bite site. These symptoms may last for a few minutes or a few hours. Thankfully, relief is as close as the kitchen.

Warning! The remedies apply to bites and stings from the insects listed above. A health provider should treat those from snakes, spiders, scorpions, ticks, centipedes, and animals.

DIETARY REMEDIES
Antihistamine. Over-the-counter antihistamines can help an itchy bite, since the itch is really a mild allergic reaction. However, do not take an antihistamine if you are sensitive to these medications, have allergies to ingredients in the products, are taking a conflicting medication, or are pregnant.

Garlic. You might not get kissed, but you might not get bitten either if you eat onions and garlic regularly. Just like humans, stinging insects are attracted or repulsed by odors in their environment. Perhaps it is to your advantage not to smell so sweet. Some people believe that by eating pungent foods such as onions and garlic, the smell of your sweat changes, sending out a signal to insects that you stink. And you do. Although this theory hasn't been proven, it can't hurt to add an extra onion to your burger or an extra garlic clove to spaghetti sauce. Just remember to have some mouthwash or gum on hand if you plan to talk to others!

TOPICAL REMEDIES
Activated charcoal. This can help draw out the toxins that cause inflammation, swelling, and itching. To make a paste, open 2 to 3 capsules of charcoal, mix with enough water to make a

paste, and apply to the affected area. After 30 minutes, wipe the paste off with a wet cloth.

Baking soda. Itching can be tamed by applying a paste of 3 teaspoons baking soda to 1 teaspoon water directly to the site. This remedy is especially good for ant bites and bee stings, both of which are acidic in nature.

Ice. Ice or any cold compress does triple first-aid duty by diminishing the itch, reducing inflammation, and easing the pain of bites/stings. Put crushed ice into a plastic bag (or use a bag of frozen vegetables), wrap it in a towel, and apply to the site for 20 minutes.

Knife, credit card, playing card, fingernail. Bees and yellow jackets leave evidence behind when they strike: their barbed stinger. It's not a pleasant sight to see this pulsating barb puncturing the skin and releasing venom. Carefully and gently remove the stinger by scraping it off with the flat edge of the object you're using. Don't reach for the tweezers or tongs. Squeezing and grabbing the stinger causes more venom to be pumped into the victim. After removing the stinger, apply a topical antiseptic such as alcohol or Betadine.

Meat tenderizer. Meat tenderizers contain the enzyme papain that, when applied immediately, degrades the venom and reduces swelling. Use an unseasoned brand, mix a few teaspoons with a few drops of water, and apply the paste to the sting. Time is of the essence with this technique. Once the venom proteins penetrate deep into the skin, it's too late for the tenderizer to reach and degrade them.

Onion. Get a tissue, a knife, and an onion for this sting remedy. An

WHEN TO CALL THE DOCTOR

Most people just yell, "Ouch!" once they've been stung or bitten. However, for the 1 or 2 people in every 1,000 who are allergic or hypersensitive to insect bites and stings, such an incident is more than an "ouch." It is life threatening. Seek medical attention immediately should any of these allergic reaction symptoms occur:

- hives
- severe itching
- swelling throughout the body
- tightness and swelling of the throat
- breathing difficulty
- a sudden drop in blood pressure
- dizziness
- unconsciousness
- cardiac arrest

Vinegar: 10,000 Years Old and Going Strong

The virtues of vinegar have long been played out in history. Hippocrates extolled its medicinal qualities, the Babylonians used it as a preservative, and the Roman legionnaires swilled it down before doing battle.

The Who and Why Behind the Sting

Stinging insects belong to the order *hymenoptera*, which includes wasps, bees, and ants. The stinger is a modified egg-laying apparatus, so only females do the dirty deed. Most hymenopterans would rather flee than fight, but when it comes to social hymenopterans, such as yellow jackets, fire ants, and honeybees, they'll fight to the end to defend the nest or hive.

onion (or garlic clove) contains antibiotic and anti-inflammatory substances that minimize infections and swelling from bites and stings. Slice the onion in half, and hold the onion on the bite site for five to ten minutes.

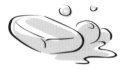 *Soap.* Besides keeping you squeaky clean, soap helps relieve the bite of the ubiquitous mosquito. Wet the skin and gently rub on soap. Rinse well. Be sure to use only nondeodorized, nonperfumed soap. Fancy, smelly soaps may irritate the bite area.

Tea bags. The tannic acid in tea helps decrease the swelling from a sting. Black tea is the most effective. Soak a tea bag in water or, after brewing tea, save the used tea bag in the refrigerator for a few days. Use it as a poultice. Apply cooled tea bags to bites/stings as needed.

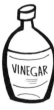 *Vinegar.* No matter which variety, vinegar may mellow the pain of an insect sting. Pour it on the affected site or mix it with baking soda to make a paste that you can apply to the bitten area. Out of vinegar? Try applying straight lemon juice instead.

Lifestyle Remedies

Cover your feet! Don't go barefoot in the grass; it's a favorite nesting, resting, and grazing ground for insects.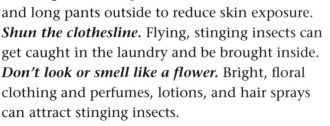
Cover up. Wear long-sleeved shirts and long pants outside to reduce skin exposure.
Shun the clothesline. Flying, stinging insects can get caught in the laundry and be brought inside.
Don't look or smell like a flower. Bright, floral clothing and perfumes, lotions, and hair sprays can attract stinging insects.

Boils
SIMMERING THEM DOWN

Boils have been a problem since the beginning of time. These painful bumps are mentioned in the Bible as one of the ten plagues used to convince the Egyptians to let the Israelites go. Even today, boils make people cringe because they are painful and unattractive. Most boils are harmless, even though they look and feel awful. Ironically enough, most of the treatments for boils have been around since the Egyptian doctors found themselves dealing with a boil epidemic.

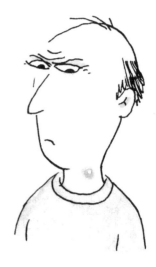

Debunking the Furuncles

Boils typically start as a red spot or pimplelike knot that turn overnight into a swollen, painful lump. Boils, or furuncles as they're known in medical circles, are a result of a bacterial infection, usually staphylococcus, setting up house in a hair follicle. The bacteria gets an open-door invitation when the hair follicle is traumatized. This can happen from a blockage, such as might occur from an oily ointment or lotion, or from irritation, as can happen when clothing rubs against the follicles. People who tend to get boils frequently are staph carriers and therefore physiologically more prone to get boils. Other problems such as acne, dermatitis, diabetes, and anemia can increase your risk of contracting the staphylococcus bacterial overgrowth. Men are more likely than women to get boils.

Boils can appear on any part of the body that has hair follicles, but they usually occur on the face, scalp, underarm, thigh, groin, and buttocks. They can vary in size from small, pimple-size sores to large, painful lumps, but they are typically larger than one-half inch in diameter.

A boil usually lasts about two weeks. During that time it will grow quickly, fill with pus, and burst. After it drains, the boil needs a little tender loving care as it begins to heal.

A cluster of boils is called a carbuncle. These are most frequently found at the back of the neck or the thigh. They are more serious than boils and are frequently accompanied by fever and fatigue. There may be whitish, bloody discharge from the carbuncle. Carbuncles require medical attention.

HERBAL REMEDIES

Burdock. Burdock helps bring circulation to the surface of the skin and is used around the world for treating boils. Put 1 ounce dried ground burdock in 1 quart water and bring it to a boil. Let simmer on low for 30 minutes. Drink 4 cups hot burdock tea each day until the boil comes to a head and drains. You can also apply a poultice of fresh boiled burdock leaves directly to the boil.

Chamomile. Chamomile contains antiseptic, antibacterial, and anti-inflammatory properties. To make a chamomile poultice, place ½ ounce chamomile flowers in a 1-pint canning jar and cover with boiling water. Cover the jar and let sit for fifteen minutes. Strain the water and apply the hot chamomile leaves directly to the boil. Cover with a cloth, and keep the cloth moist with the strained liquid. Keep the leaves on for 20 minutes; repeat every two to three hours.

Chrysanthemums. Japanese researchers have discovered that chrysanthemum flowers contain properties that inhibit staphylococcus bacteria. Try using chrysanthemum tea as a poultice and drinking it as a weapon against boils.

Tea tree oil. Tea tree leaves contain a potent oil that is antiseptic and is a very effective skin disinfectant. Research shows that tea tree oil inhibits staphylococcus, which may be why it became a traditional remedy for boils. Tea tree oil is especially useful because it doesn't irritate the skin as it cleanses. Apply directly to the boil two or three times per day.

TOPICAL REMEDIES

Bacon. The fat and salt con-tent of salt pork are believed to help bring boils to a head. Roll some salt pork or bacon in salt 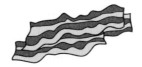 and place the meat between two pieces of cloth. Apply the cloth to the boil. Repeat throughout the day until the boil comes to a head and drains. This can be messy.

Cornmeal. The Aztecs and Cherokees used a remedy made from dried, powdered corn flour. Cornmeal doesn't have medicinal properties per se, but it is absorbent, which makes it an effective treatment for boils. Bring ½ cup water to a boil in a pot, and add cornmeal to make a thick paste. Apply the mush as a poultice to the boil, and cover with a cloth. Repeat every one to two hours until the boil comes to a head and drains.

Eggs. The whites of hard-boiled eggs were used for treating boils in the nineteenth century. After boiling and peeling an egg, wet the white and apply it directly to the boil. Cover with a cloth.

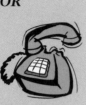

Jelly jar. "Cupping," or applying suction by placing a cup or jar over the infected area, is an age-old treatment for boils. Put a cup in a pot of water and boil for a few minutes. Using tongs, take the cup out of the pot and let it cool a bit before putting it over the boil (you don't want the cup to be too cool or there won't be any suction). As the cup cools over the boil, the suction brings blood and circulation to the area. Blot and wash pus away.

Milk. Heat 1 cup milk and slowly add 3 teaspoons salt (adding the salt too quickly can make the milk curdle). Simmer for ten minutes. Add flour or crumbled bread pieces to thicken the mixture. Divide into 4 poultices and apply one to the boil every half-hour.

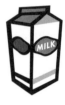

Onion. The onion has antiseptic chemicals and acts as an antimicrobial and irritant to draw blood to the boil. Cut a thick slice of onion and place it over the boil. Wrap the area with a cloth. Change the poultice every three to four hours until the boil comes to a head and drains.

MORE DO'S AND DON'TS

- Don't squeeze or break the boil open. Let it come to a head and rupture on its own. If you take matters into your own hands, you risk spreading the infection.
- Be sure to wash any towels, compresses, or clothes that have touched the boil. Otherwise, you can spread the infection.

- Don't buy over-the-counter products that say they can draw out the fluid in boils.

Bronchitis
CONTROLLING THE COUGH

That nasty cold has been hanging on much longer than it should, and day by day it seems to be getting worse. Your chest hurts, you gurgle when you breathe, and you're coughing so much yellow, green, or grey mucus that your throat is raw. These symptoms are letting you know that your cold has probably turned into bronchitis, an inflammation that causes the little branches and tubes of your windpipe to become inflamed and swollen. No wonder breathing has become such a chore—your air passages are too puffy to carry air very easily.

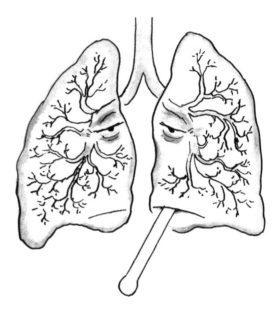

Acute bronchitis can include these other symptoms, too:

- Wheezing
- Shortness of breath
- Fever or chills
- General aches and pains
- Upper chest pain

Bronchitis is not contagious since it's a secondary infection that develops when your immune system is weakened by a cold or the flu. Some people are prone to developing it, some are not. Those at the top of the risk list have respiratory problems already, such as asthma, allergies, and emphysema. People who have a weakened immune system also are more prone to bronchitis. But anyone can develop this unpleasant condition, and most people do at one time or another.

Under most circumstances, bronchitis will go away on its own once the primary infection is cured. But in those few days when you have it, it can sure be miserable. Here are a few home remedies that can relieve some of the symptoms.

MUCUS-MAKERS TO AVOID

When you're congested, there are a few simple foods that should be avoided because they produce more mucus. Here's the list:

- Dairy foods
- Sugary products, including carbonated and noncarbonated soft drinks; sugar-coated cereal; sugary throat lozenges
- Refined cereals, bread, pasta
- Fried and fatty foods
- Red meat, including pork

Here's a handy avoidance reminder: When you're congested, skip the white stuff—milk, flour, sugar.

DIETARY REMEDIES

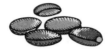

Almonds. These are loaded with vitamins and rich in potassium, calcium, and magnesium. They are often recommended for treating respiratory illnesses. Eat them in any form, except candy-coated or chocolate-covered. Drizzle a little almond cream over your oatmeal in the morning (see the Recipe Box, page 65). Or sliver some almonds and garnish your veggies. They're good in a citrus fruit salad or rubbed in a little honey, coated with cinnamon, and roasted in a 325 degree Fahrenheit oven for 10 to 25 minutes.

Honey. To relieve the cough that comes from bronchitis, slice an onion into a bowl, then cover with honey. Allow to stand overnight, then remove the onion. Take 1 teaspoon of the honey four times per day.

Lemons. These help rid the respiratory system of bacteria and mucus. Make a cup of lemon tea by grating 1 teaspoon lemon rind and adding it to 1 cup boiling water. Steep for five minutes. Or, boil a lemon wedge. Strain into a cup and drink. For a throat that's sore from coughing, add 1 teaspoon lemon juice to 1 cup warm water and gargle. This helps bring up phlegm.

Onions. These are expectorants and help the flow of mucus. Use raw, cooked, baked, in soups and stews, or as seasoning.

Water. Lots and lots of it. The more you drink, the more your mucus will liquefy. This makes it easier to cough out.

HERBAL REMEDIES

Bay leaf. Ancient Romans and Greeks loved bay leaves. They believed that this simple herb was the source of happiness, clairvoyance, and artistic inspiration. Whatever the case, it does act as an expectorant and is best taken in tea. To make the tea, tear a leaf (fresh or dried) and steep in 1 cup boiling water. Another bronchitis remedy with bay leaf is to soak some leaves in hot water and apply as a poultice to the chest. Cover with a kitchen towel. As it cools, rewarm.

Warning! Pregnant women may want to avoid bay leaf. According to one old (though unproven) theory, medicinal-strength preparations of bay leaf may stimulate the uterus.

Ginger. This is a potent expecto-rant that works well in tea. Steep ½ teaspoon ginger, a pinch of ground cloves, and a pinch of cinnamon in 1 cup boiling water.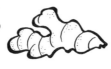

Mustard. The old-fashioned mustard plaster's warmth relieves symptoms of many respiratory

THIS MAY WORK, BUT...

Here's an old folk remedy that may relieve symptoms of bronchitis, but it's up to you if you want to try it. Keep a clove of garlic in your mouth every waking hour. Don't eat it, don't swallow it, just hold it in there. And change it twice a day. You can spit it out when you go to sleep, however.

The fact is, garlic contains compounds with antimicrobial properties, and in countries where the consumption of garlic is high, the incidence of upper respiratory tract infection is low.

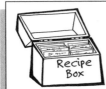

ALMOND CREAM

4 ounces whole almonds
¼ teaspoon pure vanilla extract
    (increase to ½ if you're using imitation)
honey
cinnamon (optional)

Blanch almonds by covering with ½ cup plus 2 tablespoons water, and bring to a boil. Remove the skins, then puree in the blender with the water in which they cooked. Add vanilla. Add a pinch of cinnamon (optional). Sweeten to taste with a little honey.
Makes about 1 cup.

ABOUT THAT HUMIDIFIER

More humidity usually is beneficial for a respiratory ailment because it thins out thick mucus secretions. If you have asthma or emphysema, however, talk to your doctor before using a humidifier.

If you're suffering from a simple case of bronchitis, however, steaming those lungs might be soothing. But here's a warning! Warm water quickly breeds bacteria, including Legionnaire's Disease, usually within 8 hours. And you don't want to breathe those bacteria in. So if you're using a home humidifier, here are a few tips:

- Follow the manufacturer's instructions for cleaning your humidifier or use these guidelines: Empty and wipe dry the inside of the unit every day. Every third day, wash all parts that come in contact with water, using a three-part solution of hydrogen peroxide; rinse with water several times. This eliminates the bacteria and the mineral buildup from tap water. Using bottled distilled water will prevent the mineral buildup, but it won't stop the growth of bacteria.
- Grab a new copper pot scrubber and stick it in the humidifier. Copper has a bacteriostatic property that slows bacterial growth.
- Add a capful of vinegar to the water in the humidifier. It will slow bacterial growth.
- If you have any chronic respiratory condition, check with your doctor before you use a humidifying treatment.

ailments, including bronchitis. Take 1 tablespoon dry mustard and mix with 4 tablespoons flour. Stir in enough warm water to make a runny paste. Oil the chest with vegetable shortening or olive oil, then spread the mustard mix on a piece of cloth—muslin, gauze, a kitchen washcloth—and cover with an identical piece. Apply to the chest. Keep in place until cool, but check every few minutes to make sure it doesn't burn the skin. Remove the plaster if it causes discomfort or burning.

Savory. This potent, peppery herb is said to rid the lungs of mucus. Use it as a tea by adding ½ teaspoon savory to 1 cup boiling water. Drink only once a day.

Thyme. This herb helps rid the body of mucus, strengthens the lungs to fight off infection, and acts as a shield against bacteria. Use it dried as a seasoning or make a tea by adding ¼ to ½ teaspoon thyme (it's a very strong herb, so you don't need much) to 1 cup boiling water. Steep for 5 minutes and sweeten with honey. If you have thyme oil on hand, dilute it (2 parts olive or corn oil to 1 part thyme oil) and rub on the chest to cure congestion.

TOPICAL REMEDIES

Humidity. You don't need a humidifier to get moisture into your lungs. In fact, because humidifiers can cause as many problems as they cure (see "About That Humidifier" at left), this is a better solution. Simmer a pot of water on the stove to send some steam into the atmosphere,

CHRONIC BRONCHITIS

Unlike acute bronchitis, which stays for about three to four days and then goes, chronic bronchitis doesn't know when to leave. In fact, it may keep coming back or move in permanently. About 7.6 million people have chronic bronchitis, which is diagnosed when you cough up mucus for three straight months or more, two years in a row.

Chronic bronchitis is a result of a continued irritation to the airways, from such irritants as cigarette smoke, secondhand smoke, and air pollution. Smoking, though, is the number one cause.

Symptoms of chronic bronchitis include:

• Smoker's cough, that regular morning cough that brings up mucus
• Shortness of breath, especially after the disease has progressed
• Wheezing
• In its final stages, wheezing and coughing are nearly continuous

There is no cure for chronic bronchitis, and it usually leads to other respiratory diseases such as emphysema and pneumonia. In some cases, it is fatal. Symptoms can be eased by removing the cause, however. In other words, quit smoking.

The following measures might make breathing a little easier, especially if you forgo the cigarettes:

• Get flu and pneumonia shots every year. Those with chronic bronchitis are highly susceptible to these illnesses.
• Avoid smoky rooms and stay inside on days with a high air pollution index.
• Get some exercise—moderately, however. Your lungs won't hold up to strenuous activity. Playing a wind instrument, such as a clarinet or saxophone, can strengthen the lungs.
• Boost your immune system with vitamin C. And the recommended dietary allowance (RDA) for smokers is higher than that for nonsmokers. Citrus fruit is a good way to get your RDA of vitamin C.
• Skip the dairy products, sugar, and chocolate. These promote mucus secretion.
• Eat your veggies. Studies show that those who eat at least seven servings a week have the lowest risk of developing chronic bronchitis.

WHEN TO CALL THE DOCTOR

- If symptoms last more than three to four days
- If your bronchitis keeps returning
- If the person with bronchitis is an infant or an older adult. Complications in these people can become very serious or even deadly.
- If you have a lot of greenish mucus. You may need antibiotics.
- If you have lung or heart disease, or any other debilitating chronic illness or immune problem
- If you cough up blood. Tiny bright red specks normally come from irritation to the airways, so a few specks of blood can be normal. Coughing up larger amounts or blood that is dried and brownish may require treatment.
- If your temperature lingers at 102 degrees Fahrenheit for a couple of days

which will kill germs and viruses. Better yet, use a tea kettle: It's designed to shoot out that warm, moist air. And if you have a few drops of peppermint or eucalyptus oil to add, these can relieve congestion and be quite soothing.

Water. Fill the sink with hot water, bend down to it, cover your head with a towel, and breathe in the steam. Add a few drops of eucalyptus, peppermint, or rosemary oil if you have one of them. These help clear and soothe the respiratory passages.

LIFESTYLE REMEDIES

Pamper yourself. Go to bed, read a book, listen to music, watch an old movie. Don't go about business as usual just because bronchitis isn't usually contagious or serious.

Rest up. Then rest some more. Since bronchitis is usually the second half of a double-illness whammy, your body needs all the rest it can get to build up its strength.

Stay out of harm's way. You're at risk for picking up another infection. Avoid crowds, children with colds, smoky rooms, and contact with anyone who has a cold or flu. Wear gloves or a mask if you have to, and wash your hands often.

MORE DO'S & DON'TS

- Don't take a cough suppressant unless your doctor prescribes it. Coughing is your body's way of getting rid of mucus. Mucus buildup can lead to serious respiratory complications such as pneumonia, so when you're congested, that cough is your friend!

Burns
PUTTING OUT THE FIRE

The home is one hot place. Just look at all those things heating up in your kitchen: the stove, the oven, the toaster, the microwave, and the waffle iron. Add to that electrical currents and harsh cleaning chemicals, and you have plenty of ways to get toasted.

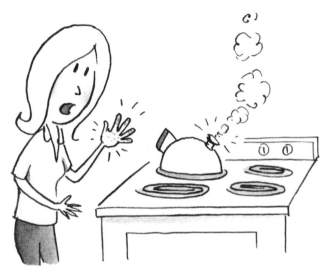

Doctors classify burns by degree. First-degree burns affect the outer layer of skin, called the epidermis. These burns cause pain and redness, but no blistering. Most household burns and sunburns are first degree, and most often they can be treated at home.

Second-degree burns go deeper, involving the epidermis and the dermis, the underlying skin layer. Fluid leaks from damaged blood vessels and causes blistering. The burns are very painful but usually aren't serious unless they are large or become infected. Some second-degree burns can be treated at home; however, if the burn is large or involves the face, hands, feet, or genitals, seek medical attention.

The most serious of all are third-degree burns, which require immediate medical attention. Deep and damaging, this burn involves the outer and inner layers of skin and leaves a path of destruction. Hair, nerves, blood vessels, glands, fat, and even muscle and bone can be damaged. The burn appears white or black and is generally painless since nerves have been destroyed. Third-degree burns often result in death, especially when they cover large areas of the body.

The following remedies only cover minor household burns. Blistering or infected burns, third-degree burns, or chemical and electrical burns require medical attention.

BUTTER ISN'T BETTER

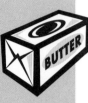

Many folk remedies have you smearing butter on burns like you would on bread. But butter, or any grease for that matter, should never be applied to burns. First, that butter in the back of your refrigerator isn't sterile. Second, the grease will insulate the burn and hold in the heat. It's best to leave butter for your toast.

TOPICAL REMEDIES

Cool water. Though ice is nice for sore muscles, cool water is the best for burned skin. Ice can restrict blood flow to the burn site and further damage delicate tissues. Instead, gently run cool water or place cool compresses over the burn site for ten minutes. Cool water not only feels good but will help stop the burn from spreading.

Honey. If you're suffering from a burn, the treatment should at least be sweet. Honey has long been a folk remedy to disinfect wounds and heal burns, and several studies show that the sticky stuff seems to be an effective salve. Everyone knows bees are attracted to honey, but did you know water is, too? When applied to a burn, honey draws out fluids from the tissues, effectively cleaning the wound. You may also apply the honey to a gauze bandage, which is less messy than direct application. Put a dollop of honey on a piece of sterile gauze, and place the bandage directly on the burn, honey-side down. Change the dressing three to four times per day.

Ice cube. A tongue burn is best treated with ice rather than cool water. Often, in great anticipation, children (and adults for that matter) sip their soup or hot chocolate before it cools down and get a tongue burn. Since it's tricky to stick a burned tongue under the faucet, try sucking on an ice cube. First rinse the cube under water so it doesn't stick to the tongue or lips.

Milk. Got milk? Then you've also got a great way to soothe a burn. For a minor burn, soak the

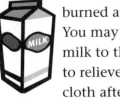 burned area in milk for 15 minutes or so. You may also apply a cloth soaked in milk to the area. Repeat every few hours to relieve pain. Be sure to wash out the cloth after use, as it will sour quickly.

Oatmeal. As minor burns heal, they can become itchy. A good way to relieve the itch is by taking an oatmeal bath. 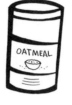 Crumble 1 cup uncooked oatmeal into a stream of lukewarm water as the tub is filling. Soak 15 to 20 minutes and then air dry so that a thin coating of oatmeal remains on your skin. Use caution getting in and out of the tub since the oatmeal makes surfaces slippery.

Plantain leaves. These are a popular remedy for treating burns among the Seneca Indians and many other practitioners of folk medicine. The major constituents in plantain leaves are mucilage, iridoid glycosides (particularly aucubin), and tannins. Together they are thought to have mild anti-inflammatory, antimicrobial, antihemorrhagic, and expectorant actions. To get the full effect of this plant, crush some fresh plantain leaves and rub the juice directly onto the burn.

 Salt. Mouth burns can be relieved by rinsing with salt water every hour or so. Mix ½ teaspoon salt in 8 ounces warm water.

Tea bags. Teatime can be anytime you suffer a minor burn. The tannic acid in black tea helps draw heat from a burn. Put 2 to 3 tea bags under a spout of cool water and collect the tea in a small bowl. Gently dab the liquid on the burn site.

WHEN TO CALL THE DOCTOR

- If the victim has experienced a third-degree burn
- If the burn is large or involves the face, hands, feet, or genitals
- If the burn blisters severely
- If someone has suffered an electrical or chemical burn
- If the pain and itching get worse after the first 24 hours
- If the victim develops chills or a fever and feels weak

Another method is to make a concoction using 3 or 4 tea bags, 2 cups fresh mint leaves, and 4 cups boiling water. Strain liquid into a jar and allow to cool. To use, dab the mixture on burned skin with a cotton ball or washcloth.

If you're on the go, you can also make a stay-in-place poultice out of 2 or 3 wet tea bags. Simply place cool, wet tea bags directly on the burn and wrap them with a piece of gauze to hold them in place.

Vinegar. Vinegar works as an astringent and antiseptic on minor burns and helps prevent infection. Dilute the vinegar with equal parts water, and rinse the burned area with the solution.

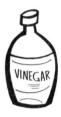

LIFESTYLE REMEDIES

Out of all areas in the home, the kitchen is number one for burns. The reasons are obvious, as are many of the precautions you can take to prevent an accident.

Lower the temperature. Set your hot-water heater below 120 degrees Fahrenheit. A second-degree burn can happen within seconds in water hotter than that.

Turn pot handles in on the stove.

Keep out of reach. Set your steaming cup of java up high, where a child can't reach it.

Cover all electrical outlets. Use specially made outlet caps if children are present.

Make the stove area off-limits to children. Put a childproof lock on the oven. Keep oven mitts and pot holders handy when cooking.

Keep 'em handy. Have a fire extinguisher and a box of baking soda nearby in case of a grease fire.

Bursitis
FOILING FLARE-UPS

You head out to the backyard after a long winter indoors to turn over your garden. The fresh air smells sweet, and you spend the afternoon pulling weeds. As the sun sets and you head inside, you feel an unfamiliar pain in your shoulder. The dull ache becomes a 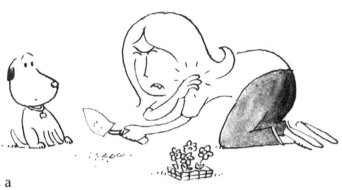 more intense pain, and you start to think you might be getting arthritis. Because it causes pain and stiffness near the joint, many people mistake bursitis for arthritis. But bursitis is a different problem altogether.

Bursitis goes by many aliases, including "Housemaid's Knee," "Clergyman's Knee," and "Baker's Cyst." Despite its nicknames, bursitis does not only affect the knee. It can hit any major joint, including the shoulder, elbow, hip, ankle, heel, or base of the big toe.

Bursitis Basics

Bursa are tiny sacks of fluid that protect your muscles and tendons from rubbing against the rough edges of your bones. There are more than 150 bursa in your body, and any one of them can become inflamed. Inflamed bursa are very painful.

Though bursitis is associated with physical activity, you don't have to be an athlete to develop the condition. Anytime you exercise too

THE ORIGIN OF ASPIRIN

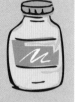

Aspirin, like many pharmaceutical drugs, has a botanical source. It was "discovered" as chemists studied plants such as willow bark, sage, and pennyroyal. Willow bark was the first plant to be studied for its pain-relieving properties. The source of willow bark's pain-alleviating power, salicin, was discovered in the 19th century. Chemists then began to look at the same properties in other plants and developed aspirin (acetylsalicylic acid) obtained from salicin in the herb meadowsweet. Those original botanical investigations ultimately led to the development of 20th century nonsteroidal anti-inflammatory agents (NSAIDs).

strenuously, especially after laying off your workout for a while, you can aggravate bursitis. You can also have bursitis problems if your work or hobbies requires repetitive physical movements, especially lifting things over your head. A bursitis attack can be triggered when you bump or bruise your bursa. And sometimes bursitis can just flare up for no good reason.

Though most people associate bursitis with the older crowd, the condition is not limited to any age group. It affects young and old alike. And once you've had one attack of bursitis, it tends to come back again and again.

Bursitis does mimic other conditions, so it's helpful to know what its symptoms are. If you have any of these symptoms, you may indeed have bursitis:

- Pain is specific and localized.
- Pain can be characterized as a dull ache or stiffness.
- Pain is predominantly in joint areas.
- Pain gets worse with movement.
- Affected area feels swollen or warm to the touch.

Most cases of bursitis clear up in a couple weeks if you stop aggravating the area, but you can do a few simple things that will speed healing and make the process more comfortable. There are also some nutritional secrets that may help prevent future bursitis flare-ups.

DIETARY REMEDIES

Orange juice. Vitamin C is a wonder nutrient. Its antioxidant properties make it an ideal addition to the diet, especially when you are recovering from an injury. Vitamin C is vital for preventing and repairing injuries and helps repair connective tissue. Not getting enough vitamin C has been found to hinder proper formation and maintenance of bursa. Men older than 19 years of age need at least 90 milligrams a day, and women older than 19 need 75 milligrams a day. However, to treat bursitis, a suggested dosage is 250–3,000 milligrams two times a day.

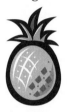

Pineapple. Pineapples contain bromelain, an enzyme that studies have shown reduces inflammation in sports injuries, such as bursitis, and reduces swelling.

HERBAL REMEDIES

Turmeric. Studies have found that turmeric, specifically the yellow pigment in turmeric called curcumin, is a very effective anti-inflammatory. In animal studies, turmeric was as effective as cortisone, and it didn't have any side effects. Take 375 milligrams three times per day for 12 weeks. Turmeric can also increase the effects of bromelain, so they are sometimes combined or taken together. Check with your doctor first before self-treating.

TOPICAL REMEDIES

Ice. Ice is a must when you're dealing with swelling. Cooling off the area slows down the blood flow and reduces inflammation. Wrap an ice pack in a 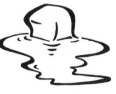 thin towel and put it on the painful area for about 20 minutes.

WHEN TO CALL THE DOCTOR

Bursitis is not life threatening, and the pain that accompanies a flare-up will usually go away on its own after a couple weeks if you go easy on the joint. However, if this is the first time you suspect you have bursitis, you may want to check with your doctor to make sure you do indeed have the condition. Seeing a doctor will also ensure you don't have a more serious problem, since bursitis can be caused by an infection, gout, or arthritis. Even if bursitis is a common occurrence, you need to talk to your doctor if you have these symptoms:

- Your pain is disabling
- Your pain doesn't go away after ten days of treatment at home
- You have excessive swelling or bruising
- You have a rash in the affected area
- Your pain is sharp or shooting

LIFESTYLE REMEDIES

Take it easy. Avoid doing the activity that caused the bursitis attack, but don't completely stop using the joint or it could become immobilized with scar tissue.

Get a new pad. If you have bursitis in your heel, make sure your shoes are well cushioned and well fitted. If your knees or elbows are the culprit, invest in some knee or elbow pads. Leaning on your knees and elbows on hard surfaces can inflame the bursa in those areas.

Look over the counter. The nonsteroidal anti-inflammatory drugs (NSAIDs) such as aspirin, ibuprofen, and naproxin will reduce swelling and ease pain. But be careful: NSAIDs can also cause bleeding in the stomach, especially with prolonged use.

Heat things up. Once you've gotten the swelling under control, applying heat will increase circulation and help get rid of excess fluid. A heating pad or heat pack also feels very good.

Make a motion. Once you're on the road to healing, start doing low-intensity exercises that will help you regain your range of motion.

MORE DO'S AND DON'TS

- Always warm up and stretch before doing any physical activity.
- Elevate the injured joint above your heart to help reduce swelling.
- When performing repetitive tasks, take frequent breaks.

Calluses and Corns
PAMPERING YOUR PIGGIES

Your poor tootsies get little respect, but they still work hard for you. They are your foundation, and without them, you wouldn't be able to chase after your toddler, walk a memo down the hall, or run in your first 5K competition. Your feet are invaluable, and they can use a little pampering. And it's better to pamper them before they start forming corns and calluses. Five percent of Americans develop corns or calluses each year, but they are avoidable. So it might be time to make sure you're treating those feet kindly.

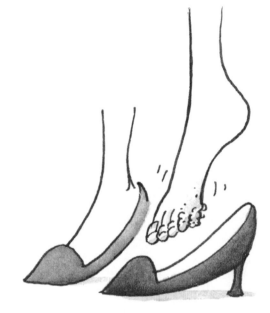

The Case for Corns and Calluses

Don't be too hard on calluses and corns. After all, their main function is protecting sensitive areas on the foot. A callus is made up of a tough protein called keratin, which is formed when dead skin cells huddle together to create a natural protection on the foot. Calluses usually form on a flat surface on the foot, such as the ball or heel. As people age, the padding on the bottom of the foot begins to thin, so a protective layer of skin naturally develops to protect the foot against too much pressure and chafing. Calluses are usually not too painful, until they get too big or too hard. Then they may start irritating the underlying skin, which can cause tenderness in the affected area.

Corns are actually a type of callus that usually forms on the toes and penetrates deeper. There are two types of corns: hard and soft. Hard corns usually form on the toe joints, such as the tops of the toes or on the outside of the pinkie toes, while soft corns form between the toes. Hard corns are described as cone-shaped because a tough core forms a tip that points

CINDERELLA FEET

Badly fitting shoes are the number one nonmedical cause of foot problems. The primary reason that corns and calluses develop is the friction and pressure caused by loose, tight, or poorly cushioned shoes. It takes some investigating to find shoes that fit like a glove, but your feet will thank you. Here are some shopping tips that will help.

- Shop late. Shop for shoes at the end of the day. Your feet swell by almost five percent during the course of a day.
- Watch the weather. Your feet will swell in hot weather and contract in cold weather.
- Take a measure. Ask the salesclerk to measure your foot. Your feet may not be the size that you think they are.
- Give them a test drive. Try on both shoes and walk around, even jog.
- Don't expect shoes that feel too tight in the store to stretch out. If they're snug, don't buy them.
- Watch the heels. A one-inch heel is about as high as you want to go in a shoe that you're going to wear often. And go for a heel that is thick.

inward. As with calluses, corns aren't always painful. But they are annoying and can become painful when they are irritated by chafing against each other or against the side of your shoe.

Causes of Corns and Calluses

Mistreating the feet by wearing shoes that don't fit well or that are too inflexible or nonporous are common causes of calluses and corns. Shoes that squeeze the toes force one toe to rub against the other, ultimately causing a corn to develop. High-heeled shoes are also major culprits, since they put pressure on the front of the foot, as can ill-fitting socks or irritation from your foot rubbing against a sock seam or shoe stitching. Shoes that are too loose cause your foot to slide, creating friction that can cause calluses.

Socks and shoes aren't the only causes of corns and calluses. You can also get them from:

- Walking on hard surfaces.
- Flat feet (People with flat feet are more likely to get calluses.)
- Thinning of the skin on the sole of the foot.
- Diabetics and others with circulatory problems should never self-treat or ignore foot problems.

TOPICAL REMEDIES

Baking soda. One tried and true way to treat corns and calluses is with a warm-water soak. This loosens the dead skin and helps with healing. Add 3 tablespoons baking soda to a basin of warm water and soak. Or massage calluses with a paste of 3 parts baking soda to 1 part water.

Chamomile tea. Soaking your feet in diluted chamomile tea can be soothing.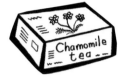

Ice. Hard corns can be particularly painful. If you find yourself with a hard-core corn, apply an ice pack to the area. This will help reduce swelling and ease the pain a bit.

Cornstarch. Sprinkle cornstarch between your toes to keep the area dry. Moisture can make a corn or callus feel miserable and can promote fungal infections.

 Lemon juice. Mix a paste of 1 tablespoon lemon juice and 5 or 6 crushed aspirin tablets. Apply the paste directly to your callus, and wrap your foot in a plastic bag. Keep your foot under wraps for ten minutes, allowing the acidity to soften your callus. Then give your callus a rub with a pumice stone.

Pumice stone. Pumice powder and stones are very useful for sloughing away dead skin. Soak your foot in warm water for about 20 minutes, then use a pumice stone to rub away corns and calluses.

Vinegar. Soak a cotton ball in vinegar and tape it to your corn or callus. Leave the vinegar-soaked cotton on overnight. In the morning, rub the area with a pumice stone.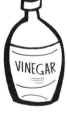

MORE DO'S AND DON'TS

- Separate your toes with cotton balls. Keeping soft corns from touching your other toes, or aggravating other corns, will speed healing and make you more comfortable.
- Don't try to remove a callus or corn yourself. Home removal can cause an infection.

WHEN TO CALL THE DOCTOR
- If a corn or callus doesn't respond to recommended treatment and grows more painful
- If you have diabetes
- If there are any signs of ulceration or infection

FASCINATING FACT
About 5 percent of the U.S. population has corns and calluses each year. Eighty-two percent of corn and callus problems are treated by podiatrists.

Canker Sores
VANQUISHING THE PAIN

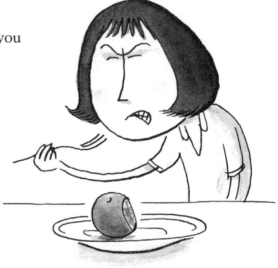

That wonderful spaghetti sauce has been simmering on the burner for hours, and you can't wait for the feast to begin. Just one last taste before culinary paradise and... Zap! It got you. It stings and your eyes tear up just a bit. All your well-planned preparations have been conquered by a painful canker, squelched by stomatitis (an inflammation of the mouth), annihilated by an apthous ulcer (the medical name for a canker). You get the point. That acidic sauce you've been craving doesn't get along with your canker, so your pasta should be served without the sauce tonight.

Cankers are small white sores with red edges that develop inside your mouth. They hurt like

Canker Sores	Cold Sores
Usually inside the mouth: on the gums, tongue, soft palate, inside the lips or cheeks	Usually outside of mouth, on or around lips or mouth
Small craterlike sores	Blisters
White, gray, or yellowish, with red halo	Red, often fluid-filled
Not contagious	Contagious
Cause: Injury to the area, stress, exhaustion, hormonal changes, menstrual period, food allergies, dietary deficiencies, medications	Cause: Herpes simplex virus, type 1

the dickens, but usually they're not serious. The most painful phase lasts about three to four days, and the sores go away in about ten days. More than 80 percent of all mouth sores are cankers, but many people confuse them with cold sores (fever blisters), which they are not (see Cold Sores, page 91). Canker sores and cold sores are two different problems altogether. The chart on the previous page will help you compare them.

Who Gets Them?

Anybody can get a canker sore, and at least 20 percent of the population does at one time or another. Women are more susceptible than men, especially during their menstrual period. The first canker sore usually occurs between the ages of 10 and 40. Some scientists believe that cankers are caused by a glitch in the immune system that causes the body to attack and damage healthy cells in the mouth and tongue. Some studies suggest that cankers are more common in people who have certain immune disorders, such as Crohn's disease. And heredity is a factor, too. If both your parents were canker sore sufferers, there's a 90 percent chance you will be, too.

Canker sores, unfortunately, can be repeaters, and some people are simply predisposed to getting them over and over. Most of the time the sores are not a major concern. They usually don't get infected, spread, or bleed if you don't bite them. But they're definitely a major pain.

You can find over-the-counter antiseptic creams, lozenges, and mouthwashes at your local pharmacy to help relieve canker sore pain. There are also some home remedies that can help.

GOLDTHREAD YOUR CANKER

Goldthread is a flower that blooms in the spring, known by its scientific name, *Coptis trifolia*. The first clue that it might cure your canker is its nickname, Canker Root. The remedy is to boil the root and rinse your mouth with the water after it cools. Some people prefer to chew the root. To find it, check a specialty market that sells herbs and natural cures.

EDIBLE NO-NOS

Some of canker's prevailing causes are said to be spicy, sour, or acidic foods. If you develop a canker after eating pineapple or a mild sandwich that you spiced up with mustard or barbecue sauce, these could be trigger foods. Only you know what you eat before cankers pop up, so if you're plagued and can't figure out why, keep a canker sore diary. Note the foods you eat before a canker erupts and also record other facts in your life such as menstrual cycle or hormonal fluctuations, medications you took, and undue stress. You may see a pattern. In the meantime, here are a few of the foods to avoid when that canker comes calling:

- Carbonated soft drinks
- Tomatoes and tomato-based products
- Citrus fruits
- Pineapple
- Spicy foods
- Foods at a hot temperature
- Chocolate
- Foods with sharp edges, such as crackers and chips
- Alcoholic beverages

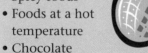

DIETARY REMEDIES

Cranberry juice. Drink this juice between meals: Many canker sufferers swear by the crimson cocktail for fast healing and pain relief.

Vitamins and minerals. Some scientists suspect that nutritional deficiencies may cause cankers. In particular, consuming too little vitamin B_{12}, folic acid, and iron may encourage growth of these mouth sores. Make sure you're eating a balanced diet that includes plenty of vitamins and minerals by checking out the food chart on page 84, or consider taking a daily multivitamin/multimineral supplement.

Stick to cool foods. Stay away from foods that are hot—either in terms of temperature or spiciness—or that are acidic. They'll burn and sting a tender canker sore.

HERBAL REMEDIES

Aloe. That beautiful aloe plant sitting on your sill has some quite potent curative powers. A little aloe juice from the juicy inner portion of the leaf rinsed over the canker several times daily could be just what you need. Don't swallow the juice, though, as it can have a laxative effect and large doses can be toxic.

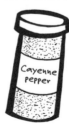

Cayenne pepper. Cayenne contains capsaicin, a constituent that temporarily desensitizes the nerves that cause pain. That's why it's in a candy recipe that will relieve canker sore pain. Use the candy for relief of mouth sores from chemotherapy and radiation, too. Be careful, though, as this may be too irritating for some people.

Sage. Used most often to spice up turkey stuffing, this herb is one that can be used to calm an angry canker. Simply add 3 teaspoons sage leaves to 1 pint boiling water. Steep, covered, for 15 minutes. Rinse your mouth with the liquid several times a day. You can also rub sage leaves into a powder and apply them directly to your sore.

TOPICAL REMEDIES

Baking soda. Make a baking soda and water paste and apply to the canker. Baking soda is also a component of a canker sore mouth rinse (see "Salt").

Honey. Mix 1 teaspoon honey with ¼ teaspoon turmeric and dab it on your canker. This one may sting a bit.

Ice. This won't make the canker disappear, but it will sure make it feel better. Simply apply ice or rinse your mouth with ice water.

Milk of Magnesia or Kaopectate liquid and Benylin or Benadryl. Several dentists swear by this homemade remedy. Mix together equal amounts of Milk of Magnesia or Kaopectate, both of which coat wet tissues like those in the mouth, and Benylin or Benadryl, which act as mild topical anesthetics and antihistamines (which reduce inflammation). Every few hours, apply the mixture to the canker sore using a cotton swab. Be careful not to swallow the stuff; you could end up numbing the reflex that keeps the windpipe closed when you swallow.

Salt. Combine 1 teaspoon salt, 1 teaspoon baking soda, and 2 ounces hydrogen peroxide. Mix and rinse your mouth

WHEN TO SEE THE DOCTOR
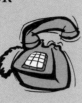
- If you have a fever of 100 degrees Fahrenheit or more, diarrhea, headache, or skin rash
- If you have general physical discomfort or feel slow, sluggish, or lethargic
- If your lymph glands are swollen
- If your canker sore persists for more than three weeks or worsens, even after home treatments
- If you think tooth or denture problems are causing your cankers, call your dentist

with it four times daily. If the taste is too strong, or the tingle uncomfortable, dilute with 2 ounces of water. You can also just rinse your mouth with lukewarm salt water. Or, if you're brave, just apply a little salt directly to your wound.

Tea. Moisten a regular tea bag and apply it directly to the canker. The tannic acid will help dry it out.

LIFESTYLE REMEDIES

Be gentle. Use a soft toothbrush and wield it extra carefully. Injury from overzealous brushing can cause canker sores.

Check toothpaste ingredients. If you see sodium laurel sulfate in the lineup, buy something else. It's a harsh detergent that can leave you with dry mouth, making your mouth vulnerable to sores. Or use baking soda to brush your teeth.

Try not to aggravate it. Biting down on a canker will prolong pain and delay healing. Chew on the opposite side of your mouth.

Canker Crusading Foods

Because a nutritional deficiency, particularly in vitamin B_{12} and minerals iron and zinc, is suspected as a cause of canker sores, it's a good plan to eat foods that are rich in those vitamins and minerals. Try to include some of each of these foods in your diet to ward off canker sores.

Iron	B_{12}	Folic Acid	Zinc
• Meat	• Liver	• Beets	• Oysters
• Fish	• Meat	• Green leafy	• Other
• Poultry	• Poultry	vegetables	shellfish
• Nuts	• Fish	• Black-eyed	• Red meats
• Seeds	• Dairy	peas & other	• Whole-grain
• Green leafy	products	legumes	cereals
vegetables	* See note	• Brussels sprouts	
		• Whole-grain	
		foods	

Note: Vegetables are rarely a source of B_{12}.

Colds
SNUFFING OUT THE SNIFFLES

Every year Americans will suffer through more than one billion colds. Colds make such frequent appearances that the infection has come to be known as the "common cold."

Small children are the most likely to catch a cold: Most kids will have six to ten colds per year. That's because their young immune systems combined with the germy confines of school and day-care situations make them prime targets for the virus. The upside of having so many colds as a child is that you develop immunities to some of the 200 viruses that cause colds. As a result, adults get an average of only two to four colds per year. By the time most people reach age 60, they're down to about one cold per year.

How Do Colds Beat a Path to Your Door?

Viruses are like the bully that torments all the kids on the playground. After entering the mucous layer of your nose and throat, the cold virus strong-arms your cells until they let the virus take over, forcing the cells to produce thousands of new virus particles.

But the virus is not the reason your throat begins throbbing and your nose starts flowing like Niagara Falls. Your immune system is responsible for that. As the virus begins replicating, the body gets the message that it's time to go into battle.

PRIME TIME FOR COLDS

Most colds happen in the fall and winter in the United States. The cold countdown starts in late August or early September, about the time the kids start school, and stays high until March or April.

You Can't Catch a Cold from the Cold

Cold weather may make you uncomfortable, but it doesn't make you more susceptible to getting a cold. There are two reasons colds tend to make more of an impact in cold weather. Number one, most people are indoors a lot more in the winter, so you've got a lot more opportunities to share the wealth of cold viruses. And number two, the heat in your house dries out the air, and cold viruses like it warm and dry. So if you throw a little wintertime soiree in your well-heated home, you've got the ideal climate for a cold virus. Scientists have done numerous tests in which they've exposed people to the cold virus in 86 degrees Fahrenheit and 40 degrees Fahrenheit temperatures, and much to the participants' chagrin, both groups ended up with a cold.

The little soldiers of the body, the white blood cells, run to the body's rescue. One of the weapons the white blood cells use in their virus war are immune system chemicals called kinins. During the battle, the kinins tell the body to go into defensive mode. So that runny nose is really your body fighting back against the cursed virus. That should make you feel a little better while you lie on the couch surrounded by tissues.

Because there are so many viruses that cause colds, the exact virus that you contracted is not easily pinned down. The most likely culprit in most colds is a rhinovirus (*rhino* is a Greek word meaning "nose"). There are more than 110 specific rhinoviruses, and they are behind 30 to 35 percent of most colds. The second most common reason for that aching head is a coronavirus. These are especially common in adults. An unknown viral assailant causes 30 to 50 percent of colds, and about 10 to 15 percent of colds are caused by a virus that will probably lead to something more serious, such as the flu.

How Colds Are Spread

The cold virus can take many routes to its ultimate destination—your cells. Most people are contagious a day before and two to four days after their symptoms start. There are typically three ways a cold virus is spread:

- Touching someone who has the virus on them. The virus can live for three hours on skin.
- Touching something that contains the virus. Cold viruses can live three hours on objects.
- Inhaling the virus through airborne transmission. If someone sitting next to you

sneezes while you are inhaling, voilà! It's likely you'll get a cold.

One study found that kids tend to get colds from more direct contact while adults tend to get colds from airborne viruses (moms of young children can expect to get colds both ways). Research has also found that emotional stress, allergies that affect the nasal passages or throat, and menstrual cycles may make you more susceptible to catching a cold.

Where's the Cold Vaccine?

Good question! One of the main reasons we don't yet have a vaccine for the cold is that it's just too hard to pin down. Viruses live inside cells, which means they are protected from most medicines in the bloodstream. So even if you took an antiviral drug, your body may not allow it to penetrate the cells. Another reason viruses are so difficult to kill is that they don't grow well in a laboratory setting. Their ultimate playground is a cool, dry place, like the inside of your nose.

Don't give up hope, though. Researchers are still on the job. Scientists have discovered the receptor sites that the rhinovirus attaches to when it invades a cell. In one study, researchers tested a drug that blocked these receptor sites, which helped slow down the time the virus actually took to develop into a cold and reduced the severity of its symptoms in people who did develop the sniffles. That offers hope that a true cure for the common cold may not be far off. But until that day comes, there are some things you can do to fend off the germs that cause colds, as well as techniques to ease your symptoms once you're sick.

HOW TO WIN THE COLD WAR

- Washing your hands is the most effective way to keep a cold at bay as well as to keep one from spreading. Antibacterial soaps don't necessarily do any more good than regular soap, and some researchers believe the prevalence of antibacterial products is contributing to the increase in resistant bacteria strains. Experts suggest washing your hands for at least 15 seconds, which is long enough to say the alphabet. So next time you're scrubbing, say those ABCs.
- When you sneeze or cough into a tissue, throw it away immediately. Sounds like a no-brainer, but how many tissues have you left sitting around the house?
- Clean any potentially virus-carrying surface of your home with a heavy-duty cleanser or disinfectant.
- Try to limit your exposure to others when you have a cold.

DIETARY REMEDIES

Chicken soup. Science backs up your mom—chicken soup does help a cold. Scientists believe the warm fumes release the 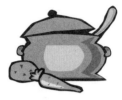 mucus in your nose and help your body better fight its viral invaders. Chicken soup also contains cysteines, which are good at thinning mucus. And soup provides easily absorbed nutrients.

Honey. Make your own cough syrup by mixing together ¼ cup honey and ¼ cup apple cider vinegar. Pour the mixture into a jar or bottle and seal tightly. Shake well before using. Take 1 tablespoon every four hours.

Peppers. Hot and spicy foods are notorious for making your nose run and your eyes water. The hot stuff in peppers is called capsaicin and is pharmacologically similar to guaifenesin, an expectorant found in some over-the-counter cough syrups. This similarity leads some experts to believe that eating hot foods can clear up mucus and ease that stuffy nose.

Tea. A cup of hot tea with honey does the same trick as chicken soup: It loosens up your nasal passages and makes that stuffy nose feel better. Folk healers often suggest drinking tea with spices and herbs that contain aromatic oils with antiviral properties. Try tea with elder, ginger, yarrow, mint, thyme, horsemint, bee balm, lemon balm, catnip, garlic, onions, or mustard.

Vitamin C. Vitamin C won't prevent a cold, but research shows it can help reduce the duration of symptoms. But to reap the benefits, you've got to take a lot of "C." The RDA for men age 19 and older is 90 mg and 75 mg for women age 19 and older, but studies show that you'd need to take upward of 1,000 mg to 3,000 mg to get the cold-symptom-sparing rewards of vitamin C. For the short term, experts believe that wouldn't be harmful, but taking too much vitamin C for too long can cause severe diarrhea. Before loading up on vitamin C, check with your doctor.

Water. Don't stop hydrating yourself even if you lose your appetite. Dehydration will make your cold last longer, and you'll be more uncomfortable to boot. Drink eight ounces of water—or some other fluid—every two hours. This will keep your mucus flowing and easier for your body to expel, along with the viral particles trapped in it.

Yogurt. One study found that participants who ate ¾ cup yogurt per day before and during cold season had 25 percent fewer colds. But you've got to start early and maintain your yogurt eating throughout the peak cold season.

Zinc. Studies have found that zinc may help immune cells fight a cold and may ease cold symptoms. The most effective zinc lozenges are those that contain 15 to 25 mg of zinc gluconate or zinc gluconate-glycine per lozenge. You can get the most out of your zinc lozenges if you start using them at the first sign of a cold and continue taking them for several days.

HERBAL REMEDIES

Echinacea. This herb has immune-stimulating properties and it is used in contemporary herbal

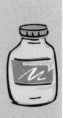

WATCH THE MEDICINES

During cold season, you'll find tons of commercials for over-the-counter cold remedies. They may make you feel better temporarily, but they may also make your cold stick around longer. That runny nose and cough are your body's way of getting rid of all the virus. But if you desperately need some relief, avoid multi-symptom cold medicines. Stick with medicines that treat your specific symptom, such as a stuffy nose or a dry cough.

WHEN TO CALL THE DOCTOR

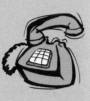

Colds generally have to run their course, typically about 2 to 14 days. In rare cases, they can lead to a more serious infection. Call your doctor if you have:

- High fever
- Severe pain in the chest, ears, head, or stomach
- Enlarged lymph nodes (glands in the neck)
- A fever, sore throat, or severe runny nose that doesn't get any better in a week
- A headache and stiff neck but no other symptoms (could be meningitis)
- A headache and sore throat but no other symptoms (could be strep throat)
- Typical cold symptoms and pain across your nose and face that sticks around (could be a sinus infection)
- Lessening cold symptoms but then the sudden onset of fever (could be pneumonia)

treatments in Britain, Australia, and the United States. In Germany, where botanical products are prescribed just like pharmaceutical medicines, doctors recommend it for treating colds. Scientists still debate the benefits of echinacea, but one review of several studies recently found that preparations containing the herb can help prevent colds and reduce the severity of symptoms. For the best results, take it at the onset of cold symptoms—but not for longer than two weeks.

TOPICAL REMEDIES

Salt. Make your own saline drops by adding ¼ teaspoon salt to 8 ounces water. This same recipe can be used as a gargle to ease a painful throat.

Sesame oil. A 2001 study compared saline drops to sesame oil. The researchers found that more than 80 percent of people with dry nasal passages who used a spray containing pure sesame oil for two weeks said their symptoms had disappeared or improved; just 30 percent of the subjects who used saline spray got relief. It may not be a good idea to shoot sesame oil up your nose (it could get into the lungs), so try rubbing a drop around the inside of your nostrils.

LIFESTYLE REMEDIES

Rest. Extra rest helps when you have a cold.

Keep your chin up. Having a positive attitude can help you win the war against your cold.

MORE DO'S AND DON'TS

- Don't smoke. Smokers tend to have longer colds, and they are more likely to have complications, such as bronchitis.

Cold Sores
MINIMIZING THE MISERY

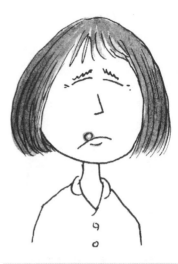

You know it's coming when you feel that notorious tingling on your lip and the accompanying itching and burning. You can't help stressing out about it; all you can think about is the pain and embarrassment those ugly cold sores cause. But there's not a darned thing you can do to stop a cold sore, also known as a fever blister, from erupting.

Many people get confused about whether they have a cold sore or a canker sore. But that confusion is easily cleared up. (See Canker Sores/Cold Sores chart, page 80.) If the sore is on your external lip or near your mouth or nose and looks like a fluid-filled blister, chances are it's a cold sore. Caused by a virus called herpes simplex type 1, herpes blisters are very contagious. They also love company, so where there's one there are usually many. Within a few days to a week, the blisters break, ooze, and form an ugly yellow crust that can stay around for weeks. When it finally sloughs off, though, there's nice, healthy pink skin underneath. Best of all, cold sores leave no scars.

You can't cure cold sores, and they like to keep coming back, usually to the scene of a previous visit. When a cold sore's not making itself a huge lip ache, it's snoozing in the nerves below your skin, just waiting for a reason to wake up. And what sets off its alarm clock?

FACTS ABOUT HERPES

- It's estimated that at least half of the U.S. population suffers from cold sores.
- After the tingling starts, the blisters appear within 24 to 48 hours.
- The viral infection typically lasts 10 to 14 days.
- Herpes blisters can last from two to six weeks.
- Symptoms may take up to three weeks to appear after the initial exposure to the virus, and this first onset can make you good and sick, too. Symptoms include fever, swollen glands, bleeding gums, dehydration, and painful sores around the mouth. These symptoms require immediate attention from your physician!

FOODS THAT FIGHT COLD SORES

There's a good amino acid, lysine, that helps block the herpes virus. So try some foods high in this cold sore warrior, such as:

- Meats
- Milk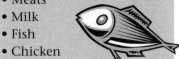
- Fish
- Chicken
- Eggs
- Beans & bean sprouts
- Cheese

Foods rich in bioflavonoids can help prevent or speed up the course of the blisters that flare up, too. These include:

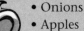

- Onions
- Apples
- Grapes
- Tea

Foods packed with vitamin C are also valiant in their quest to rid you of your herpes foe. Eat a lot of these foods that are rich in vitamin C:

- Oranges, grapefruits, seedless berries (they all make great smoothies)
- Peppers
- Green leafy vegetables
- Sweet potatoes and potatoes

- Fever
- Infection, colds, flu
- Ultraviolet radiation, such as a sunburn
- Stress
- Fatigue
- Changes in the immune system
- Trauma
- Food allergies
- Menstruation
- Dental work

Who's Prone?

Anyone who comes in contact with the herpes simplex virus can catch it. It is spread in air droplets and by direct contact with fluid from the blister. Those at highest risk have a weakened immune system and a family history of cold sores.

Conventional medicine does have a few tricks in its little black bag, including antiviral lotions and creams. But they don't cure, just treat. So take a look around your house. You might just find some useful treatments there, too.

DIETARY REMEDIES

Avoid salty or acidic foods. These will hurt and irritate the cold sore, so skip them until it's healed.

Licorice. Studies show that glycyrrhizic acid, an ingredient in licorice, stops the cold sore virus cells dead in their tracks. So try chewing a licorice whip. Just be sure it's made from real licorice, as most candy in the United States today is flavored with anise. If the ingredient list says "licorice mass," the product contains real licorice. You could also try buying some licorice powder and sprinkling it on the sore. Or mix up a cream with a pinch of licorice power and a smidgen of pure vegetable shortening, then apply to the sore.

TOPICAL REMEDIES

Ice packs. If you ice a cold sore when it first arrives, you may cut down on the amount of time it hangs around. Ice packs and cold compresses will provide some temporary relief. A tasty popsicle will feel good, too, but skip the juice bars. Their acid content may irritate that major irritation even more. Super-cold drinks such as slushes or smoothies are another tasty way to provide comfort.

Milk. This remedy doesn't involve drinking. Soak a cotton ball in milk and apply it to the sore to relieve pain. Better yet, if you feel the tell-tale tingling before the cold sore surfaces, go straight to the cold milk. It can help speed the healing right from the beginning.

OTC anesthetic. Applying an over-the-counter anesthetic ointment containing benzocaine can help numb the pain temporarily. Check your local drugstore for the ointment or ask your pharmacist to recommend one, then follow the package directions.

Petroleum jelly. Coating the cold sore with petroleum jelly will speed healing and help protect from secondary infection with bacteria.

LIFESTYLE REMEDIES

Change toothbrushes. Once when the blister has formed and once when the attack has cleared up. Toothbrushes can harbor the virus.

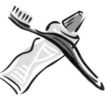

FOODS TO AVOID

During a herpes simplex episode, anything with arginine, an amino acid, is on the no-no list. Arginine causes the herpes virus to multiply. Foods containing arginine include:
- Chocolate
- Peanuts and other nuts
- Raisins
- Seeds
- Wheat and wheat products
- Oats
- Coconut
- Soy beans

Several foods that don't contain arginine can also make the episode worse. Stay away from sugar, coffee, fried foods, alcohol, and hot spices. And if you're prone to cold sores, stay away from tobacco, too, as it suppresses the immune system.

WHEN TO CALL THE DOCTOR

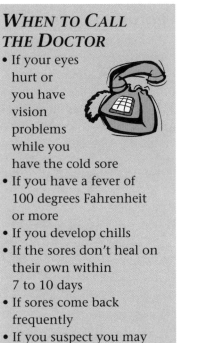

- If your eyes hurt or you have vision problems while you have the cold sore
- If you have a fever of 100 degrees Fahrenheit or more
- If you develop chills
- If the sores don't heal on their own within 7 to 10 days
- If sores come back frequently
- If you suspect you may have infected your genitals

Reduce your stress. Once you've been infected with the herpes virus, it can become reactivated and stress can be a trigger. Exercise, meditate, do yoga, or read a good book to keep stress at bay.

MORE DO'S AND DON'TS

- Don't kiss. Whether you're the one with the cold sore or it's your partner, don't give any smooches. In fact, don't even make skin contact when blisters are present.
- Don't share drinks, foods, utensils, towels or anything that may have come in contact with a moist secretion from the blister.

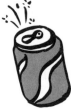

- Don't touch other parts of your body (or anybody else's body) without first washing your hands. Cold sores can spread to your eyes and your genitals, so wash those hands frequently or that little lip sore could turn into something much worse.
- Use a lip balm with a strong sun-block. Products with the highest sunburn protection factor (SPF) provide the most protection.

- Don't hide your boo-boo with makeup. The chemicals can make the sore worse. And don't share your lipstick or other makeup either.
- Don't squeeze, pinch, or pick a blister. These actions can cause a bacterial infection.
- Suck on zinc lozenges. During stressful times they can boost the immune system, and some studies suggest that zinc may help prevent cold sores.
- Carry hand sanitizer in case you accidentally scratch and there's no wash basin handy.

Colic
COPING WITH CRYING

Bringing home a newborn baby is one of life's greatest joys. Yet it can also be one of life's greatest trials, especially if that cute little bundle of joy cries constantly. That's the number one symptom of colic: nonstop crying combined with bouts of irritability and fussiness that last a total of more than three hours per day on more than three days of the week. Colic, if it happens, typically begins at around two weeks of age and tapers off around three months. It generally is more pronounced during the evenings. Parents will be pleased to know that despite the crying, most colicky babies are healthy, well-fed infants, and the condition isn't life threatening or classified as a disease.

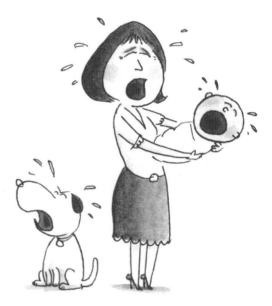

It's a Mystery
Unfortunately for both baby and parents, doctors don't know what causes colic, what the disorder is, or how to cure it. They don't even know if colicky babies are in pain. Fortunately for everyone involved, there are many tried-and-true ways to soothe a baby. Experiment with a few, determine what works, and stick to it.

DIETARY REMEDIES
Basil. This aromatic herb contains large amounts of eugenol, which, among other things, may reduce intestinal spasms and ease digestion. Place 1 teaspoon dried basil leaves in a cup and fill it with boiling water. Cover and let stand for ten minutes. Strain and, while warm or at room temperature, give it to the infant in a bottle. A nursing mother may also drink the tea. However, never use straight basil oil to make tea. It is too potent for a baby.

WATCH WHAT YOU EAT

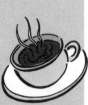

Many experts suggest nursing mothers look to recent dietary changes for the cause of colic. Nursing mothers should try to avoid eating the following:

garlic
onions
broccoli
cauliflower
cabbage
peanut butter
fish
eggs
berries
coffee
tomatoes
apricots
chocolate
If colic persists, avoid dairy foods and grains.

Mint. Mint may also help reduce intestinal spasms in colicky infants. Place 1 teaspoon dried mint in a cup and fill with boiling water. Let stand for ten minutes. Strain well and, while warm, feed to the baby in a bottle. Nursing mothers may want to have a cup of mint tea, too. A peppermint stick soaked in water may be used as an alternative, but note that many sticks contain sugar. Never use straight peppermint oil to make tea. It's too potent for a baby.

Soy products. That carton of cow's milk looks innocent enough, but it can be the problem source for 5 to 10 percent of colicky babies. Many studies have shown an improvement in colic after dairy products have been eliminated from babies' diets. The culprit seems to be the proteins in cow's milk. (Don't think milk is the only villain. This protein lurks in many infant formulas containing dairy and is also found in the milk of breast-feeding mothers who consume dairy products.) Talk to your pediatrician about eliminating dairy products and switching to soy products. A two-week trial, both for baby and for you if you're breast-feeding, could provide the necessary evidence of a dairy problem. If you don't notice any improvement, milk probably isn't the culprit.

HERBAL REMEDIES

Chamomile tea. Chamomile eases digestion and has sedative properties and may relieve intestinal cramping and induce relaxation at the same time. In

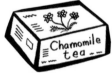

fact, chamomile contains a number of different constituents that may relieve intestinal spasms and act as sedatives. To make a cup of tea: Place 1 teaspoon chamomile flowers in a cup and fill with boiling water. Cover and let stand for ten minutes. Strain and, while warm or at room temperature, give to the infant in a bottle. A nursing mother may also drink the tea, unless she is allergic to pollens. Prepackaged chamomile tea bags may be used instead of flowers.

TOPICAL REMEDIES

Warm water. Put warm (not hot) water in a hot water bottle and place it against your baby's stomach. This can be soothing.

LIFESTYLE REMEDIES

Running water. Water soothes the savage beast...and the screaming baby. One of the simplest calming techniques is to place a bowl in the sink and turn on the faucet. Hold your baby next to the sink so he can hear the water cascading into the bowl. If the kitchen sink doesn't produce enough volume, perhaps try the bathroom sink. An enclosed space, like a bathroom, may accentuate the soothing sounds of water.

MORE DO'S AND DON'TS

- Try holding your baby face down across your lap and rubbing his back.
- Motion and vibrations some- 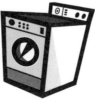 times help. Put your baby in a car seat and go for a ride, or put her in a stroller and go for a walk. If you can't get out, hold your baby on top of a running dishwasher or washing machine or dryer—or put her in a baby swing.

WHEN TO CALL THE DOCTOR

- If the crying continues past three months of age
- If bouts of colic are accompanied by fever, diarrhea, vomiting, or constipation
- If your baby sounds like he's in pain, not fussy
- If your infant fails to gain weight or isn't hungry
- If you have reached your breaking point

AN ALL-AROUND SPICE

In ancient times, caraway, an aromatic seed related to the parsley family, did more than flavor cheeses and breads. This versatile spice was thought to cure colic in the young and gout in the old. The spice also had some, well, guard-dog quali- ties: Caraway was believed to protect objects from theft.

Constipation
GETTING A MOVE ON

Nothing's moving, even though you know you have to move your bowels. Everything in your body is sending you that signal. You feel bloated and uncomfortable pressure, but when you try to go, nothing happens. Or, if you do finally go, it hurts.

Constipation occurs for many different reasons. Stress, lack of exercise, certain medications, inadequate water intake, eating large amounts of dairy products, and a diet that's lacking fiber or fluids can each be the culprit. Certain medical conditions such as an underactive thyroid, irritable bowel syndrome, diabetes, and cancer also can cause constipation. Even age is a factor. The older we get, the more prone we are to the problem.

And constipation is a problem, although it's not an illness. It's simply what happens when bowel movements are delayed, compacted, and difficult to pass.

What's Normal?

Some people mistakenly believe they must have a certain number of bowel movements per day or per week or else they are constipated. That couldn't be further from the truth, although it's a common misconception. What consti-

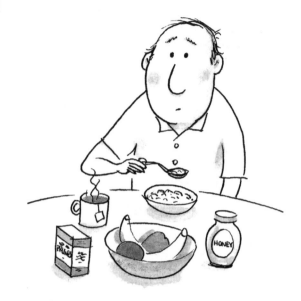

tutes "normal" is individual and can vary from three bowel movements per day to three per week. You'll know if you're constipated because you'll be straining a lot in the bathroom, you'll produce unusually hard stools, and you'll feel gassy and bloated.

Laxatives Aren't Number One

It's not a good idea to use laxatives as the first line of attack when you're constipated. They can become habit-forming to the point that they damage your colon. Some laxatives inhibit the effectiveness of medications you're already taking, and there are laxatives that cause inflammation to the lining of the intestine.

Conventional thinking on laxatives is that if you must take one, find one that's psyllium- or fiber-based. Psyllium is a natural fiber that's much more gentle on the system than ingredients in many of the other products available today, although for some people, these laxatives cause bloating and abdominal pain. Or, simply look to home remedies for relief. There are many.

DIETARY REMEDIES

Apples. Especially with the peels on, these are a good source of fiber.
Apple juice, apple cider. These are natural laxatives for many people. Drink up and enjoy!

Bananas. These may relieve consti- pation. Try eating two ripe bananas between meals. Avoid green bananas because they're constipating.

Barley. It can relieve constipation as well as keep you regular, and it has cholesterol-lowering properties too. What more could you ask of a simple grain? Buy some barley flour, flakes, and grits. Add some barley grain to vegetable soup or stew.

Blackstrap molasses. Take 2 tablespoons before going to bed. It has a pretty strong taste, so you may want to add it to milk, fruit juice, or for an extra-powerful laxative punch, prune juice.

Fiber. Sometimes all you need to ensure regularity is some extra fiber in your diet. Fiber is the indigestible part of plant foods, and it adds mass to the stool and stimulates the colon to push things along. It's found naturally in fruits, vegetables, whole grains, and legumes. The current recommendations for daily dietary fiber are 20 to

THE SCOOP ON CASTOR OIL

Castor oil is a constipation cure that's been used for 5,000 years. And it was so popular 50 years ago that some people were even dosed on a regular basis just for the sake of regularity. Castor oil works quickly, in 4 to 5 hours. However, it's generally not recommended any longer because it's a very strong laxative that can interfere with the body's ability to absorb certain vitamins and minerals. As with other laxatives, your intestinal muscles may be weakened, and your body may become dependent on the oil, only making matters worse.

Children younger than 12 and women who are pregnant should never take castor oil.

GETTING A LUBE JOB

Agar-agar, a dried seaweed extract, has laxative properties that may make you want to run to your nearest health food store and grab some. It is a natural intestinal lubricant and is best combined with fruit juices, fresh fruits, or fruit gelatin desserts.

LAXATIVE TIMETABLE

Most laxatives are to be taken overnight, so relief will come in the morning. Or so the instructions say. The problem is, our bodies don't necessarily respond to those instructions, and the laxative you're taking, or making, may have its own timetable. When you take any laxative, consider the timing of the dose or you could end up missing an activity or being late for work if the remedy kicks in at the wrong time. Better yet, if you can wait until you have a day off, or a weekend, you'll save yourself the stress of guessing.

35 grams per day, but most people eat only 10 to 15 grams. Fiber supplements may be helpful, but you're better off getting your fiber from foods, which supply an assortment of other essential nutrients as well. To avoid getting gassy, increase the fiber in your diet gradually, and be sure to drink plenty of water so the fiber can move smoothly through your digestive system.

Garlic. In the raw, it has a laxative effect for many. Eat it mixed with onion, raw or cooked, and with milk or yogurt for best results.

Honey. This is a very mild laxative. Try taking 1 tablespoon three times per day, either by itself or mixed into warm water. If it doesn't work on its own, you may have to pep it up by mixing it half and half with blackstrap molasses.

Oil. Safflower, soybean, or other vegetable oil can be just the cure you need, as each provides a lubricating action in the intestines. Take 2 to 3 tablespoons a day until the problem is gone. If you don't like taking it straight, mix the oil with herbs and lemon juice or vinegar to use as salad dressing. The combination of the oil and the fiber from the salad ought to fix you right up.

Raisins. Eat a handful daily.

Rhubarb. This is a natural laxative. Cook it and eat it sweetened with honey or bake it in a pie. Or, create a drink with cooked, pureed rhubarb, apple juice, and honey.

Vinegar. Mix 1 teaspoon apple cider vinegar and 1 teaspoon honey in a glass of water and drink.

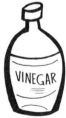

Sesame seeds. These provide roughage and bulk, and they soften the contents of the intestines, which makes elimination easier. Eat no more than ½ ounce daily, and drink lots of water as you take the seeds. You can also sprinkle them on salads and other foods, but again, no more than ½ ounce. Sesame is also available in a butter or paste and in Middle Eastern dips, such as tahini. **Walnuts.** Fresh from the shell, they may be just the laxative you need.

Herbal Remedies

Flaxseeds. These provide natural bulk and will relieve constipation. Wash 2 teaspoons seeds in cold water. Add to 1 cup boiling water. Let steep for ten minutes, then drink. Do not strain out the seeds.

Lifestyle Remedies

Fluids. Drink at least eight glasses of water a day.
Exercise. A nice, brisk, 30-minute walk can lead to regularity.
Keep the daily routine. Train yourself. Pick a time, possibly after a meal, and retire to the bathroom. Do that every day, whether you have to go or not, and soon it may become your time.

More Do's and Don'ts

- Don't rush things. It takes time for your bowels to move, so allow sufficient time.
- Don't take mineral oil unless prescribed by your physician.
- Keep a food diary to see which foods are clogging you up.
- Cut back on refined foods, such as processed cereals, white flour, and sugar.
- Don't delay! Go when nature calls.

When to Call the Doctor

- If you have a fever or lower abdominal pain with constipation
- If you have blood in your stools
- If constipation develops after you start taking a new medication. This includes vitamins and minerals.
- If you're elderly or disabled and you've been constipated for more than a week
- If you experience sudden weight loss in addition to constipation
- If the problem persists, off and on, for more than two weeks
- If you have gone long enough without a bowel movement that you're experiencing extreme pain and discomfort
- If constipation is causing a problem with normal daily activities
- If you experience à marked change in your normal bowel habits

Cough
HAMPERING THE HACK

Annoying, loud, and disruptive, a persistent cough can put a damper on your daily routine. Coughs can be defined by how long they last. A brief cough is caused by such factors as breathing cold air, irritating fumes, or dust; or drawing food into the airways. A persistent cough, however, typically results from mucus and other secretions brought on by respiratory disorders such as the cold, the flu, pneumonia, asthma, tuberculosis, lung cancer, or emphysema.

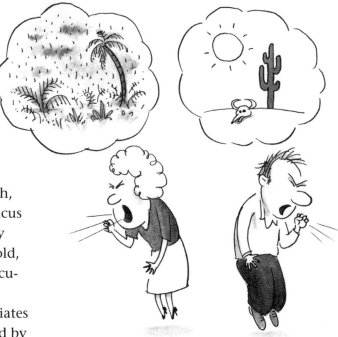

Moisture content also differentiates coughs. Some are dry, accompanied by a ticklish or sore throat. Others are accompanied by a thick phlegm and are called wet coughs.

A Beneficial Reflex

A cough is produced when viruses, bacteria, dust, pollen, or other foreign substances irritate respiratory passages in the throat and lungs. The cough reflex is the body's effort to rid the passageways of such intruders, and it spares no power in the expulsion. A cough reflex can expel a foreign substance at velocities as high as 100 miles per hour.

Determine what kind of cough you have and search out cures specific to that type. Some remedies aim to moisten dry throats, while others are expectorants, helping you cough up and get rid of mucus and irritants. Most of these cures aim to battle both coughs unless otherwise noted.

DIETARY REMEDIES

Chicken soup. Take some advice from your grandma: Sip a bowl of chicken soup. It doesn't matter if it's homemade or canned. Chicken soup is calming for coughs associated with colds. Although scientists can't put a finger on why this comfort food benefits the cold sufferer, they do believe chicken soup contains anti-inflammatory properties that help relieve a cold's miserable side effects, one being the cough. Plus, chicken soup contains cysteine, which thins phlegm. The broth, chock-full of electrolytes, keeps you hydrated, and the steam helps soothe irritated mucous membranes and air passageways. Last, but not least, it tastes yummy.

Honey. Honey has long been used in traditional Chinese medicine for coughs because it's a natural expectorant, promoting the flow of mucus. This is the simple recipe: Mix 1 tablespoon honey into 1 cup hot water and enjoy. Now how sweet is that? Squeeze some lemon juice in if you want a little tartness. Before bedtime, adults may add 1 tablespoon brandy or whiskey to aid in sleep.

Licorice. If you love licorice, you're in for a treat with this remedy. Many folk remedies use licorice root to treat coughs and bronchial problems. It serves not only as a flavoring agent but also as a demulcent (a substance that soothes inflamed or irritated throats) and an expectorant. Licorice or candy that's made with real licorice (look for "licorice mass" on the label) works best. Most licorice candy made in the United States contains no licorice root, however. Reach into your candy jar and slice up 1 ounce licorice sticks. Add 1 quart boiling water and steep for 24 hours. Drink throughout the day, adding 1 teaspoon honey for sweetness. Don't overdo it, because in

THE GOODS ON GARLIC

One of the oldest cultivated plants, garlic's virtues have long been extolled. It has been used for centuries to treat everything from the plague to toothaches. The ancient Egyptians valued the little white orb for its medicinal qualities, Greek Olympians chewed on it before competing, and Louis Pasteur acknowledged it as an effective bacteria fighter. Even today, entire Western towns celebrate the garlic harvest with lavish festivals.

large amounts, a compound in licorice root called glycyrrhizin can cause high blood pressure, salt and water retention, and low potassium levels. Large amounts may cause preterm labor, so pregnant women should choose licorice products that don't contain glycyrrhizin.

HERBAL REMEDIES

Garlic. Eating garlic won't have you winning any kissing contests, but who wants to kiss you when you sound like a seal? Since kissing isn't on your agenda, you can indulge in one of nature's best cures for coughs: garlic. It's full of antibiotic and antiviral properties, plus garlic is also an expectorant, so it helps you cough up stubborn bacteria and/or mucus that are languishing in your lungs.

Some experts advise that to reap garlic's full cold- and flu-fighting benefits, you have to eat it raw. Yet swallowing 4 to 8 raw garlic cloves per day (the recommended amount) is hard for most people to stomach. Cheat a little by mixing the cloves into plain yogurt and putting a dollop on your soup. If you make a pasta sauce, put the garlic in at the last moment, or toss garlic slices into your salad.

A cup of garlic broth may do the trick for your cough, too, and it is easy to prepare. Smash 1 to 3 cloves garlic (depending on how strong you like your garlic), add them to 2 quarts water, and boil on low heat for one hour. Strain and sip slowly.

You can also chop up some garlic cloves and toss them into that pot of chicken soup (see Dietary Remedies, pages 102–103).

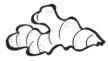

Ginger. Ginger, which has antiviral properties, shares the limelight with licorice in this cough remedy. To make ginger-licorice (anise) tea, combine 2 teaspoons freshly chopped gingerroot, 2 teaspoons aniseed, and 1 teaspoon dried licorice root (if available) in 2 cups boiling water. Cover and steep for ten minutes. Strain and sweeten with 1 or 2 teaspoons honey. Drink ½ cup every one to two hours, but no more than 3 cups per day.

Mustard seed. An irritating but useful spice for wet coughs, mustard seed has sulfur-containing compounds that stimulate the flow of mucus. To get the full effect of the expectorant compounds, the mustard seeds must be broken and allowed to sit in water for 15 minutes. Crush 1 teaspoon mustard seeds or grind them in a coffee grinder. Place the seeds in a cup of warm water. Steep for 15 minutes. This concoction might be a little hard to swallow, so take it in ¼-cup doses throughout the day.

Pepper. Pepper is an irritant (try sniffling some), but this characteristic is a plus for those suffering from coughs accompanied by thick mucus. The irritating property of pepper stimulates circulation and the flow of mucus in the airways and sinuses. Place 1 teaspoon black pepper into a cup and sweeten things up with the addition of 1 tablespoon honey. Fill with boiling water, steep for 10 to 15 minutes, stir, and sip.

Thyme. Store-bought cough syrups are often so medicinal tasting that it's hard to get them down without gagging. Here's a sweet, herbal version, made of thyme, peppermint, mullein, licorice, and honey, that's guaranteed to go down the hatch easily. Thyme and peppermint help clear congested air passages and have antimicrobial and antispasmodic properties to relieve the

A SOOTHING CHEST RUB

When the chest hurts from coughing fits and breathing is congested, a soothing remedy to loosen and lighten things up is a homemade eucalyptus-lavender chest rub. Eucalyptus, a common ingredient in store-bought vapor balms, opens congested airways and acts as an antimicrobial. Lavender, long regarded as a soothing herb that eases anxiety, also aids slightly in the battle against bad germs and microorganisms. To make a chest rub, combine 10 drops lavender essential oil, 15 drops eucalyptus essential oil, and ¼ cup olive oil or vegetable oil. Mix and massage on your upper chest before going to bed.

If you'd rather not have an oily chest but want the same benefits, try taking a bath instead. Add 3 drops eucalyptus oil and 3 drops lavender oil to a full warm bath. Soak for ten minutes.

WHEN TO CALL THE DOCTOR

- If you have a persistent cough that doesn't improve after ten days of treatment, especially an unexplained cough or one that's dry and hacking
- If you have a cough that produces thick, foul-smelling rusty or greenish phlegm
- If you experience chest pain when you breathe
- If you cough up blood

hacking. Mullein and licorice soothe irritated membranes and help reduce inflammation.

To make the syrup, combine 2 teaspoons each dried thyme, peppermint, mullein, and licorice root into 1 cup boiling water. Cover and steep for half an hour. Strain and add ½ cup honey. If the honey doesn't dissolve, heat the tea gently and stir. Store in the refrigerator in a covered container for as long as three months. Take 1 teaspoon as needed.

TOPICAL REMEDIES

Salt. A saltwater gargle is a simple solution to a cough, although you have to remain devoted to gargling to get results. Mix ¼ teaspoon salt into 4 ounces warm water. Mix and gargle. Repeat this every one to two hours each day for best results. The salt, combined with soothing warm water, acts as an astringent to help ease irritated and inflamed throat tissues and loosen mucus.

Steam. One of the kitchen's best remedies for a cough is also one of the easiest. Inhaling steam helps flush out mucus, and it moisturizes dry, irritated air passageways. Fill a cooking pot one-quarter full with water. Boil, turn off the heat, and if available, add a couple drops essential oil of eucalyptus or a scoop of Mentholatum or Vicks VapoRub. (These work as decongestants and expectorants.) Carefully remove the pot from the stove, and place it on a protected counter or table. Drape a towel over your head, lean over the pot, and breathe gently for 10 to 15 minutes. Don't stick your face too far into the pot or you'll get a poached nose.

Cuts, Scrapes, and Sores
OVERCOMING "OWIES"

It could be a scene in a National Lampoon movie. One balmy afternoon on the way back to work, you're trying to juggle a large coffee and your purse while navigating the stone pathway that leads to your office. As you're slipping your keys into your purse, a stone you've never seen before jumps up and trips you. As you fall to the ground, you catch yourself with your hands and knees. And before you can say "bloody mess," you've got your belongings thrown back into the purse and are headed for the nearest bathroom. Once you reach the bathroom, you look down to see a trickle of blood heading down your leg from cuts on your knee and dirt-engraved scrapes on your hands. If it's any consolation to your bruised ego and skin, you've just had one of the most common accidents. Americans have millions of lacerations a year. Now your biggest concern is figuring out how to take care of yourself without alerting the whole office to your fiasco.

Accidents Happen

The sidewalk scenario is replayed thousands of different ways every day. Especially if you take care of small children, cuts and scrapes are so common you probably have a stockpile of supplies to treat

MAKE YOUR OWN DISINFECTANT

Rosemary is known in folk medicine for its disinfectant properties. To make a disinfectant, put 1 ounce rosemary leaves in a 1-pint jar and fill with boiling water. Cover tightly and let stand until the tea reaches room temperature. Wet a cloth with the solution and apply to the wound three to four times per day.

GUNG HO FOR GARLIC

Galen, the noted Roman doctor, used flour infused with garlic to stop the bleeding in gladiators with serious sword wounds. Roman soldiers showed the British how to dress wounds with a garlic-soaked moss. This method of treating serious wounds was used until the early 20th century.

them. Both cuts and scrapes can hurt like the dickens, even if they are usually only minor injuries. But they hurt for different reasons. Cuts are incisions in the skin, made accidentally, say from the jagged edge of an aluminum can, or surgically. Although cuts may be bloody, they don't affect as many nerves as scrapes do, so they actually hurt less. Scrapes hurt so badly because they basically slough away a layer of skin on a rough surface, such as the pavement, and leave raw nerve endings hanging underneath. Scrapes often damage some blood vessels, so they are prone to bleeding but usually not as heavily as cuts do.

Cuts and scrapes should be attended to immediately because of the risk of infection. Skin is the body's shield against germs. When a foreign body invades the skin, germs have an open invitation to raid healthy cells. Left untreated, cuts and scrapes can become painful sores, which are wounds that are slow to heal, or they can become infected. Sores can also come from acute or chronic bacterial or fungal infections or from diseases that affect the body's ability to heal, such as diabetes or AIDS.

HERBAL REMEDIES

Aloe. The sap from an aloe vera plant can be used to treat sores. Break off an aloe vera leaf and apply the sap to the sore. Repeat every few hours.

 Garlic. Garlic is an old folk remedy for healing cuts, scrapes, and sores. It contains an antimicrobial agent called allicin that protects against infection. But be careful, as fresh garlic can be irritating to the skin and should never be left on the skin for more than 20 to 25 minutes. Mix 3 cloves garlic with 1 cup wine in a blender. Let it stand for two to three hours, then strain. Apply to the well-cleaned wound with a clean cloth one to two times per day. Discontinue if the treatment is irritating.

Plantain leaves. The leaves of this plant (*plantago major*) are well known in folk medicine for their cleansing and anti-inflammatory properties. Crush the leaves to get the potent juice. Apply the leaves to the cleaned wound.

TOPICAL REMEDIES

Honey. If you think bees are attracted to honey, you should see germs flock to the stuff when it's applied to a cut, scrape, or sore. Honey dehydrates the bacteria in a wound, making it clean and free from infection. Place honey on sterile gauze and apply it directly to the cleaned wound area.

Onion. Allicin, the same antimicrobial component in garlic, is found in onions. And onions don't irritate the skin like garlic does. Grind half an onion in a food processor. Mix with honey and apply to a sore. Do not leave in place more than one hour. Repeat three times per day.

Water. The first step to treating a cut or scrape is cleaning it. So rinse the injury thoroughly with water. Clean it with soap, then rinse it again.

White vinegar. Use a mixture of 1 tablespoon white vinegar to 1 pint water to soak off scabs. This will help kill bacteria and get rid of the scab gently without picking. Just remember: Vinegar stings!

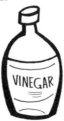

TO BANDAGE OR NOT TO BANDAGE?

Letting a scab form is not the best way for a cut or scrape to heal. Scabs interfere with the body's ability to make new skin cells. The new skin cells are what heals the injury. Just as important, the new cells reduce the risk of scarring, while a scab actually increases the chances of a scar forming. A bandage can prevent further damage (especially if you tend to be a magnet for accidents). A basic generic bandage will do fine. Avoid bandages with antibiotic creams, aloe, or vitamin E on the pads. They won't help with healing and may cause allergic reactions in some people.

WHEN TO CALL THE DOCTOR

- If there are signs of infection, such as redness, red streaks, swelling, pus, fever, or enlarged lymph nodes
- If you haven't had a tetanus shot in ten years and a dirty object was responsible for your injury
- If your face is the site of injury
- If your cut or scrape is too dirty or too deep to clean properly at home
- If your cut is wider than ¼ inch or has ragged edges that can't be closed evenly
- If you cut yourself in an area full of tendons and nerves and you can't feel or move the area
- If bleeding is severe. If blood is spurting out of the cut, cover it with a cloth, elevate it above heart level, and get to an emergency room immediately.
- If the injury is the result of a bite from a dog or human

MORE DO'S AND DON'TS

- Don't use hydrogen peroxide to clean your wound. Recent research shows that it damages healthy tissue around the wound and can slow the healing process. And it's not a great germ fighter, despite its reputation.
- Wash the wound every day with soap and water to keep it clean and prevent infection.
- Lick the wound if you can't wash it. Research has found that saliva can help kill bacteria.
- If you've been injured by a rusty object or have a puncture wound or animal bite, find out when you last had a tetanus shot. Adults need to be reimmunized every ten years.
- Use tincture of iodine or povidone-iodine for minor cuts and bruises. Iodine effectively kills bacteria and viruses.

MAKING THE POINT ABOUT PUNCTURE WOUNDS

Puncture wounds can happen anytime. You walk through a construction site and step on a nail, or you accidentally staple your finger. Since puncture wounds often don't bleed much, they seem less serious than they are. Follow these rules about treating puncture wounds:

- Put the pressure on. Because they don't bleed much, puncture wounds sometimes don't get rid of dangerous bacteria through the blood flow. Squeeze the area and help blood and bacteria leave the wound.
- Give it a thorough examination. Use your tweezers to get rid of any dirt or any other foreign objects. Then clean the wound with soap and water.
- Stop the invaders. Because it's hard to tell how deep a puncture wound traveled, you might want to check with your doctor about antibiotic treatment to prevent infection.

Dehydration
GETTING FLUSH AGAIN

Every cell in your body needs water in order to function properly. In fact, an adult's body weight is 60 percent water while an infant's is as much as 80 percent water. Other than oxygen, there's nothing that your body needs more than water. Water is so important because it has many critical functions in the body. Among other activities, water

- Lubricates your joints and connective tissues
- Helps digest food
- Liquefies mucus when you've got a cold. This makes it easy to blow and cough it out.
- Eliminates body heat through sweat
- Carries oxygen, carbohydrates, and fats to working muscles, then carries away wastes such as carbon dioxide and lactic acid
- Flushes wastes from the body through urine
- Boosts endurance during prolonged exercise
- Dilutes and disperses medications and vitamins so they won't give you a bellyache
- Fights flight fatigue, often caused by dehydration from the dry air on the plane
- Wards off bladder infections by washing out harmful bacteria
- Helps curb your appetite

FASCINATING FACT
By the time you feel thirsty, you've already lost 1 percent of your body's total water.

DEHYDRATION IN SENIORS
Older adults have a decreased sense of thirst, so they are even less able to tell when they need to drink than younger people. Indicators of dehydration in older adults include:
- Decreased urination
- Dry tongue
- Dry gums, or the inside cheeks are dry
- Upper-body weakness that's out of the ordinary
- Mental confusion
- Difficulty speaking
- Sunken eyes

FASCINATING FACT
A person can live several weeks without food but only a few days without water. It is second only to air in importance to life.

- Plumps up wrinkles. We have water in and around every cell in our bodies, and when water around those cells decreases, wrinkles happen.
- And yes, water quenches thirst. Thirst is our body's mechanism to alert us that we have insufficient fluids. If you're thirsty, it's time to restock.

The Great Escape

Each and every time you exhale, water escapes your body—up to as much as 2 cups per day. It evaporates invisibly from your skin—another 2 cups per day. And you urinate approximately 2½ pints every 24 hours. Add it up, and you could be losing up to 10 cups of water every day, and that's before you break a sweat.

Because water has so many life-sustaining functions, dehydration isn't just a matter of being a little thirsty. The effects depend on the degree of dehydration, but a water shortage causes your kidneys to conserve water, which in turn can affect other body systems. You'll urinate less and can become constipated. As you become increasingly more dehydrated, these symptoms will develop:

- diminished muscular endurance
- dizziness
- lack of energy
- decreased concentration
- drowsiness
- irritability
- headache
- tachycardia (galloping heart rate)
- increased body temperature
- collapse
- permanent organ damage or death

How Much Is Enough?

Obviously, you don't want to develop the problems listed above, so you have to ask: How much water do I need each day? Under normal conditions, the standard of 64 ounces per day is sufficient. That amount includes water from sources other than the tap. If you're an athlete or someone who spends a lot of time out in the sun sweating, you'll probably need more. A good way to tell if you're adequately hydrated is by observing the color of your urine. If it's dark yellow or amber, that's a sign that it's concentrated, meaning there's not enough water in the wastes that are being eliminated. If it's light (the color of lemon juice) that's normal.

Here are more facts about your urine:

- Some medications change the color, which means you can't keep an eye on your hydration level. Ask your physician about the medications you take, including over-the-counter drugs, vitamins, and minerals, that could change the color of your urine.
- Urine is normally darker and more concentrated in the morning, but with adequate hydration it lightens to lemon juice color and remains that way throughout the day.
- Bathroom breaks should happen every two to three hours. If you don't need to urinate for longer periods of time, you're not drinking enough water.

The simple cure for dehydration comes from the tap. Turn it on and drink. But there are other helpers that will keep you hydrated too.

DIETARY REMEDIES

Bananas. They have great water content and are especially good for restoring potassium that has

WATER-LOSS FORMULA

Here's how to tell how much you've lost and how much you'll need to drink to replace it.

- Weigh yourself nude before activity.
- Weigh yourself nude after the activity.
- Every one-pound weight loss equals a half liter (about 16 ounces) of water that must be replaced.

FASCINATING FACT

About 45 percent of all Americans are always mildly dehydrated.

JET LAG CURE

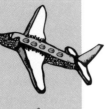

Some experts believe jet lag is caused by dehydration. But even if dehydration isn't the main cause of jet lag, it certainly is part of the jet-lag package. The air on board a plane is desert-dry, and you don't have access to fluids the way you do on land, unless you plan ahead. Those who are worried about making trips to the cramped airplane bathroom may consciously or subconsciously cut down on liquids.

Here's how to avoid that jet lag:

- One hour before flying, drink a cup of ginger tea to soothe your nerves and get last-minute hydration.
- On the plane, drink 2 to 3 cups water every couple of hours. Airlines may provide sufficient water, but to be sure you have a supply when you want it, take an empty bottle and fill it with water after you pass through security. Skip the caffeinated drinks and alcohol. They are diuretics, which cause the body to lose water.
- After you arrive, continue drinking fluids.

vanished with dehydration. (See "Banana Basics," page 16.)

Bland foods. If you've experienced dehydration, stick to foods that are easily digested for the next 24 hours because stomach cramps are a symptom and can recur. Try soda crackers, rice, bananas, potatoes, and flavored gelatins. Gelatins are especially good since they are made primarily of water.

Decaffeinated tea. Just another tasty way to get fluids in your body. Don't drink caffeinated tea, however, as caffeine is a mild diuretic.

Fruit juice. It's liquid and has essential vitamins and minerals that need to be replenished. Add water if the juice itself is too sweet.

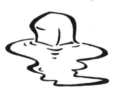

Ice. Suck on it, or rub it on your body when you're overheated. This will help cool you down and prevent excess evaporation, which may lead to dehydration.

Lime juice. Add 1 teaspoon lime juice, a pinch of salt, and 1 teaspoon sugar to a pint of water. Sip the beverage throughout the day to cure mild dehydration.

Popsicle. A great way to restore water to your body. It's an easy way to get fluids into kids too.

Raisins. They're packed with potassium, a body salt lost during dehydration.

Salt. Most Americans get plenty of salt. But if you're experiencing symptoms of mild dehydration or heat injury, or you're just plain sweating a lot, make sure you replace your salt. Eat salty foods such as salted pretzels, salted crackers, or salty nuts.

Sports drinks. Not only will they add water back into your system, they'll restore potassium and other essential electrolytes (a salt substance, such as potassium, sodium, and chlorine, found in blood, tissue fluids, and cells that carry electrical impulses). For children, these adult drinks may be too harsh, so talk to your pharmacist about pediatric rehydration drinks now on the market.

Watery fruits. Bananas are the number one fruit for rehydration, but watery fruits are a delicious and nutritious way to restore fluids. Try cantaloupe, watermelon, and strawberries. Watery vegetables such as cucumbers are good too.

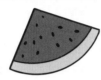

TOPICAL REMEDIES

Salt. To slough off the dry, flaky skin that comes from dehydration, try this: After you bathe and while your skin is still wet, sprinkle salt onto your hands and rub it all over your skin. This salt massage will remove dry skin and make your skin smoother to the touch. It will also invigorate your skin and get your circulation moving.

Also, if your skin is itchy as a result of dehydration, soaking in a tub of salt water can be a great itchy skin reliever. Just add 1 cup table salt or sea salt to bathwater. This solution will also soften skin and relax you.

Vinegar. Since achy muscles are a side effect of dehydration, this can bring relief. Add 8 ounces apple cider vinegar to a bathtub of warm water. Soak in tub for at least 15 minutes.

WHEN TO CALL THE DOCTOR

- If you're experiencing excessive thirst, no matter how much you drink. This can be a sign of diabetes. (See Diabetes, page 131.)
- If you can't stop the diarrhea flow. Diarrhea causes dehydration. Ride it out for a couple days and drink plenty of fluids, but if it doesn't stop, dial the doc. (See Diarrhea, page 141.)
- If you suffer chronic constipation
- If mild fever, which can cause dehydration, lasts more than a couple of days. Also, if fever spikes above 104 degrees Fahrenheit. (See Fever, page 171.)

LIFESTYLE REMEDIES

Drink even when you're not thirsty. You're losing body fluids every second of the day, and they must be replaced.

Water. Drink your daily requirement at home or on the go. Start your day with 16 ounces, and end your day with 16 ounces. That's a great way to prevent mild dehydration.

MORE DO'S & DON'TS

- Don't cut back if you're retaining fluids. Water retention that's caused by salt needs to be addressed by increasing water consumption to flush salt from the body.
- Don't depend on sport drinks or soft drinks for all your fluid requirements. They can come with side effects and calories. Plain old water is the best choice.
- Don't skip water if what comes from the tap tastes terrible. Bottled brands are available everywhere.

Dental Decay
CHERISHING YOUR CHOPPERS

We take those choppers for granted, don't we? Except for that first year or two of life, they've always been there, ready to take on the grueling task of chewing. We douse them with sugar that erodes their enamel, require them to work overtime on foods hard enough to be called petrified, and then we forget the basics our parents taught us: Brush after every meal, and don't eat so many sweets.

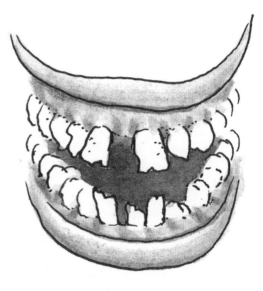

Our teeth serve us well when they're in good order, but when something goes wrong, ouch! First comes that off-and-on-again little twinge, the one we ignore and hope will disappear. Next comes the sensitivity to hot and cold. And finally the full-out throb that hurts so bad that pulling the tooth out with a piece of string tied to a doorknob doesn't seem like such a bad way out.

Tooth problems hurt like a . . . toothache, and ultimately the solution comes in a dentist's chair, the drill screaming in your ear, your teeth clenching against the needle being jabbed into your mouth.

Yes, we do abuse our teeth. And what's amazing about that is that overall, we're not neglecting our dental health. On average, 60 percent of all American adults visit their dentist once a year. So what's the deal? Why the toothache?

- Poor food choices
- Bacteria
- Bad brushing technique
- Not enough flossing
- Heredity
- Lack of professional care

Take your pick, the list is long. But there are also home remedies that can solve some of your dental dilemmas, from toothache to tooth care.

MORE BAKING SODA TIPS

- To clean your toothbrush, soak it overnight in a solution of baking soda and water.
- Clean your dentures by scrubbing or soaking them in baking soda and water.

RUB THAT ACHE AWAY

For a toothache in the upper jaw, place your thumb in the middle of your ear and slide it slowly to about an inch in front of the ear, where you'll feel an indentation in the bone. Then apply hard pressure for a minute.

For a toothache in the lower jaw, place your thumb in the spot where the jawbone turns toward the front of the head, and massage briskly.

DIETARY REMEDIES

Cheese. You know those nasty bacteria that's just waiting to take a whack at your tooth enamel? Cheese is their sworn enemy. First, it stimulates the salivary glands to clean the mouth. According to studies, just a few ounces of hard cheese eaten after a meal may protect against decay. There's also evidence to suggest that fatty acids in cheese may have antibacterial properties. And finally, cheese proteins may actually coat and protect tooth enamel. So, here's another reason to "say cheese"!

Green Tea. A 2009 study indicates that regularly drinking green tea may promote periodontal health and ward off gum disease.

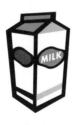

Milk. Milk is alkaline, which doesn't erode tooth enamel like acidic fruit juices and soft drinks do. It's also calcium-rich, which is vital for strong teeth and bones. Check your fridge for these other calcium-packed foods while you're there: yogurt, broccoli, Swiss chard, and salmon.

Orange juice. Add ½ teaspoon natural sugar and a pinch of cumin to 1 cup fresh orange juice to help bleeding gums. Rinse with water afterward.

Salsa. The spicier the better. Foods that make your mouth water actually fight dental decay. They stimulate the salivary glands, and all the extra saliva cleans your teeth and gums. And if that salsa is too hot, the water you'll drink to cool the burn will clean your mouth too.

HERBAL REMEDIES

Allspice. It helps relieve toothache, though it's not as effective as cloves because it contains less eugenol. Wet your finger and dip it into the spice, then rub it along the gum line near the aching tooth. You can also steep some in a glass of warm water, then rinse your mouth with it. Not only does this rinse relieve pain, but it also freshens your breath.

Cloves. Cloves contain eugenol, a chemical with natural antiseptic and anesthetic properties. That explains why ground cloves have been used to relieve toothaches for thousands of years. Moisten 1 teaspoon powdered cloves in olive oil and pack it into an aching cavity. Or use a few drops of clove oil or eugenol from your pharmacy to help deaden pain temporarily. Follow the directions on the bottle. Dentists still use a mixture of eugenol and zinc oxide before applying amalgam when filling teeth.

Coriander. This spice, as well as thyme and green tea, has antibacterial properties. Brew a tea from your choice of the three and use as a mouth rinse after meals.

Sage. Add 2 teaspoons sage to 2 cups water, then boil. Cool for 15 minutes, then swish in your mouth for several minutes. Sage has an antibacterial property that may reduce decay.

Sesame seeds. Chew a handful slowly but don't swallow. Brush your teeth with a dry toothbrush, using the chewed seeds as you would a toothpaste. They will both clean and polish.

TOPICAL REMEDIES

Coconut oil. Massage this into sore gums for relief.

THE ANATOMY OF A TOOTHACHE

Most toothaches result from dental decay, which is a destruction of the tooth enamel. The destruction process is simple. You consume carbohydrates such as candy or soft drinks and don't clean your mouth of the leftover particles immediately. The bacteria that normally live in your mouth jump on this feast you've left behind and have a party. What they leave behind for you is acid that will, over time, eat right through the enamel, causing a cavity and, when the acid invades the nerve-filled and very sensitive pulp inside your tooth, a great big pain in the mouth.

Be aware, too, that all the dental preventatives won't stop those annoying little bacteria from invading your tooth if it's cracked or a filling is loose. To them, these are open invitations to go on in.

ENAMEL BUSTERS

Fruits containing citric acid, such as oranges and grapefruit, can erode the enamel in teeth, so eat them only with meals.

If you do eat them as a snack or drink fresh citrus fruit juice, swish your mouth out with water afterward. Do the same when you drink colas and other carbonated beverages.

FROZEN FRUIT JUICE FIASCO

We all love these treats, especially in the summer when it's hot and they're so refreshing. And they seem like such a healthy treat too. But these chilly goodies are rotting your teeth.

How? The acid content in these juice bars is so high that the normally protective saliva fails to clean your teeth. To make matters worse, you suck on the bars or hold them in your mouth until they melt, prolonging the acidic exposure. Definitely not tooth friendly. So after you eat the treat, swish with some water.

Ice. That's the last thing you want to stick on an aching tooth, isn't it? Well, don't stick it on your tooth. Rub an ice cube in the soft spot between your thumb and first finger. This acupressure treatment may stop tooth pain. If your jaw is really throbbing and swollen, though, an ice pack to the face for about ten minutes every hour will help relieve both the pain and the swelling. Just be careful, as rapid cooling can increase pain. If that doesn't work, try moist heat.

Rhubarb. It's high in potassium and calcium, which are both tooth protectors. But don't eat it. Instead, crush fresh rhubarb to extract the juice, then rub your teeth with the juice to protect the enamel. Apply once every other day.

Salt. Dissolve 1 teaspoon salt in 1 cup warm water, and rinse your mouth with it to help treat bleeding gums, canker sores, and toothache. Salt makes a great whitening toothpaste too. Pulverize salt in a blender, food processor, or coffee grinder, or spread some on a cutting board and roll it with a pastry rolling pin to crush it into a fine sandlike texture. Mix 1 part crushed salt with 2 parts baking soda, then dip a dampened toothbrush into the mixture and brush your teeth. Keep the powder in an airtight container in your bathroom. This mixture also helps remove plaque.

Sesame oil. Gargling with warm sesame oil is an Ayurvedic treatment for gum disease. Take a mouthful and swish it around twice a day, then rinse. It's also said that this simple gargle can reduce cheek wrinkles. What a great bonus!

Strawberries. They're a wonderful tooth whitener. Rub the juice on the teeth and leave for five minutes. Then rinse off with warm water that has a pinch of baking soda dissolved in it.

Tea bag. Black tea contains fluoride that can suppress the growth of bacteria that cause decay and dental plaque, the sticky white film that forms on your teeth. (When it hardens, it's called tartar.) Drop a tea bag of black tea into a cup of hot water, and let it brew for six minutes. This will allow the maximum amount of fluoride to escape into the water. Squeeze the tea bag into the water before discarding it to get that last little bit of fluoride. Use the tea as a rinse to prevent plaque buildup after you eat sweets.

Vinegar. Here's an easy but temporary toothache fix: Try rinsing your mouth with a mixture of 4 ounces warm water, 2 tablespoons vinegar, and 1 tablespoon salt.

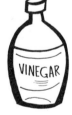

LIFESTYLES REMEDIES

Floss regularly. Also, if pain or pressure suddenly comes on, it may be caused by some lodged-in-tight food. Try to floss that pain away first before seeking other treatment.

Scrape your tongue. Brushing or scraping your tongue is an important part of your oral hygiene routine. It rids your mouth of bacteria and food particles, and it stimulates your salivary glands to wake up and get to work. Use a spoon to scrape from the back of the tongue to the front, repeating until you've covered the entire area.

FASCINATING FACT
Tooth enamel is the strongest substance in the body, but unlike bone, it will not heal or regenerate when broken.

A DENTAL MARVEL
Who ever would have guessed that something as common as sugarless gum could work dental wonders? Sugar-free gum with a sweetener called xylitol may prevent plaque buildup by helping remineralize teeth. But it offers other key benefits too. Xylitol increases the production of saliva, cutting down on the number of bacteria in the mouth, and it seems to increase the efficiency of fluoride toothpastes. Other sweeteners, such as sorbitol and mannitol, do not support the growth of oral bacteria either.

WHEN TO CALL THE DENTIST

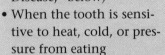

- When gingivitis or periodontitis might be present (see the list in "Gum Disease," below)
- When the tooth is sensitive to heat, cold, or pressure from eating
- If pain is severe
- If there's pus or an abscess
- If the tooth is cracked or broken

MORE DO'S & DON'TS

- Try an over-the-counter pain reliever, such as acetaminophen or ibuprofen, if the pain is too severe.
- Keep your head upright to decrease the pressure in the painful area if you have a toothache.
- Don't apply aspirin to the tooth. Aspirin is an anti-inflammatory medication that works only if it's taken internally. And it's acidic, which can cause local gum erosion and more pain.
- Keep the air out if your tooth is sensitive. Cover it with gauze or sugarless gum until you can get professional treatment.

GUM DISEASE?

Gum disease is an infection in the tissues surrounding the tooth. Although it often goes unnoticed, it is the major cause of tooth loss in adults.

Gum disease is called gingivitis in its early stage. The gums are red and swollen, and they bleed. Gingivitis is usually easily reversed by daily brushing and flossing.

If the infection progresses, it becomes periodontitis. Periodontitis damages both the gums and the bones surrounding the teeth. Teeth become loose and often fall out. Or, they may have to be pulled by the dentist.

Look for these signs of gum disease:
- Bleeding gums when you brush
- Gums that are painful, swollen, and red
- Gums that are pulling away from the tooth
- Persistent bad breath
- Loose teeth

If you suspect gum disease, call your dentist. In the meantime, brush and floss!

Denture Discomfort
MAKING THE ADJUSTMENT

Anyone who has donned a set of dentures knows discomfort is part of the process. There are two periods when discomfort is at its peak: the initial days of wearing the new device and several years later when the dentures may no longer fit properly.

The cause of the discomfort isn't a mystery. After the teeth are extracted, the dentures sit on the bony ridge that's leftover. Without the stability of permanent teeth, this bony ridge changes and shrinks over the years while the dentures remain fixed. Slipping and sliding dentures cause sore spots, which is the reason for much of denture discomfort.

Dentures may not fit like a glove, but you shouldn't suffer. There are a variety of ways to prevent and resolve denture discomfort.

DIETARY REMEDIES
Soft foods. Eat like a baby during the adjustment period. You don't have to mash peas in a blender, but you should stick to soft, easy-to-chew foods such as soups, stews, and pastas (macaroni and cheese). If you chew on hard foods, such as carrots and pretzels,

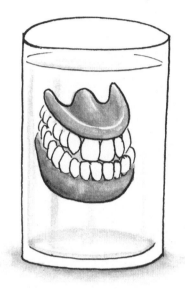

you'll risk damaging tender gum tissues that are still reeling from the shock of losing their natural teeth. For dessert, enjoy puddings, gelatin, and applesauce.

HERBAL REMEDIES
Aniseed. This gentle herbal mouth rinse is perfect for sensitive mouths. Combine 2 teaspoons crushed aniseed, 1 tablespoon peppermint leaves, and 2 cups boiling water. Cover and steep for eight hours. Strain and add 1 teaspoon myrrh tincture, which acts as an antiseptic and preservative. Use

AMAZING MYRRH

The antimicrobial effects of myrrh are so strong that ancient Egyptians used this plant for the process of embalming their dead for the afterlife. In the contemporary world, myrrh does a mouthful of things. It stimulates circulation to mucosal tissues, especially in the bronchial tubes, throat, tonsils, and gums. Myrrh's antiseptic qualities help bleeding gums, gingivitis, tonsillitis, and sore throats.

A HEALTHY RINSE

Use a 3-percent solution of hydrogen peroxide as a rinse to keep mouth and gums healthy. A solution stronger than 3 percent is dangerous. Hydrogen peroxide rids the mouth of food particles, and the oxygenating agent helps boost the fighting properties of good bacteria. The rinse also acts against bad bacteria, although on a more limited basis.

For gargling, dilute hydrogen peroxide with an equal amount of water, and swish around your mouth for 30 seconds. Don't swallow the rinse. If a drop or two sneaks down your throat, body heat and stomach acid should dissipate it.

2 tablespoons twice a day for rinsing. The remainder of the rinse can be stored in a glass bottle. Shake before using.

Cloves. The clove has been used as a remedy for aching mouths since antiquity. The clove remedy started in Asian folk medicine, and the concept traveled along trade routes to Europe and the Mediterranean along with the spice itself. By the 3rd century B.C. the clove was the universal folk remedy for mouth and dental pain in the Mediterranean. Cloves' medicinal use continued into the 19th century, when dentists used clove oil to relieve dental pain. Even today dentists use eugenol, a major ingredient in clove oil, as a pain reliever and to disinfect dental abscesses. Perhaps cloves' timeless popularity stems from the fact that they not only eliminate pain but also smell terrific. There's nothing like having a fresh and pain-free mouth all in one. To tap into these healing properties, blend 1 teaspoon cloves into a powder using a coffee grinder or use ½ teaspoon prepackaged ground cloves. Moisten with olive oil and dab around a mouth or gum sore.

TOPICAL REMEDIES

Salt. Gargling with warm salt water may help denture wearers breeze through the adjustment phase sans mouth sores. Prevent sore spots from becoming infected or inflamed by rinsing every three to four hours. The salt water cleans out bacteria, shrinks swollen tissue, and helps toughen the tender tissue. Make a saltwater rinse by adding ½ teaspoon salt to 4 ounces warm water. Gargle and spit. Do this twice daily.

Soap. After teeth are extracted and new dentures fit, it's of prime importance to keep your new choppers sparkling clean. 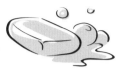 Excess bacteria buildup on dentures can retard the gum's healing process. Plain old soap, warm water, and a hand brush do a grand job at cleaning. Scrub at least twice a day and rinse well.

LIFESTYLE REMEDIES

Give your mouth a rest. Always remove your false teeth at night. You may also want to remove dentures for 24 hours should you develop a red spot on the gums.

MORE DO'S AND DON'TS

- Have your dentures checked yearly.
- Have your dentures relined every two to three years.
- Replace dentures every five to six years, depending on the amount of wear and tear and the shrinkage of the gums.

WHEN TO CALL A DENTIST

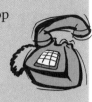

- If you develop soreness that doesn't improve within a week
- If an area on your gum bleeds spontaneously or is filled with pus
- If you notice extra tissue growing, particularly between the upper lip and the gum
- If a white sore persists for more than a week.
- If you have a mouth sore that doesn't heal completely within 10 to 14 days

Depression
BATTLING THE BLUES

There are many times in the course of life that you may feel overwhelmed and distraught. If you didn't feel like singing the blues now and again you wouldn't be human. It's actually healthy to get down from time to time. It's when that down-in-the-dumps feeling begins to stick around longer than a couple of weeks that you might be suffering from a more serious condition, such as clinical depression. If you are experiencing a bout of depression, don't feel alone. Mental health experts say at least 30 million people deal with mild depression every year, and 14.8 million Americans are diagnosed with a more serious form of depression annually.

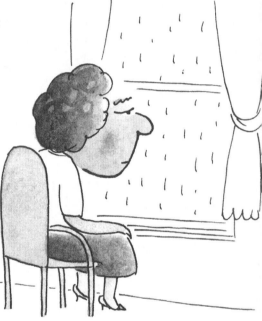

Major or Minor?

Though it'd be nice to go through life pretending that you're in a *Brady Bunch* episode, it's not realistic. There are going to be times when life throws you a few curveballs. Perhaps you suddenly lose a parent or your spouse is diagnosed with a major illness. Feeling depressed during tough times is normal. Mild depression is something everyone encounters. But sometimes stressful situations can cause more than a few days of sadness.

If your hopeless feelings begin to become more intense and last more than a couple of weeks, you could be experiencing clinical

> ### *FASCINATING FACT*
> Women are twice as likely to suffer from depression as men. Approximately 9.8 million women and 5 million men are diagnosed with clinical depression each year.

depression. Major depression, one form of clinical depression, may only happen once in your lifetime, or it may come back several times. Major depression usually lasts weeks or months and is disabling. It can cause you to lose interest in work, sleep, eating, or going out to dinner with a friend. A less severe form of clinical depression is dysthymia. Dysthymia isn't as emotionally crippling as major depression. With dysthymia you go about your life, attending soccer games and birthday parties, but it feels as though there's a gray cloud hanging over you. Dysthymia is a chronic condition. And people with dysthymia may suffer bouts of major depression throughout their lives.

Causes of Depression

Researchers have discovered that depression can run in the family. That doesn't mean that you'll definitely suffer bouts of depression if your parents did. But if you encounter a stressful situation, such as losing your job, you'll be more likely to slip into a major depression than someone who doesn't have a genetic link to the condition.

Physiologically most types of depression are related to a malfunction in neurotransmitters in the brain. Researchers have discovered that if there is a glitch in the way neurotransmitters communicate, you can experience problems with mood, sleeping, and eating. Also, people who are more susceptible to depression physiologically tend to overreact to stress.

Other causes of depression include:

• Major stresses, such as going through a serious illness or losing someone close to you.

EAT TO LIVE, HAPPILY
What you eat affects how you feel, but what you don't eat may do the same. Depression has been linked to low levels of many nutrients, such as biotin, calcium, copper, iron, magnesium, pantothenic acid, potassium, pyridoxine, riboflavin, thiamin, vitamin C, vitamin E, and zinc. So if you are dealing with mild depression, take a look at what you're eating. Some changes in your diet may make a difference in your mood.

- Hormonal changes. As hormones fluctuate—after having a baby, before and during menstruation, and during menopause—women tend to suffer more depression.
- Medications. Check with your doctor if you've recently started a new medication and are feeling symptoms of depression.

DIETARY REMEDIES

Brazil nuts. Selenium, a trace mineral found abundantly in Brazil nuts (100 mcg in one nut), can help ease depression. Studies have shown that people who had low levels of selenium tended to be more anxious, depressed, and tired. Once they ate foods containing selenium, however, they felt better. Other selenium-rich foods are tuna, swordfish, oysters, and sunflower seeds.

Chicken. Low levels of vitamin B_6 may be an instigator of depression, especially in women on birth control pills. Vitamin B_6 is necessary for the body to make serotonin, a neurotransmitter. The RDA for vitamin B_6 is 1.3 mg for men and women up to age 50; after age 50 the amount increases to 1.7 mg. There are 0.5 mg of vitamin B_6 in 3 ounces of chicken.

Coffee. If you're a regular morning coffee drinker, you know what life can be like if you don't have your morning cup. You get a headache, you're cranky, and you feel bad. Well, researchers are finding that caffeine can indeed alter your mood. It makes you less irritable and helps you feel better. Experts do think that having a cup or two of coffee a day may indeed help ease mild depression. But don't go overboard. Downing too much caffeine can make you jittery and may even make you more anxious.

Fish. The brain is one of the richest sources of fatty acids in the body. And research is finding that depressed people have lower 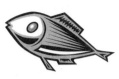 levels of omega-3 fatty acids. This polyunsaturated fat is found mostly in fatty fish. Researchers believe that getting enough omega-3 fatty acids is essential to ensure the brain is at its healthiest. And a healthy brain is less likely to become seriously depressed.

Spinach. Studies are finding that a folic acid deficiency is a major cause of depression. Scientists began to suspect a link between this B vitamin and the brain when they discovered that people diagnosed with depression have lower levels of folic acid than the general population. It seems that folic acid deficiency causes serotonin levels to fall, which can lead to feelings of depression. Ironically enough, folic acid deficiency is one of the most common nutrient deficiencies in women. But the good news is you only need about 200 mcg a day to meet your folic acid needs. That adds up to about ¾ cup of cooked spinach.

HERBAL REMEDIES

 Garlic. German researchers studying garlic's effect on cholesterol discovered that participants being treated with garlic experienced an elevation in mood. So try a little garlic therapy if you're feeling down.

LIFESTYLE REMEDIES

Abstain from alcohol. Alcohol is known to aggravate a depressed mood.

WHEN TO CALL THE DOCTOR

Occasional mild depression is normal, but clinical depression is not and should be taken more seriously. If you've felt five or more of these symptoms, and they've lasted more than two weeks, call your doctor.

- You are always sad, anxious, numb, or empty
- You have become pessimistic and feel hopeless
- You feel helpless, guilty, or worthless
- You've lost interest in things you enjoy
- You have less energy and feel tired
- You can't concentrate or remember things
- You have trouble making decisions
- You can't sleep or you sleep too much
- You don't have any appetite or you eat too much
- You dwell on death and think about suicide. Call a medical professional immediately!
- You are increasingly restless and irritable
- You have physical symptoms that don't respond to conventional treatment

Get some R & R. Be sure you are getting plenty of sleep and are taking time to stop and smell the flowers.

Energize with exercise. Runner's high is caused by an increase in endorphins—the feel-good brain chemicals. But you don't have to run a marathon to get the same mood-lifting feeling. Try taking a walk around the block or walking the dog for 10 or 15 minutes. You'll feel good the rest of the day.

Junk the junk food. Sure that sugar high feels good, but when you go through detox a couple of hours after that cupcake, you can feel terrible. Try skipping the sugary stuff and eating something more nutritious.

See a therapist. A trained counselor can help you make changes in the way you think and act that may have an impact on your depression. If necessary, a therapist can refer you to a doctor who can prescribe antidepressants.

MORE DO'S AND DON'TS

- Focus on friends and family. Leaning on others is one of the healthiest things you can do to get through a tough time in your life.
- Learn to laugh. Laughing actually triggers the same endorphins that are affected by exercise. Read some cartoons, watch your favorite Three Stooges movie, and if possible, try to find humor in your situation.
- Think happy thoughts. A recent study found that people who learn to have a more optimistic attitude are less likely to become depressed—even if they were naturally pessimistic. Changing your perception of life can have a huge affect on your mental health.

Diabetes

CONTROLLING BLOOD SUGAR

Diabetes is a disease that reduces, or stops, the body's ability to produce or respond to insulin, a hormone produced in the pancreas. Insulin's role is to open the door for glucose, a form of sugar, to enter the body's cells so that it can be used for energy. When the body has a problem metabo- lizing glucose, it builds up in the blood, and the body's cells starve.

There are two major types of diabetes·

Type 1. The body produces no insulin at all, and daily insulin shots are required. This disease used to be called juvenile diabetes because there is a higher rate of diagnosis among chil- dren ages 10 to 14. It is also referred to as insulin-dependent diabetes because injections of insulin are required to control blood glucose. The cause isn't known, but type 1 tends to run in families. Only 5 percent of people with diabetes have type 1.

Type 2. This is the most common form of diabe- tes, and it occurs when the body is insulin resis- tant. That could be either because the body fails to make enough insulin or because it doesn't properly use the insulin it does produce. The cause is often poor dietary habits, sedentary lifestyle, and obesity. Those with type 2 may or may not need oral medication or insulin, depend- ing on how their body responds to changes in diet and exercise.

FASCINATING FACT
As fruits are dehydrated, the sugar in them becomes con- centrated. Limit your intake of dried fruit to two or three times per week or less.

AN INFORMATIVE TEST

A simple blood test called hemoglobin A1C (also called HbA1C) can measure your cumulative average blood sugar levels for the past three months. It's the best test to find out whether your blood sugar is under control. People with diabetes should have a hemoglobin A1C test at least every six months. A test result of 6 percent or less is normal. If your result is above 7 percent, it means your diabetes control may not be as good as it could be. A major diabetes study has found that those whose results were 7 percent or lower had a much better chance of delaying or preventing diabetes complications related to the eyes, kidneys, and nerves than those whose levels were 8 percent or higher.

Here's the risk list for diabetes. Do any of these describe you?

- Older than age 45
- Family history of diabetes
- Overweight
- Don't exercise regularly
- Low HDL cholesterol (see High Cholesterol, page 255) or high triglycerides
- Member of an at-risk ethnic group (see "Top Ten Diabetes Stats," page 136)

Symptoms

In children, symptoms of the onset of type 1 diabetes may be similar to flu symptoms. They also may include these:

- Frequent urination
- Unusual thirst
- Extreme hunger
- Unexplained weight loss
- Extreme fatigue
- Irritability

Symptoms of type 2 diabetes include:

- Any of the type 1 symptoms
- Frequent infections, including those of the skin, gums, and bladder
- Blurred vision
- Sores that are slow to heal
- Tingling or numbness in hands or feet
- In women, recurring vaginitis

Treatment

There is no cure for diabetes, but it can be controlled. And control is essential because diabetes can lead to heart disease, stroke, kidney disease and failure, blindness, and amputation if not treated. This profile will not address diabetic medical treatment, including prescribed diabetic diets. Those specifics must be left up to your physician and dietitian. It will, however, cover the go-alongs—things that can make the diabetic experience easier, as well as alternative practices that might help. Before you try any alternative practice, consult your physician. Nothing contained in this profile is intended to stop or replace your prescribed diabetic care!

Diabetes is a complex disease, affecting many parts of the body. Some of the problems of the disease can be relieved with simple things, though. And for a person with diabetes, a little relief never hurts.

DIETARY REMEDIES

Asparagus. This vegetable is a mild diuretic that's said to be beneficial in the control of diabetes. Eat it steamed and drizzled with olive oil and lemon juice.

Lemon. A tasty substitute for salt. It's great squeezed into a diet cola too. It cuts the aftertaste.

Olive oil. Studies indicate this may reduce blood sugar levels. Use it in salad dressing or wherever cooking oils are indicated. For an inexpensive and easy no-stick olive oil spray-on coating, buy an oil mister in any department store kitchen supply area and use it to spray your pans before cooking.

Oolong tea. Drinking oolong tea combined with taking hypoglycemic drugs may be an effective treatment for type 2 diabetes. Participants in a 2003 study of Taiwanese adults with diabetes were given either six cups of oolong tea or water per day, along with blood glucose-lowering medications. After one month, the

FACTS ABOUT MEN AND WOMEN WITH DIABETES

Men
- Approximately 12 million men aged 20 or older in the United States have diabetes. Fifty to 60 percent of those older than age 50 are impotent.

Women
- Approximately 11.5 million women in the United States have diabetes.
- Birth control pills may affect blood glucose levels.
- Diabetic complications include increased risk of vaginal yeast infections and serious pregnancy problems.
- Four percent of all pregnant women who don't have diabetes develop gestational diabetes, which is a form of diabetes that occurs with pregnancy and usually goes away afterward. Fifty percent of women with gestational diabetes will develop diabetes in the next five to ten years.

glucose levels of those given the oolong tea were significantly reduced compared to those given water alone.

Peanut butter. After you've experienced an episode of low blood sugar and corrected it, follow up with a protein and carbohydrate snack. Peanut butter on a couple of crackers supplies both, and it's easy to fix when you may still feel a little jittery. Just avoid brands that contain added sugar, glucose, or jelly.

Salt. Set the saltshaker aside, put it back in the cupboard, hide it. High blood pressure is a side effect of diabetes, and that means salt's a no-no. So don't cook with it, and don't make it handy to grab when you eat a meal or snack. If it's out of sight, or inconvenient to get, you might just skip it. Instead, reach for an herb or spice blend that's sodium free. Make one yourself with your favorite spices, or buy one at the store.

Sugar. Yes, even people with diabetes need it occasionally when their blood sugar goes too low. A spoonful of straight sugar will work, as will a piece of hard candy. Just be sure it's not sugarless.

Vinegar. Muscle cramps, especially in the legs, can affect people with diabetes. For relief from the ache, add 8 ounces apple cider vinegar to a bathtub of warm water. Soak for at least 15 minutes.

HERBAL REMEDIES

Parsley. Steep into a tea and drink. This may act as a diuretic as well as lower blood sugar.

Watercress. This is said to strengthen the natural defense systems of people who have diabetes. It's also a mild diuretic. Wash the leaves thoroughly, and add them to a salad. Or smear a little cream cheese on a slice of bread, then top with watercress for a delicious open-faced sandwich.

TOPICAL REMEDIES

Salt. Dry, itchy skin is a side effect of diabetes, and soaking in a tub of salt water can be a great itchy skin reliever. Just add 1 cup table salt or sea salt to your bathwater. This solution will also soften skin and relax you. To exfoliate, after you take a shower or bath and while your skin is still wet, sprinkle salt onto your hands and rub it all over your skin. This salt massage will remove dry skin and make your skin smoother to the touch. It will also invigorate your skin and get your circulation moving. Try it first thing in the morning to help wake up or after a period of physical exertion.

LIFESTYLE REMEDIES

Eat foods with a low glycemic index. They release sugar slowly into the bloodstream.
Exercise. It lowers blood sugar and, combined with weight loss, can minimize the disease to easily manageable levels.

Lose weight. If you carry extra pounds, try to get rid of them.
Maintain a regular eating schedule. Your body needs it.

FASCINATING FACT
According to a Dutch study, fish eaters are half as likely to get type 2 diabetes as people who don't eat fish. The amount consumed was small—1 ounce per day. Most likely the omega-3 oil found in fish helps the pancreas handle glucose.

WHEN TO CALL THE DOCTOR

If you have not been diagnosed with diabetes, call if one or more of the symptoms outlined on page 132 are present. Otherwise call if:

- You've been vomiting or have diarrhea for more than 24 hours
- You can't eat or drink
- Your blood sugar is more than 240 or less than 80 for more than 48 hours
- You run a fever of 101 degrees Fahrenheit or more for two days
- Your vision goes blurry
- You experience other unusual physical symptoms such as weakness or difficulty when speaking
- You have an open sore on your legs or feet

MORE DO'S AND DON'TS

- Monitor your glucose levels regularly via finger sticks. That's the only way you can accurately gauge how you're doing. Record the results for your doctor and dietician.
- See your eye doctor at least once a year. Diabetes is the leading cause of blindness.
- Don't despair. Diabetes is treatable, and there are many options to control the disease other than "the needle." Seek emotional support from friends and family, or call a counselor if necessary.

TOP TEN DIABETES STATS

According to the National Diabetes Education Program:

1. 23.6 million people have diabetes.
2. 5.7 million of these people are not aware they have it.
3. 4,384 new cases of diabetes are diagnosed every day, totaling about 798,000 people a year.
4. Diabetes is the 7th leading cause of death in the United States.
5. People with diabetes have double the risk of premature death of those without diabetes.
6. Type 1 diabetes accounts for 5 to 10 percent of all diagnosed cases of diabetes.
7. Type 2 diabetes accounts for 90 to 95 percent of all diagnosed cases of diabetes.
8. Total health care and related costs for the treatment of diabetes is $174 billion annually.
9. 0.2 percent of people younger than 20 years of age have either type 1 or type 2 diabetes.
10. Type 2 diabetes is increasingly being diagnosed in children and adolescents.

THE DIABETIC FOOT

Even though it looks much the same as any other foot, the diabetic foot requires special attention. Why? Nerve damage is common with diabetes, especially in the lower extremities. Blood vessels are damaged as a result of the disease and circulation is decreased. When this happens, feet and legs tend to be cold and sores heal slowly, in some cases taking years to heal. This can easily lead to infection. Nerve damage can also decrease your ability to feel sensations in your feet, such as pain, heat, and cold. That means you may not notice a foot injury until you have a major infection.

Here are some general guidelines for diabetic foot care:

- Don't think a foot injury will heal on its own. It may not. If you develop a sore—even a blister—call your doctor immediately.
- Don't be tempted to warm your cold feet with a heating pad or hot water bottle. If you have neuropathy, you may burn yourself without even feeling it. Instead, wear warm socks, or indulge in a gentle foot massage. See the instructions on page 200, and make sure that after the massage you clean away any remaining oil from between your toes. A mild solution of vinegar and water will do it.
- Wear good shoes. Specialty diabetic shoes are available. Check with your health insurance carrier to see if your plan covers them.
- Always wear socks with your shoes to prevent blisters. Never go barefoot.
- Inspect your feet daily.
- Don't let your physician overlook your feet during a physical. Take off your shoes and socks, and remind the doctor to take a look.
- Expect dry skin. The nerves that control sweating in your feet may no longer work. So, after a bath, dry your feet and coat them with a thin layer of moisturizer. DO NOT use oils or creams between your toes. Moisture there can cause an infection such as athlete's foot.
- DO NOT soak your feet. The more you do, the more you put yourself at risk for infection.
- If you have a callus, don't cut it off. Use a pumice stone to rub it off. Oil down the callus with olive oil before you begin, then dab a little more on the spot when you've finished. If the callus becomes thick and too difficult to care for, it can cause an ulcer. Before it gets to this stage, call your podiatrist.
- Keep your toenails trimmed. Carefully cut them straight across to prevent an ingrown toenail, and file off the rough edges.

Diaper Rash
BABYING THE BUTTOCKS

One of life's earliest discomforts—diaper rash—is more of an annoyance than a serious medical problem. A baby's skin is sensitive, and no matter how much the baby is pampered, an irritating red rash can develop in diaper regions.

Diaper rash is a type of irritant dermatitis, or inflammation of the skin. The moist, warm, and enclosed environment of a diaper, combined with loads of bacteria, make a baby's bottom the perfect place for a rash to pop up. Other factors that can contribute to rash development include hot and humid weather, skin allergies, poor laundering of diapers, new materials in diapers that irritate sensitive skin, and infrequent diaper changes.

The causes aren't pleasant, but the solutions to stopping this rash are straightforward. You can cure the rash in a few days and, with a little effort, keep baby rash free for the remainder of diaperhood.

DIETARY REMEDIES
Cranberry juice. When urine soaks the diaper region, the result is a high pH that irritates the skin and promotes diaper rash. A solution for older infants is to give them 2 to 3 ounces of cranberry juice. Cranberry juice acidifies the urine, making it less friendly to bacteria growth and perhaps reducing irritation. Constituents in the juice also prevent bacteria from sticking to the bladder, which also helps prevent infection.

TOPICAL REMEDIES
Baking soda. If baby's bottom is very raw, try giving a sitz bath for 10 minutes, 3 times per day. Add 2 tablespoons baking soda to the tub of warm water.

Cornstarch. A nice patting of cornstarch helps dry up damp areas and reduces friction caused by elastic in diapers. When applying, first shake the cornstarch into your hand far from the baby's face. Avoid store-bought talcum powders, as recent studies have shown that talcum is dangerous for babies to inhale.

Maalox. This medicine does more than treat heartburn and stomach upset in adults. It can prevent diaper rash on babies by cooling irritated skin and neutralizing acid. With a cotton ball, apply a small amount of the liquid to baby's bottom. Allow to dry before diapering.

Oatmeal. Add 1 tablespoon dried oatmeal to your baby's bath. It is soothing and helps protect the skin.

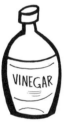

Vinegar. Urine is an extremely acidic solution and can burn the skin. To balance out the equation, try adding ½ cup white vinegar to the rinse water when you wash the baby's diapers. The vinegar helps neutralize the ammonia found in urine, gets rid of any soap buildup, and gets rid of diaper smells. You can also go directly to the source by wiping the baby's bottom with a solution of 8 parts water to 1 part vinegar.

LIFESTYLE REMEDIES

Take it off. Airing out a baby's bottom is one of the most natural ways to prevent diaper rash. Of course, there is the risk of a mess happening, but that's easy to prevent. Lay your baby on a rubber mat covered by a soft, washable towel. An hour or two a day of aeration can help those nether regions see the light of day and flourish!

Wipe it up naturally. Store-bought baby wipes are convenient, but many are full of alcohol and

FROM OIL RIG TO BABY'S BOTTOM

If there's one ointment found in most nurseries, it's petroleum jelly (or the brand-name version, Vaseline).

You might think a wise mom came up with this versatile, soothing spread, but alas, the jelly was invented by a fellow who was as far removed from a nursery as they come. A 22-year-old chemist named Robert Augustus Chesebrough discovered the oddly named substance in 1859.

While working in the petroleum industry in Pennsylvania, his scientific eye noticed a peculiar, colorless substance that collected around the pump rods on the oil wells. The stuff was a bit of a nuisance, since it clogged up equipment, but the hardened, tough workers didn't mind. They noticed that when they applied it to their cuts and burns, it appeared to help them heal.

Curious to examine this medicinal gel, Chesebrough returned to his home in Brooklyn with a sample and spent months creating a clean form, which he appropriately dubbed petroleum jelly. No news if his wife used it on their children.

WHEN TO CALL THE DOCTOR

- If the rash is accompanied by red, pimplelike dots along the edges
- If the rash is accompanied by blisters or pus-filled sores
- If your child is taking an antibiotic and the rash is bright red
- If you have tried everything and, after two to three days, the condition doesn't improve
- If it is very painful

other chemicals that can irritate or dry baby's sensitive skin. Try using a soft cotton towel, lukewarm water, and plain, nonperfumed soap to clean the diaper area.

Keep on checking. Routine checking and changing of baby's diapers will make diaper rash a distant memory. Change the diaper once per hour, if possible. This keeps the area dry and allows for regular air circulation.

Once a rash appears, treat it immediately. Apply a small dab of petroleum jelly, zinc oxide, or lanolin to the affected area three times a day. These substances protect the skin, blocking irritants and promoting healing.

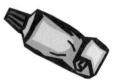

Diarrhea
RIDING OUT THE RUNS

It's got all kinds of colorful nicknames, including "Greased Lightning," "Turkey Trots," and "Montezuma's Revenge." You may even have heard your 11-year-old singing a catchy little ditty about it. But just saying the word diarrhea gets a reaction from most people—they either giggle or turn pale. Diarrhea is probably one of the most unpleasant problems that plagues us, and it's a common malady. Americans usually suffer from diarrhea a couple times a year. For most adults, diarrhea isn't serious. And it does give you a chance to ponder some redecorating ideas for the bathroom.

The Rundown on Diarrhea

On a typical day, you eat a hoagie and drink an iced tea and your meal makes its way through the digestive system without any problems. By the time it reaches the intestines, your food is mostly fluid with bits of solid material. The intestines reabsorb most of the fluid, and the solid stuff is excreted in the usual fashion. But when you've got diarrhea, something blocks the intestine's ability to absorb fluid. You've got loads of watery fluids mixed in with your stool, and you get that "gotta go" feeling.

There are essentially two types of diarrhea: acute and chronic. Thankfully, the vast majority of diarrhea is acute, or short term. This type of diarrhea keeps you on the toilet for a couple of days but doesn't stick around long. Acute diarrhea is also known as noninflammatory diarrhea. Its symptoms are what most people associate with the condition: watery, frequent stools accompanied by stomach cramps, gas, and nausea.

NO MORE EXCUSES TO BE A BRAT

Although the classic BRAT (bananas, rice, applesauce, and toast) diet is touted as the best for refeeding after a bout with diarrhea, the American Academy of Pediatrics considers that diet too low in energy density, protein, and fat for children. Although those foods can be tolerated, the Academy suggests introducing complex carbohydrates (rice, wheat, potatoes, bread, and cereals), lean meats, yogurt, fruits, and vegetables. Research shows these foods are also well tolerated.

Foods to avoid giving your children include those that are high in fat, salt, or sugar (including juice and soft drinks).

MILK'S NOT ALWAYS GOOD FOR YOU

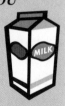

Between 80 and 100 percent of Asian, African American, and Native American adults lack the enzyme lactase, which is responsible for digesting lactose, a sugar found in milk. Lactose intolerance is the most common reason for chronic diarrhea.

Acute diarrhea usually has a bacterial or viral culprit. Gastroenteritis, mistakenly called the "stomach flu," is one of the most common infections that cause diarrhea. Gastroenteritis can be caused by many different viruses. Eating or drinking foods contaminated with bacteria can also cause diarrhea. Other causes of acute diarrhea are lactose intolerance, sweeteners such as sorbitol, over-the-counter antacids that contain magnesium, too much vitamin C, and some antibiotics.

If you have chronic, or long-term, diarrhea that comes on suddenly and stays for weeks, you may have a more serious condition such as irritable bowel syndrome or a severe food allergy.

Dehydration Dangers

With any kind of diarrhea, you lose a lot of fluids. One of the quickest ways you can end up going from the bathroom to the emergency room is to take a pass on liquids while you're sick. Fluids not only keep things running smoothly in your body, they also keep electrolyte levels balanced. Your body needs electrolytes such as sodium, potassium, and chloride salts for proper organ function. An electrolyte imbalance can cause your heart to beat irregularly, causing life-threatening problems. Though drinking or eating anything while you're running back and forth to the bathroom might sound grotesque, it will help make you more comfortable and get you back on your feet more quickly.

Though experts don't see eye to eye on what fluids are best during a bout with diarrhea, they do agree that getting two to three quarts of fluid per day is a good idea. When you drink, it's easier on the tummy if you sip instead of gulp (who has the energy for gulping?) and if you drink cool, not cold or hot, fluids. Here are some tried-and-true fluids that should get you through the rough days:

- Decaffeinated tea with a little sugar
- Sports drinks
- Commercially available electrolyte replacement drinks for children
- Bouillon
- Chicken broth
- Orange juice diluted with water

Though it may not sound logical to put diarrhea and food in the same sentence, if you don't put something in your body while you're enduring tummy troubles, you might end up getting sicker. There are loads of good things from the kitchen that will ease your grumbling stomach, and there are a few things that will prevent those diarrhea-causing agents from coming back for a return engagement.

DIETARY REMEDIES

Banana. Long known as a soother for tummy trouble, this potassium-rich fruit can restore nutrients and is easy to digest.

Blueberries. Blueberry root is a long-time folk remedy for diarrhea. In Sweden, doctors prescribe a soup made with dried blueberries for tummy problems. Blueberries are rich in anthocyanosides, which have antioxidant and antibacterial properties, as well as tannins, which combat diarrhea.

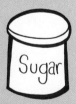

BABIES AND SENIORS NEED SPECIAL CARE

Because their blood volume is smaller than adults, babies can dehydrate in minutes and children can dehydrate in hours. And many elderly people have slower circulatory systems because of hardening of the arteries and can't afford to be low on fluids.

Call the doctor as soon as the baby has a loose stool. Though diarrhea may be hard to identify in a breast-fed baby, since their stools are already loose, err on the side of caution. The same is true for seniors; call the doctor as soon as a senior has a loose bowel movement. The diarrhea may be the side effect of a medication, such as an antibiotic, and it needs to be remedied without delay.

Call the doctor or go to the emergency room if your baby

- has fewer wet diapers
- has dark yellow urine
- has dry, pale skin that's cool to the touch
- has a dry tongue
- is not drooling
- is thirsty
- has a rapid pulse
- has sunken eyes
- cries but has no tears
- has a sunken soft spot

Cooked cereals. Starchy foods, such as precooked rice or tapioca cereals, can help ease your tummy. Prepare the cereal according to the directions on the box, making it as thick as you can stomach it. Just avoid adding too much sugar or salt, as these can aggravate diarrhea. It's probably a good idea to avoid oatmeal since it's high in fiber and your intestines can't tolerate the added bulk during a bout with diarrhea.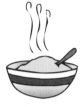

Orange peel. Orange peel tea is a folk remedy that is believed to aid in digestion. Place a chopped orange peel (preferably from an organic orange, as peels otherwise may contain pesticides and dyes) into a pot and cover with 1 pint boiling water. Let it stand until the water is cooled. You can sweeten it with sugar or honey.

Potatoes. This is another starchy food that can help restore nutrients and comfort your stomach. But eating french fries won't help. Fried foods tend to aggravate an aching tummy. Other root vegetables such as carrots (cooked, of course) are also easy on an upset stomach, and they are loaded with nutrients.

Rice. Cooked white rice is another starchy food that can be handled by someone recovering from diarrhea.

 Yogurt. Look for yogurt with live cultures. These "cultures" are friendly bacteria that can go in and line your intestines, providing you protection from the bad guys. If you've already got diarrhea, yogurt can help produce lactic acid in your intestines, which can kill off the nasty bacteria and get you feeling better, faster.

HERBAL REMEDIES

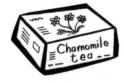

Chamomile tea. Chamomile is good for treating intestinal inflammation, and it has anti-spasmodic properties as well. You can brew yourself a cup of chamomile tea from packaged tea bags, or you can buy chamomile flowers and steep 1 teaspoon of them and 1 teaspoon of peppermint leaves in a cup of boiling water for 15 minutes. Drink 3 cups per day.

Fenugreek seeds. Science has given the nod to this folk remedy, but only for adults. Mix ½ teaspoon fenugreek seeds with water and drink up.

LIFESTYLE REMEDIES

To ease stomach pain, try resting with a heating pad on your belly.

Don't take antidiarrheal medications at the onset of your illness. Let your body rid itself of whatever's causing the problem first.

Wash your hands thoroughly before preparing food. You don't want to pass your illness to everyone in the household.

WHEN TO CALL THE DOCTOR

Most diarrhea has to run its course. However, diarrhea can be a sign of a more serious problem. If you're concerned, here are some symptoms that warrant a trip to the emergency room or a call to your family physician.

- Your diarrhea symptoms last more than 48 hours
- You have severe stomach cramps
- You have blood or pus in your stool
- You start showing any signs of severe dehydration such as dizziness when you stand, infrequent or reduced urination, dark yellow urine, increased thirst, and dry skin
- You have fever or chills

Diverticular Disease
PREVENTING PROBLEMS

Diverticulosis is a common condition in which small pouches, called diverticula, develop in the colon. No one is sure what causes diverticulosis, but it appears to occur when the inner lining of the large intestine is forced, under pressure, through weak spots in the outer layer of the colon. Eating a low-fiber diet and getting too little exercise have been shown to put you at greater risk. The diverticular pouches are present in about 50 percent of people older than age 60, and they themselves are not much of a problem. However, diverticula can become inflamed and cause a more serious illness called diverticulitis. What causes this inflammation isn't clear, but it may arise because waste material lodges in diverticula, leading to an infection. Diverticulitis can range from a mild infection to a severe one requiring hospitalization and even surgery.

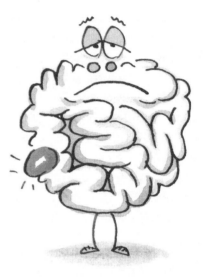

Symptoms
Diverticulosis usually causes no symptoms. Most people won't even know they have the condition unless it has shown up on a routine colonoscopy or developed into diverticulitis. But diverticulitis does have symptoms, including the following:
- Abdominal cramping, usually more severe on the lower-left side
- Abdominal pain triggered by touch
- Nausea
- Gas, belching, bloating
- Fever

> ### FACTS ABOUT DIVERTICULOSIS
> - Ten percent of people older than age 40 have diverticulosis
> - Fifty percent older than age 60 have diverticulosis
> - Almost everyone older than age 80 has diverticulosis
> - About 20 percent of those with diverticulosis will develop diverticulitis

- Diarrhea, constipation, or very thin stools
- Blood in the stools
- General feeling of being tired or run-down

If you have any of these symptoms, don't self-diagnose. Call a doctor or, if the symptoms are severe, go to the doctor's office or an emergency room. Diverticulitis that's untreated can lead to perforation of the colon; formation of an abscess; peritonitis, a life-threatening infection of the lining of the abdominal cavity; and other serious complications.

Diverticula don't go away. Once you have them, you're stuck with them. It's a good idea to adjust your lifestyle to avoid flare-ups, and for mild symptoms, there's some relief to be found at home.

Warning! The following tips are intended to help prevent the development of diverticulitis or to ease the mildest of symptoms. For all other symptoms, see a doctor!

DIETARY REMEDIES

Barley. This grain may act as a digestive anti-inflammatory. And it's a top source of fiber, which is critical to preventing diverticulitis. Add some to vegetable soup or stew. Or buy some barley flour, flakes, and grits.

 Brown rice. It's easy on the digestive system, rich in fiber, and may help calm inflammation and spasms in the colon. Eat it plain or as a dessert with a little honey, mix it with vegetables for a stir-fry, try it in the morning as a breakfast food instead of oatmeal, or boil it for a tea and drink the liquid in addition to eating the rice. There are no limits to the ways you can serve up brown rice.

FABULOUS FIBER (AKA BULK)

Fiber, also known as bulk, is essential to alleviating problems associated with diverticulitis and for having a healthy colon. Everyone needs 25 to 30 grams per day. The problem is, even though we think we're getting plenty of fiber, most of us are getting less than half of what we need.

Remember, though, to add fiber to your diet slowly at first. Try a little one day, skip a day, then add a little more the next. Too much too soon can lead to constipation. And be sure to drink plenty of water as you're adding fiber—at least 8 glasses per day. That helps push all that added fiber on through the digestive system. The faster it's gone, the less likely that it, or any other foods, will get lodged in one of the diverticula and cause a problem.

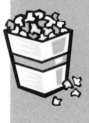
Fiber. Studies show that people who eat little fiber have the highest risk for diverticulitis, so ramping up your intake of roughage may be the most important dietary change you can make. Aim for 25 to 35 grams per day—that's about twice as much fiber as the typical American consumes. Adding fiber to your diet couldn't be simpler: Just be sure to eat plenty of fruits, vegetables, whole grains, and beans and other legumes. And be sure to increase your fluid intake when you increase your fiber intake to keep things moving along.

Papaya. This cool fruit may help soothe diverticulitis. Find a nice, ripe, red-tinged papaya, cut it open, toss away the seeds, and eat. Use it in a fruit salad—it's especially good with melons. Or put it in the blender and make juice. Add a little honey to sweeten it up, if necessary. Papaya has an unusual but enjoyable flavor.

Pear. Another fruit that may help soothe inflammation, pears don't need any doctoring to eat. Simply find one that's ripe and enjoy.

HERBAL REMEDIES

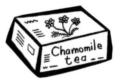

Chamomile. This herb acts as a mild anti-inflammatory and is often recommended for digestive problems. Drink it as a tea or use the essential oil, mixed with lavender oil, to massage the abdomen, especially over the lower-left area when it's tender. Add it to bathwater, too.

Dandelion. Doctors in Germany sometimes prescribe preparations containing extract of this backyard weed for various digestive problems.

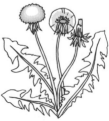

Dandelions can be prepared in a variety of ways:

- Steep fresh tender leaves for a tea.
- Scrub and steam the root and add it to steamed, mixed vegetables.
- Make a salad by tossing 2 cups mixed lettuce leaves with ½ cup dandelion greens. Add 3 tablespoons olive oil and the juice of ½ lemon. Toss well.

If you pick your own dandelion leaves, be sure to harvest them from an area that is free of pesticides and fertilizers and away from roadways.

Garlic. The "stinking rose" may help prevent infection. Eat 1 clove, three times per day. Chop it into a salad or add it to soup or stew. Pasta sauce, however, is not a good choice since tomato-based, spicy, and acidic foods can exacerbate symptoms.

Marigold. These have strong anti-inflammatory properties and may help heal digestive woes. Pick the flowers, dry them, and use in a tea. Or add fresh or dried petals to salads, vegetables, and brown rice. Be careful if you have pollen allergies.

Teas. Any of these may help relieve the symptoms of diverticulitis: fenugreek seed, marshmallow root, slippery-elm bark. If you don't have them on hand, try the health food store.

LIFESTYLE REMEDIES

Exercise. Everything in your body works better, including your digestive tract, when you exercise.

Skip the caffeine. It can cause digestive upset.

Don't rush things. It takes time for your bowels to move, so allow sufficient time.

Cut back on red meats. Diets rich in red meat have been linked to a high risk of diverticulitis.

WHEN TO CALL THE DOCTOR

- If you experience severe abdominal pain along with fever, swelling, chills, and nausea or vomiting, go to the emergency room immediately. Your symptoms can't wait for a call to the doctor.
- If there's blood in the stool or your stool is black and tarlike. You may be bleeding internally.
- If pain persists in spite of treatment

Dry Hair
RESTORING THE SHINE

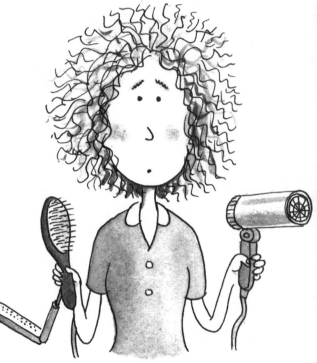

Oily hair is a drag, but dry hair is no picnic, either. Dry hair is dull hair, and it looks the same after you wash it as it did before. Everyone has bad hair days, but with dry hair you may have those days more often than not.

Along with dry hair, you may also have a dandruff problem. Although it's more often a condition associated with oily hair, people with dry hair get dandruff, too. Common dandruff is simply a layer of skin shedding from your scalp. When the skin cells get trapped on your scalp by your hair and clump together, you have dandruff. And dandruff can make your hair look dull.

Why Dry?

Dry hair can result from external factors, such as exposure to harsh chemicals such as hair dye or the chlorine in swimming pools, or from internal causes, such as an illness.

These are the primary external factors for those lackluster locks:

- Harsh shampoo
- Shampooing too often
- Hair dye
- Hair perms
- Chlorine in swimming pools and hot tubs
- Overuse of the blow-dryer or curling iron
- Too much exposure to sun and wind
- High mineral content in local water supplies

External factors are easy to remedy. You just need to be careful about how you treat your hair, cutting back on activities that cause it to become dry. Switch products. Wear a cap when swimming. Cover your head when you're outside in the sun for prolonged periods. And try the cures in this profile.

Internal factors, though, don't quite have such a quick fix. Internal factors that cause dry hair include

- Cancer treatment
- Certain medications
- A nutritional deficiency
- Prolonged illness

If your hair has the moisture content of the Mojave Desert and nothing short of dipping your mane in a bucket of oil seems to correct the problem, here are a few simple repairs that can make brittle hair supple and shiny again.

DIETARY REMEDIES

Nuts and seeds. Try snacking on some seeds and nuts. They contain essential fatty acids that can pop that sheen right back into your hair.

TOPICAL REMEDIES

Avocado and banana. Mash a little overripe banana and avocado together, spread in your hair, and leave it there as long as an hour. Then rinse with warm water.

Beer. After your shampoo, rinse your hair with a little beer. This can help restore shine.

Eggs. To clean hair and give it a super shine, whip an egg into lukewarm water (not too hot or you'll be dealing with a poached egg), then lather it into your hair. Rinse it out with lukewarm water or that egg will poach right on top of your head. To deep-treat damaged hair, give it a healthy sheen, and cure dryness

MINIMIZING THAT GRAY

Gray hair is often dry and dull looking. But two different rinses may help minimize that gray.

1. Use 1 tablespoon apple cider vinegar in 1 gallon water as an after-shampoo rinse.
2. Treat your hair to a sensational rinse that can cover gray or help it blend in. Follow these steps:

   • Combine 2 cups fresh sage and 1 cup fresh rosemary leaves in a pan.
   • Add just enough water to cover the herbs.
   • Bring the mixture to a boil, then simmer for 6 hours. Make sure the water doesn't boil away.
   • Remove from heat, and let mixture steep overnight.
   • Strain, then add enough water to make 5 cups.
   • Add 2 teaspoons apple cider vinegar, and store in a plastic bottle.

   To use, thoroughly rub mixture into scalp, then lightly rinse.

right down to the roots, use this preshampoo conditioning treatment: Mix together 3 eggs, 2 tablespoons olive oil or safflower oil, and 1 teaspoon vinegar. Apply it to your tresses, cover with a plastic cap, and leave it on for 30 minutes. Then shampoo as usual.

Mayonnaise. You'll need the full-fat kind, not a diet or low-fat version. Slather 1 tablespoon or so onto your hair, rub it in down to your scalp, then cover with a plastic cap and wait about 30 minutes. Rinse it out thoroughly or you'll be craving tuna salad the rest of the day.

Oil. Rub a little oil into your scalp. Olive oil works well, as does coconut oil. After you rub it on, cover your hair with a cap, leave it on overnight, then shampoo and rinse out the oil in the morning.

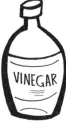

Vinegar. There are several ways you can help your dry hair with vinegar. Vinegar is a great conditioner and can improve cleanliness and shine. Just add 1 tablespoon vinegar to your hair as you rinse it. Keep a travel-size plastic bottle of vinegar in your shower for this purpose, and take one when you travel, too. Since dandruff can make your hair look dull, use vinegar to make dandruff disappear. Massage full-strength vinegar into your scalp several times per week before you shampoo. A brief soak in vinegar and water before you shampoo can help control dandruff as well as remove the dulling buildup from sprays, shampoos, and conditioners. Add ¼ cup apple cider vinegar to a small basin of water and drape your hair into it. As an alternative, you can put the concoction in a spray bottle and apply it to your hair. A conditioner that controls dandruff and gives your hair a healthy shine can be made by mixing 2 cups water and ½ cup vinegar. Apply the conditioner after rinsing out your shampoo, and let it stay on your hair for a few minutes before rinsing thoroughly with water. If you need a stronger treatment for dandruff control, use this same method, but keep the rinse on your hair for 1 hour, covered with a shower cap. Then rinse it out. This vinegar rinse will also help control frizziness in dry or damaged hair.

LIFESTYLE REMEDIES

Shampoo at least every three days with a gentle shampoo. This will stimulate the oil glands.

MORE DO'S & DON'TS

- Minimize your use of heated styling treatments, such as hot rollers, blow dryers, and curling irons. Hot rollers and hot combs are especially damaging because they stretch the hair while the heat shrinks it. If you use these styling methods every day, your hair is destined to be dry. When you do use them, make sure to keep them on a low setting and avoid pulling or stretching the hair.
- Don't go for 100 strokes when you brush your hair. Use a soft-bristled brush and be gentle and sparing. And never brush when the hair is wet.
- Don't use unnecessary chemicals, such as dyes. And if you use them, do so sparingly. Chemicals damage both scalp and hair.

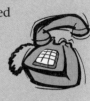

WHEN TO CALL THE DOCTOR

- If you've tried everything and nothing restores luster to your locks
- If you're experiencing these symptoms: hair loss, lethargy, sluggish thinking, weight gain, tingling or numbness in the hands, hypersensitivity to cold, dry skin, and constipation—along with dry hair. These symptoms could indicate a thyroid problem.
- If you're experiencing these symptoms: hair loss, weight loss, fatigue, vomiting, diarrhea, brownish skin, and mood swings—along with dry hair. These symptoms could indicate a problem with your adrenal glands.
- If you can't get dandruff to clear up or if the falling flakes don't look like normal, tiny white dandruffy specks
- If your scalp is inflamed or sore

Dry Mouth
TURNING ON THE TAP

Do loud mouths get dry mouths? Unfortunately, dry mouth isn't caused just by yapping too much or too loud, although you can run your throat and vocal chords ragged. Dry mouth, also known as xerostomia, is a condition in which saliva production shuts down.

When working at full capacity, saliva has many duties. This versatile fluid helps us talk, chew, and spit. It acts as a natural cavity fighter by washing away food particles and plaque, and it helps to digest food, works to buffer acids, and remineralizes those pearly whites. Saliva is vital in maintaining a healthy mouth, so when production decreases or stops, there is more than a dry mouth to pout about. Teeth and gums become more prone to decay and infection, and your taste buds might suffer, too.

What Causes Dry Mouth?

Dry mouth is caused by several factors, most commonly by the use of medications. Look on almost any label of nonprescription and prescription drugs, and you'll find that dry mouth is typically listed as a possible side effect. Some of the worst offenders are the drugs designed to dry out your mucous membranes, such as antihistamines and many allergy medications. Other drugs contributing to dryness are those used to treat high blood pressure, depression, and heart disease.

BLAME IT ON YOUR BIRTHDAY

Dry mouth is associated with aging. An estimated 25 to 50 percent of Americans older than 65 suffer from dry mouth.

Dehydration is an obvious cause of dry mouth. However, dehydration doesn't always arise from obvious reasons, i.e., not drinking eight glasses of H_2O a day. You can become dehydrated through fever, extensive exercise, vomiting, diarrhea, burns, and blood loss. Other causes of xerostomia are radiation therapy, menopause, surgical removal of the salivary glands, and cigarette smoking.

The primary symptom of xerostomia is, of course, a dry mouth. But this can be punctuated by myriad other conditions, including excessive thirst, a raw tongue, lip sores, difficulty swallowing, sore throat and hoarseness, bad breath, difficulty speaking, dry nasal passages, and dry lips.

But here's something to smile about: Most cases of dry mouth are easy to solve.

DIETARY REMEDIES

Celery sticks. Munching on water-logged snacks helps stimulate the saliva glands and adds moisture to your mouth. Should your sweet tooth strike, suck on sugar-free candies.

Stay away from sugar-filled treats since they promote decay in an already vulnerable mouth.

Liquids. If the salivary glands are down for the count, you'll need all the reinforcements you can muster to help get food down. Try to complement each dish with sauce, gravy, broth, butter, or yogurt. Another option is to stick to soft, liquidy foods, such as stews, soups, and noodle dishes.

Parsley. A dry mouth often brings out bad breath. This can ruin just about any social situation. Luckily, battling bad breath is easy. The restaurant may put parsley on your plate for decoration, but

MOUTHWATERING NEWS

The nervous system controls the secretion of saliva, both in volume and in the type of saliva secreted. A good way to get the nervous system stimulated and increase salivation is to visualize a luscious dessert, smell the aroma of a barbeque, or see a buffet overflowing with treats. On the less palatable side of salivation, the nervous system will increase saliva production if an irritating substance enters the mouth, such as a gnat.

NOT JUST FOR COLDS

Echinacea, an herb that's been touted as a remedy for colds and flu, also contains a saliva stimulant. Unfortunately, echinacea isn't famous for making a tasty tea, so try disguising the taste. Mix a dropperful of echinacea tincture into your favorite juice (several times per day if necessary). Or, if it's available, chew the root of the fresh plant. Just don't expect to find it delicious.

THE ORIGIN OF SALIVA

There are three major salivary glands in your mouth and throat. The largest is the parotid gland, with ducts located near the upper teeth. The submandibular gland has ducts under the tongue, and the sublingual gland has ducts on the floor of the mouth. This threesome is complemented by hundreds of tiny minor salivary glands in the lips, inner cheek, and lining of the mouth and throat.

it can serve a more useful purpose. This herb is a natural breath sweetener, and it provides ample amounts of vitamins A and C, calcium, and iron. So, chew on some.

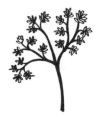

Sugar. Since dehydration is a major cause of dry mouth, it is vital to restore electrolytes to the body. This kitchen-made elixir works like a commercial sports drink but is much less expensive and doesn't require a trip to the grocery store. Mix 1 teaspoon salt, ½ teaspoon baking soda, and 1 tablespoon sugar into a cup of water. Mix in a dash of lemon, lime, or orange for added flavor. Drink 1 cup per day or more following heavy exercise, vomiting, or a bad case of diarrhea.

Water. To keep your system well-lubricated, it's recommended you down eight 8-ounce glasses of water each day. Cut back on other refreshments such as coffee, sugary sodas, and alcohol, all of which can exacerbate dry mouth. Accompany every meal with a glass of water.

HERBAL REMEDIES

Aniseed. Munching on aniseed can help combat the bad breath that accompanies dry mouth. In fact, many Indian restaurants have a bowl of anise and fennel (see "Fennel," next page) available to remove pungent food odors from your breath. Mix a few teaspoons of these seeds, place in a covered bowl, and keep on the table.

Cayenne pepper. A dry mouth can inhibit taste buds from distinguishing between sour, sweet, salty, and bitter flavors. Stimulate saliva production and bolster those buds by sprinkling red pepper (cayenne) on your food or mixing it into some tomato juice. Or, prepare an entire meal around red peppers. Go south of the border with spicy salsas, or make that all-American favorite, chili, and start drooling!

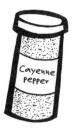

Fennel. Munching on fennel seeds mixed with aniseed (see previous page) can help combat bad breath that accompanies dry mouth. In addition, fennel seed can be combined with other herbs to make a mouthwash (see "Rosemary," below).

Rosemary. Store-bought mouthwash overflows with germ-killing alcohol, which is also a drying agent. Read labels and don't purchase any that contain alcohol. Better yet, make your own refreshing herbal mouthwash. Combine 1 teaspoon dried rosemary, 1 teaspoon dried mint, and 1 teaspoon aniseed with 2½ cups boiling water. Cover and steep for 15 to 20 minutes. Strain and refrigerate. Use as a gargle. The rosemary helps fight germs, while the mint and aniseed freshen breath.

LIFESTYLE REMEDIES

Close that trap. Sleeping with the mouth wide open invites a dry mouth in the morning. Make a conscious effort to breathe through your nose.

Breathe steam. It helps moisturize nasal passages and airways.

Practice good hygiene. Without saliva, the mouth and teeth are more susceptible to decay and infection. Brush and floss regularly. During the day, rinse the mouth out with water or a saltwater rinse.

Cut down on coffee and alcohol consumption. Both are diuretics and can leave your mouth feeling as dry as the Sahara.

WHEN TO CALL THE DOCTOR OR DENTIST

- If you suspect a medication is causing dry mouth. Your physician may have you try an alternative drug.
- If the condition lasts more than a week
- If you have sudden dental problems
- If taste is impaired

Dry Skin
REMOVING THE ROUGHNESS

You could sand a cabinet with your palm. Your legs look like you're molting. And you're afraid if you shake hands with your new boss, he'll think you're part alligator. If only you could shed your itchy, scaly, rough skin and get a new supple, soft covering every year. Unfortunately, people have to keep the skin they're in for a lifetime.

Millions of people cope with dry skin every year, helping to make the skin care business a billion-dollar industry. There are no magic ways to give you baby soft skin, but knowing why your skin gets dry and learning simple ways to hydrate it will help.

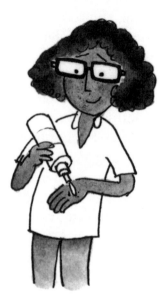

Super Skin

Your skin is much more than a covering for your bones. It is a shield, protecting you from disease-causing bacteria. The skin carries blood vessels and is a home for your nerve endings (that's why you're so ticklish). And the on/off nozzle for your sweat glands is found in the surface of your skin. It's also the part of your body that faces the harshest outside obstacles, so it gets a lot more wear and tear.

Dry skin is one of the more frustrating skin problems. Ideally, your skin gets saturated with moisture from your sweat glands and tissues that lie beneath the skin, and oil produced by the skin's sebaceous glands seals the deal by holding onto that moisture. But when your body has trouble holding in the water and oil it needs to keep skin moist, you end up with dry skin.

Why You're So Dry

There are lots of reasons why skin loses moisture. Sometimes you inherit the tendency to have parched skin—your skin may not be able to hold onto water very well or your sweat glands may not produce as much moisture as other people. And as you get older, your skin produces less oil, which means you can't retain water on your skin as you once could.

Besides genetics and getting older, there are environmental reasons skin gets so dry. These include:

- The air out there (or in there). The main reason you get scaly skin is low humidity. Though Old Man Winter is the one to blame for most climate-related dry skin problems, he's not the only culprit. Anywhere you encounter low humidity, you'll encounter dry skin. That includes heat or air conditioning, both of which can dry out your skin.
- You aren't Daffy. Water may roll off a duck's back, but human skin doesn't work that way. Too much water, especially from hot showers or baths, or from hot tubs, makes your skin less able to retain water because it removes oils that keep your skin moist.
- Cleaning up can leave you dry. Cleaning house with harsh products can cause you to develop alligator hands.

TOPICAL REMEDIES

Baking soda. Instead of using an abrasive dishwashing cleanser, try sprinkling baking soda in your dishwater. A baking soda sponge bath is a skin-friendly alternative to jumping in a hot shower. Use 4 tablespoons baking soda to 1 quart water. A baking soda soak is a folk remedy to relieve itching. Add 1 cup baking soda to a tub of hot water. Soak for 30 minutes and air dry.

Cornstarch. This can help ease itchy, dry skin. Sprinkle a handful in the bathtub and have a soak.

GETTING THE MOST FROM MOISTURIZERS

The shelves at your local drugstore are packed with lotions, cold creams, moisturizers, and oils. How can you tell what's best for your skin? It takes a little label reading and some background on how these products work. Just don't expect a miracle cure. Most products ease the symptoms of dry skin, such as itching, flaking, and tightness. But they can't get below the skin to treat the reasons behind dryness.

The American Academy of Dermatology suggests looking for products with urea, alpha hydroxy acids, lactic acid, or ammonium lactate. These reduce scaliness and help the skin to retain water, though some may irritate the skin. Talk to your doctor about which lotion is best for you. Petroleum jelly mixed with a little water is a top-notch skin protector.

Lotions have more water and less oil, while cold creams have more oil and less water. If your skin is very dry, choose an oilier moisturizer.

The more expensive moisturizers aren't necessarily better, either. *Consumer Reports* looked at more than 30 moisturizers and found that the cheapest (Vaseline Intensive Care Dry Skin Formula) was the overall best.

Oatmeal. Adding instant oatmeal to your bath will soothe your skin. The oats are packed with vitamin E, a nutrient vital to healthy skin. Oatmeal is also used as a folk remedy for treating dry, chapped hands. Rub your hands with wet oatmeal instead of soap. Dry your hands with a towel, then rub them with dry oatmeal.

Salt. Massage a handful of salt onto wet skin after a shower or bath. It will remove dry skin and make your skin smooth.

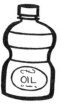

Vegetable oil. Coating yourself with vegetable oil may make you feel like a french fry, but your skin will love you. In fact, experts say that any oil, from vegetable to sunflower to peanut, offers relief from dry skin.

Vinegar. Try this folk remedy for chapped hands: Wash and dry hands thoroughly, then apply vinegar. Put on a pair of soft gloves and leave them on overnight.

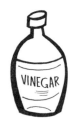

LIFESTYLE REMEDIES

Be cool. Take lukewarm or cool showers. Hot water draws out skin's valuable oils, which will dry out your skin.

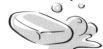

Be selective about soap. Pretty, perfume-laden soap may look and smell nice, but it can leave your skin screaming. Try soaps with fat or oil in them, such as Dove or Basis. Liquid soaps tend to be milder than bar soaps.

Douse while damp. Slathering lotion on damp skin is your best bet for retaining moisture. When you get out of the bath or shower, pat, don't rub, to get rid of just enough water so you don't leave a wet trail to the sink. Then spread on your lotion while you've still got droplets clinging to your skin. This will help seal in the moisture.

Wear vinyl gloves. Whenever you wash dishes, clean the bathroom, or dust the furniture, wear vinyl gloves to protect your hands from chapping, chaffing, and harsh chemicals.

MORE DO'S AND DON'TS

- Avoid alcohol. That means both the kind you drink and the kind you use to clean. Drinking alcohol can cause your body to soak up water from skin. Limit yourself to no more than 2 ounces per day to keep your skin healthy. Alcohol-based cleansing products (such as astringents) dry out your skin, too. It's best to skip them altogether.

- Watch the sun. You put your wet tennies outside to dry out. Well, just as the sun evaporates moisture from your water-soaked shoes, it evaporates moisture from your skin. Though a little bit of that evaporation is healthy (sweat evaporating keeps you cool when you exercise), too much can be a problem. So protect your skin by wearing sunscreen and moisturizing lotions if you spend lots of time in the sun.

- Rehydrate your skin with lotion after using any degreasers or solvents when painting around the house.

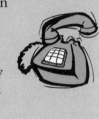

WHEN TO CALL THE DOCTOR
- If you develop a rash
- If you begin blistering
- If you develop thick, scaly patches on your skin

SEAL IT WITH GLYCERIN
Lotions containing glycerin and rosewater are still available at some pharmacies and are good for relieving dry skin. Glycerin is a humectant, which means it helps hold water in.

Eye Puffiness
REDUCING SWELLING

Do you wake up looking as though you cried all night? Are your eyes so swollen when you come home from work that your significant other thinks you spent the day at the pub instead? Swollen, red eyes can make life miserable, not to mention cause others to misinterpret your lifestyle. Using a little insight, however, can help determine the cause of marshmallow eyes. Two common reasons for eye puffiness are a diet dominated by salty foods and allergies or chronic sinusitis.

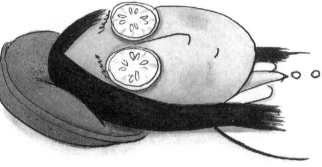

Oftentimes, what you can't see can bother you. Irritants and chemicals found in makeup, perfumes, and detergents can have inflammatory effects on eyes. And eyes definitely don't take kindly to today's computer-focused workplace; they rebel with redness.

Look at it this way: Puffy eyes are only a temporary problem for most people. Many cases can be cured by simple home remedies and/or by eliminating substances that may cause swelling.

DIETARY REMEDIES
Drinking water. Water is the saving grace when it comes to reducing eye puffiness. Be sure you drink at least eight 8-ounce glasses of water each day, and don't substitute sodas, coffees, or sugary drinks. When the body is dehydrated, it acts much like a camel, storing water for the long haul across the desert. Instead of a camel's hump, you'll develop water reserves around the eyeballs. By keeping yourself adequately hydrated, the body isn't put into survival mode and won't puff up in all the wrong places.

TOPICAL REMEDIES
Cold water. Eyes seem to puff up on workday mornings when you have 30 minutes to get ready. There's no time to luxuriate with tea bags and cucumber slices—but don't despair.

Cold water will work in a pinch. Rise, shine, and rinse your face with several splashes of cold water. This may be a rude awakening, but the coldness will constrict blood vessels and reduce swelling. Plus, it only takes ten seconds. Repeat throughout the day if possible. Just remember to wear water-proof eye makeup.

Cucumbers. From the vegetable bin comes the well-known cucumber remedy. Cucumbers aren't only deliciously cool and soothing to the touch, but their astringent properties cause blood vessels to constrict. Lean your head back, rest a slice on each closed eye, and relax for five to ten minutes while the cukes cure your puffiness.

Egg whites. Call this kitchen cure a soufflé for the face. Whip up 1 or 2 egg whites until stiff and apply with a brush or soft cloth underneath your eyes. The skin will feel tighter and look less like puff pastry.

Potato. The common potato also pampers puffy eyes. Tubers are tried and true in European folk medicine as a means to soothe painful joints, headaches, and other inflammatory conditions. Potato starch acts as an anti-inflammatory agent to ease irritated eyes. Start by pretending you're making hash browns. Peel one potato, wash and dry it. Grate the potato as fine as possible, then instead of frying it up with butter, place the pulp in a clean cloth and fold to make a poultice. Place the poultice on your eyelids for 15 minutes.

 Salt. Jumbo fries, pepperoni pizza, and other salt-infested foods can cause puffy eyes. However, salt by itself does the eyes good. Get rid of the puffy eye facade by mixing ½ teaspoon salt into 1 quart warm water. Dip cotton balls or facial pads into the solution, then lie down and apply pads to the eyelids. Rest in this position for at least ten minutes while keeping the pads in place. You'll arise with deflated eyes.

Spoons. Teaspoon-size spoons are just the right utensils for temporarily helping your eyes reduce to normal propor- tions. Place 4 (or 6) spoons in the refrigerator. When you need to deflate those eyeballs, lie down, close your eyes, and place one spoon (curved side down) on each eye. As the spoon warms, replace it with a cold one from the fridge.

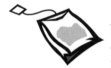

Tea. Green tea or black? Both work well to soothe puffy, irritated eyes. The difference? Not much. Caffeinated teas help constrict blood vessels and reduce swelling, while herbal teas (especially chamomile) contain anti-irritants that soothe redness and inflammation. Steep 2 bags of your choice of tea in hot water for three to five minutes. Let cool until the bags are comfortably warm to the touch. Lie down, close your eyes, and place a tea bag over each eye; then cover with a soft cloth. During hot months, put the cooked tea bags in the refrigerator and apply to eyes when needed for a refreshing, eye-opening experience.

LIFESTYLE REMEDIES

Give your eyes a break! For every hour you are on the computer, take a five- to ten-minute rest. Stare out the window, close your eyes and meditate, or stroll to the water cooler. While working on the computer, try to look away every few minutes.

Sleep with two pillows. These will keep your head elevated while sleeping so that fluid won't accu- mulate underneath the eyes.

Leave them alone. Don't rub your eyeballs in the morning. Avoid touching them during the day.
Go free. Use hypoallergenic soaps and fragrance- and color-free detergents.

MORE DO'S AND DON'TS

- Cut down on allergens. Allergy sufferers often emerge from bed with swollen eyes and faucet noses. If you're allergy prone, keep your bedroom free from dust, pollen, and animal dander. Remove dust-collecting objects, wash sheets in very hot water, cover the mattress and pillows with dust-mite protective coverings, and bar pets from the bed. During pollen season, wash your hair before hitting the pillow, and use air conditioning instead of opening the window.

- A light self-massage can help relieve puffy eyes. Close your eyes and gently press your ring finger underneath one eye, moving in an arc-shape from the inside corner to the outside corner. Massage 10 to 15 times. Then repeat on the other eye. This is great to do before jumping out of bed.

- Watch what you wear. Do your eyes puff up midday? It could be from your fancy fingernails or at your hairdo or face. Many fingernail 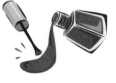 polishes, hair sprays, and makeups contain formaldehyde, which can cause eyes to swell. Luckily, new formaldehyde-free beauty products are hitting the shelves. Use the process of elimination, avoiding each product for a week or two, to find the culprit.

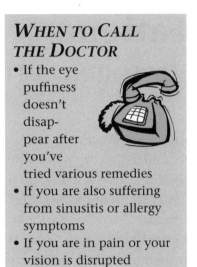

WHEN TO CALL THE DOCTOR

- If the eye puffiness doesn't disappear after you've tried various remedies
- If you are also suffering from sinusitis or allergy symptoms
- If you are in pain or your vision is disrupted

Fatigue
RESTORING VITALITY

Americans are all too familiar with being tired. Consider: Twenty percent of us today sleep fewer than six hours a night, up from 13 percent in 2001, according to the 2009 Sleep in America Poll conducted by The National Sleep Foundation. Furthermore, fewer Americans are getting the recommended eight hours or more of shut-eye per night—just 28 percent—compared to 38 percent eight years ago. Not getting enough sleep is sure to contribute to fatigue, but it also increases the risk for diabetes, obesity, and other health problems, as well as for dangerous drowsiness behind the wheel. And people who are sleep deprived are more than twice as likely to miss family events, leisure activities, or work functions due to sleepiness or a sleep problem, according to the study.

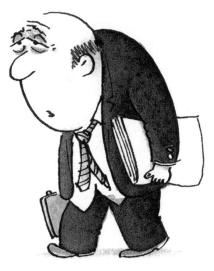

What Type of Tired Are You?
There are two types of fatigue: emotional and physical. Emotional fatigue is a tiredness of the mind. It happens when stress piles up, such as having to meet multiple deadlines at work or dealing with the death of a parent. Physical fatigue happens when you spend the day working in the garden and at the end of the day you can't even lift your little toe. Both types of tiredness can cause you to feel lethargic. And they both require rest and relaxation.

How do you know what type of tired you're experiencing? If you wake up tired in the morning but start feeling better as the day goes on, take a look at what's going on in your life emotionally. The key to your fatigue may be in your head. If the morning finds you energized and raring to go, but you start to lose your spark as the afternoon appears, you're probably dealing with a physical problem.

Reasons for emotional fatigue:

- Doing too much. You're a room mother, a Girl Scout leader, and a volunteer tutor, and now you've decided to take on the school's annual fund drive. And you wonder why you're wiped out?
- Doing too little. Sounds strange, but boredom makes you tired. Being motivated to accomplish goals adds a spark to your life. The secret is finding the right balance.
- Stressful situations. Major turmoil such as changing jobs or moving to a new city can make you feel exhausted.
- Mental maladies. People who are lonely or depressed are prone to tiredness.

Reasons for physical fatigue:

- Skipping needed nutrients. Low-calorie diets, fasting, or just missing meals because of meetings or too-busy schedules can wipe you out.
- Not sleeping enough. There's no perfect number of hours you should sleep. Different people have different sleep needs. But if you wake up feeling exhausted morning after morning, you might need to add more sleeping hours in your day.
- Getting no exercise. Exercise is essential to feeling better—physically and mentally.

UNCOVERING CHRONIC FATIGUE SYNDROME

Occasional fatigue is normal, ongoing fatigue is not. Chronic fatigue syndrome (CFS) has gotten a load of press lately, mostly because it is such a mystery. Unlike normal tiredness, chronic fatigue syndrome starts out feeling like the flu. Sufferers feel tired and generally yucky, and they have muscle and joint aches, sore throat, low-grade fever, and swollen lymph nodes. The problem is these symptoms don't go away after a few days or even a few weeks.

No one knows what causes CFS, and a doctor can't tell you for sure that's what's ailing you. The verdict of chronic fatigue syndrome is given after eliminating other conditions that may have the same symptoms.

The good news is that with increased numbers of CFS, doctors are finding out more keys to understanding and treating the disease. Though there is no cure, you can learn to deal with your symptoms and get on the road to feeling better. Your first destination if you think you have CFS is your doctor's office.

SAY SI TO SIESTAS

Many cultures have long known the benefits of grabbing an afternoon nap. The Amish are fond of saying that a half-hour nap in the afternoon is worth two hours of sleep at night. And scientific studies are confirming what the Amish have known all along. One study found that nodding off for as little as ten minutes can make you more alert and energized.

• Dodging drinks. Dehydration is an energy zapper. Drinking and eating go hand-in-hand in giving your body the fuel it needs to feel good.

Fatigue as a Symptom of Disease

Fatigue that is brought on by an unexpected loss of sleep or a stressful situation, like being a new parent, is usually easily remedied simply by taking good care of yourself. But ongoing fatigue can be the signal that something more serious is going on in your body. Ongoing fatigue can often be a symptom of

- anemia
- arthritis
- a slower-than-usual thyroid (hypothyroidism)
- an underlying sleep disorder
- cancer
- chronic fatigue syndrome
- diabetes
- heart disease

DIETARY REMEDIES

Coffee. Caffeine is a known pick-me-up. And the American Dietetic Association says there's no harm in drinking the stimulating stuff, as long as you do so in moderation. Studies confirm that caffeine does perk up the brain and get those mental faculties humming. But be careful—the ADA says a couple of cups per day should do you fine. More than that and you risk anxiety and insomnia.

Eggs. This is a folk remedy that is backed by sound nutrition. One of the most important ways you can

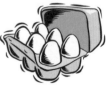

battle fatigue is to eat a well-balanced diet, and eggs are loaded with good things such as protein, iron, vitamin A, folate, riboflavin, and pantothenic acid. Eat one egg per day, however you like it, and you may be feeling better in no time.

Fluids. Drink plenty of water, juice, milk, or other beverages to keep yourself hydrated. Dehydration can contribute to fatigue.

Skim milk. Mixing a little protein with your carbohydrates can keep you energized. Eating only carbohydrates, such as a doughnut or a pancake slathered in syrup, can cause serotonin, a neurotransmitter, to build up in the brain, making you feel drowsy. Eating protein with your carbohydrates can block that sleepy feeling and leave you feeling energized. A good meal to start your day—cereal covered with a good dousing of skim milk.

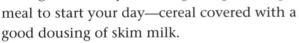

HERBAL REMEDIES

Ginseng. Ginseng is an age-old energy booster. This root has a sweet licorice taste and has been used for thousands of years to treat weakness and exhaustion. Be cautious: Don't take ginseng unless you are really fatigued. It can be too stimulating if you're feeling fine. In America you're probably wise to buy Asian ginseng. Another variety, Siberian ginseng, may not be as potent as the Asian variety. Both Asian and Siberian varieties of the herb have been labeled "adaptogens." Herbalists use this term to describe compounds that help you adapt to stresses in your environment. You can buy ginseng powder at a reputable herb shop. Take 2 grams of ginseng powder per

COMBING CENTURIES OF CAFFEINE

Caffeine is a mild stimulant and is found naturally in foods such as chocolate, coffee, and tea. It's been around for thousands of years and was once so valuable that coffee beans were used as currency in Africa. Many early physicians wanted caffeine banned from common use because they were afraid the stimulant would be too powerful for your average Joe. Around the 15th century, coffee finally made its debut in Europe, both pharmaceutically and in coffeehouses (the Starbucks of the Middle Ages). And coffee is now the number one source of caffeine in the United States.

**WHEN TO CALL
THE DOCTOR**
• When you
  have
  ongoing,
  unresolved
  fatigue that
  lifestyle
  changes—such as eating
  a balanced diet, getting
  more rest and exercise,
  and reducing stress—
  haven't helped improve.

day for a six-week stint. Then take at least a two-week break before using the energizing herb again.

LIFESTYLE REMEDIES

Take some time for yourself. Try taking a walk or simply sitting in the garden and meditating on your blessings. Play some soothing music. Focusing on what's important can restore your energy.

Get moving. Exercise at least 30 minutes on most days of the week. Walk up and down the stairs in your office building or take a dance class at your local gym. Exercise releases endorphins and other important chemicals in your brain that make you feel better and give you more strength mentally and physically to face anything that life throws at you.

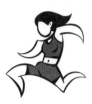

Take off a few pounds. If you're carrying around a spare tire or two, you can get tired faster. Taking off the weight slowly and nutritiously can restore your energy.

Nix the television. Instead of turning into a vegetable, choose something that will keep those brain cells stimulated, such as playing a game with your sweetie or picking up that novel you keep meaning to finish.

Fever
FEELING THE HEAT

Fever is a good thing. It's your body's attempt to kill off invading bacteria and other nasty organisms that can't survive the heat. The hypothalamus, which is the body's temperature regulator, senses the assault on the body and turns up the heat much the way you turn up the thermostat when you feel cold. It's a simple defense mechanism, and the sweat that comes with a fever is merely a way to cool down the body.

It used to be standard medical practice to reduce fever as quickly as possible. Not anymore. The value of fever is recognized, and since a fever will usually subside when the infection that's causing it runs its course, modern thinking is to ride out that fever, especially if it stays cooler than 102 degrees Fahrenheit in adults. However, if a fever is making you uncomfortable or interfering with your ability to eat, drink, or sleep, treat it. Your body needs adequate nutrition, hydration, and rest to fight the underlying cause of the fever.

Fever is a symptom, not an illness, and so there's no specific cure. But there are some fever-relievers in the home that may make you feel better for the duration. Be aware that the most significant side effect of fever is dehydration. Specific ways to deal with it can be found in the Dehydration profile, pages 111–116.

FASCINATING FACT
Shivering makes your body produce as much as five times more heat.

DIETARY REMEDIES

Apple water. It tastes good, relieves the miseries of fever, and keeps the body hydrated. To make it, peel, skin, core, and slice 3 sweet apples. Put them in a pan with 3¾ cups water. Bring to a boil, then simmer until the apples are barely mushy. Remove, strain without pressing apple puree into the liquid, and add 2 tablespoons honey. Drink and enjoy.

Blackberry vinegar. This is a great fever elixir, but it takes several days to prepare. Pour cider vinegar over a pound or two of blackberries, then cover the container and store it in a cool, dark place for three days. Strain for a day, since it takes time for all the liquid to drain from the berries, and collect the liquid in another container. Then add 2 cups sugar to each 2½ cups juice. Bring to a boil, then simmer for 5 minutes while you skim the scum off the top. Cool and store in an airtight jar in a cool place. Mix 1 teaspoonful with water to quench the thirst caused by a fever.

Cream of tartar. Try this fever tea. Combine 1½ teaspoons cream of tartar, ½ teaspoon lemon juice, 2½ cups warm water, and ½ teaspoon honey. Drink 4 to 6 ounces at a time.

Fruit juice. It will replace the fluids lost through sweating. Lemonade is a good choice, too.

 Lettuce. Pour a pint of boiling water over an entire head of lettuce and let it steep, covered, for 15 minutes. Strain, sweeten the liquid to taste, and drink. In addition to keeping you hydrated, this lettuce infusion may help you sleep better.

Pineapple. Fresh is best. It's one of nature's anti-inflammatory agents that can fight fever. Pineapple is also packed with juice that can prevent dehydration.

Popsicle. These can reduce the risk of dehydration. Fruit juice bars are good too. This can be an especially handy way to keep small children hydrated.

Raisins. Put ¾ cup chopped raisins in 7½ cups water. Bring to a boil, then simmer until the water has been reduced by one-third. Drink a little of this several times a day to keep yourself hydrated during a fever.

RAISINS

Tea. A cup of hot tea is just another way to take fluids, which are essential when you have the flu. Just be sure to choose decaffeinated varieties. Caffeine is a mild diuretic, which is counter-productive when you have the flu, and you certainly don't want to be awakened with the need to use the bathroom when you need your rest!

Water. Drink lots of it to prevent dehydration. Sponging the body with lukewarm water can relieve fever symptoms, but it's recommended that you use fever-reducing medication first to reduce the possibility of chills and shivering. Do not use cold water or ice on the body.

HERBAL REMEDIES

Basil. Mix 1 teaspoon basil with ¼ teaspoon black pepper. Steep in 1 cup hot water to make a tea. Add 1 teaspoon honey. Drink two to three times per day.

Oregano. A tea made from a mixture of some spice-rack staples can help reduce fever. Steep 1 teaspoon each of oregano and marjoram in 1 pint of boiling water for 30 minutes. Strain, and

WHEN TO CALL THE DOCTOR

- In infants younger than 3 months, 100 degrees Fahrenheit or above
- Infants 3 to 6 months, 101 degrees Fahrenheit or above
- In children and adults younger than 60, 104 degrees Fahrenheit
- In adults older than 60, 102 degrees Fahrenheit
- In adults and children, 101 degrees Fahrenheit for more than three days
- In children, if febrile seizures develop
- If pain, diarrhea, swollen joints, rash, or stiff neck occur with fever

FASCINATING FACT

You may call that unsightly sore on your lip a fever blister, but it's not caused by a fever. These painful blisters are actually caused by the herpes virus. For more information, see page 91.

drink warm a couple times per day. Refrigerate unused portion until needed, then gently warm.

LIFESTYLE REMEDIES

Skip the alcohol and caffeine.
They're diuretics, and you don't need to lose more fluid.
If you don't feel like eating, don't.
Just make sure you get sufficient

fluids. Do reintroduce yourself to foods gradually, though, if you haven't been eating very much.

MORE DO'S & DON'TS

- Do not sponge alcohol on the body to reduce fever. It can cause chills and increased fever.
- Use analgesics if necessary. Acetaminophen will reduce a fever, as will aspirin. However, NEVER give aspirin to children younger than 18 without first consulting the doctor. The result can be Reye's syndrome, a potentially fatal disease.
- Use only light clothing and blankets. Heavy clothing and blankets will make the fever go higher.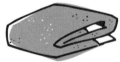

FEBRILE SEIZURES

They look frightening, especially when you see them happening to your child. But as bad as they look, febrile, or fever, seizures are not usually harmful and rarely cause permanent damage. The seizures most typically happen in children between the ages of six months and five years when body temperature rises quickly.

Symptoms include:

- jerking arms or legs
- fixed stare or eyes rolling back
- drooling
- heavy breathing
- blue-tinged skin, especially on the face

Febrile seizures normally last only a few minutes and rarely cause permanent damage. Here's what to do if your child experiences one:

- Lay him on a flat surface on his side or stomach.
- Turn his head to the side to keep him from swallowing vomit and so that saliva doesn't choke him.
- Remove clothes, sponge the body with lukewarm water to reduce temperature. Do not use cold water; it can cause a chill.
- If the seizure lasts more than a few minutes, seek emergency help immediately. For a mild and short seizure, call the doctor.

HYPOTHERMIA

Just as the body can heat up too much, it can cool down too much too. This is called hypothermia, and it develops when the body's temperature drops below 95 degrees Fahrenheit. It's most common in infants, whose small bodies aren't large enough to generate heat, and in seniors who may experience circulatory problems. Those who are exposed to prolonged cold conditions may experience hypothermia, as may those who take a plunge into chilly water for a nice swim.

Here's what to look for if you suspect hypothermia:

- confusion
- slurred speech
- irrational behavior
- lack of coordination
- rigidity of the body
- loss of consciousness
- loss of heartbeat

To treat hypothermia immediately, begin these warming steps:

- Get the person into a warm environment
- Wrap in dry, unheated blankets
- Then call 9-1-1.

Fibrocystic Breast Disease
DECREASING DISCOMFORT

Although the term fibrocystic breast disease may sound ominous, it actually describes a benign condition of the breasts that more than 60 percent of all women experience. If your breasts feel lumpy and you have intermittent breast discomfort, such as tenderness, swelling, and pain, you may have fibrocystic breast disease.

How can you tell? Symptoms include a dense, irregular, and bumpy consistency of the breast tissue. During a self-exam, you may feel a thick area of irregularly shaped tissue with a lumpy or ridgelike surface, or you may encounter a beadlike texture to your breast tissue. Fibrocystic breasts typically become swollen, tender, heavy, and lumpier a week or two before the menstrual period. You also may experience changes in nipple sensation, and the nipples may itch.

Symptoms can range from mild to severe, and they usually improve after menstruation. Some women, however, have persistent rather than intermittent symptoms. The condition tends to subside with menopause.

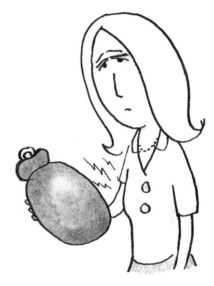

What's Behind the Pain...and What's Not

No one understands the causes of this condition, but some researchers believe that breast lumps are inherited. What we do know is that the condition is related to how the breast responds to hormonal changes during the monthly cycle. Hormonal stimulation causes milk glands and ducts to swell and the breast to retain water. The condition is more common in women aged 30 to 50, most likely because of years of repeated hormonal stimulation, which can harden lumps.

What's usually not behind the pain is breast cancer. Fibrocystic conditions do not increase breast cancer risk. Unlike the lumps associated with fibrocystic breast disease, which are tender and move freely, cancerous lumps most often are not tender and don't move freely.

If you think you have fibrocystic breast disease, be sure to check it out with your physician, who should always examine any lump(s) in the breast. You'll be pleased to discover that breast tenderness and other symptoms can usually be managed through diet.

DIETARY REMEDIES

Fish. The best fish for female health include those high in the omega-3 fatty acids such as salmon, trout, and mackerel. These fish are also high in iodine, a deficiency of which may be a factor in the development of breast lumps. Eating moderate amounts of fish may help prevent lumps.

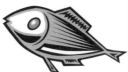

Kelp. Kelp and other sea vegetables, such as nori and dulse, are good sources of iodine. Studies suggest that an iodine deficiency may predispose women to having breast lumps. You can find these vegetables in some food markets, and kelp and dulse are also available in powdered form and can be used in cooking as a salt substitute.

Meats. Cut back on meat consumption. Before heading to the butcher's block, cows, chicken, and other livestock are often pumped full of hormones. Your body doesn't need the additional influx, especially during the hormone high time of your period. If meat needs to be on the menu, purchase hormone-free meats and poultry at a health food store.

THE BREAST SELF-EXAM

Only by getting to know your breasts through regular monthly breast self-exams will you be able to learn what's normal for you and what's not. Familiarity will allow you to discover a new lump or suspicious area and get it checked out with your doctor.

The best time in your cycle to do a breast exam is one week after your period. (Try marking your calendar or programming your e-mail to send you a message each month.) The exam is best performed lying down, not standing up.

Here's how:

- Use the opposite hand for the opposite breast; i.e., left hand for the right breast.
- Press firmly with your fingers and move the fingers in a circle covering the entire breast and the armpit.
- Check the other breast in the same manner.
- After your shower, check your breasts in a mirror for any dimpling, discharge, or other changes.
- Immediately report any lumps, knots, or changes to your doctor.

Salt. Two weeks before your period, hide the saltshaker. During the menstrual cycle, women tend to retain water, which in turn causes their breasts to feel heavy and become sensitive. Salt only increases this uncomfortable bloating. Be aware of the hidden salts in processed foods, too, and save that pizza order until after your period.

Vegetables. Diuretics help flush excess fluids from the body and reduce breast swelling. Unfortunately, many store-bought diuretics can also deplete your potassium reserves, unbalance your electrolyte count, and cause your blood sugar to rise. Turn to natural diuretics instead. Parsley, cucumbers, and cabbage are healthy for you and will keep you naturally flushed.

Vitamin A/Beta-carotene. Some studies have shown that vitamin A can reduce breast pain in women with moderate to severe symptoms. There is a risk to taking high doses of vitamin A, how- ever, because it can be toxic. It's safer to eat a diet high in beta-carotene, the precursor to vitamin A, with yellow, orange, red, and dark green vegetables and fruits.

Whole-grain foods. Increasing your intake of fiber may help control the hormonal fluctuations behind fibrocystic breast disease. Eat whole-wheat bread, brown rice, beans, and fruits.

TOPICAL REMEDIES

Hot compresses. Less shocking than ice packs, but equally soothing to swollen breasts, is the hot compress. Run hot water over face towels and place them on your chest for a few minutes. Rewarm when necessary. A heating pad will hold the heat longer, as will a homemade rice bag. To construct a rice bag, fill a clean, thick sock with a cup of rice, close the opening with a knot, and place in the microwave for 30 seconds or so. (Watch it carefully, since you don't want popped rice!) Remove, test the temperature, and place on your breasts.

Ice compresses. Ice packs may be a bit of a shock to delicate breasts. However, a cold compress can give breasts some relief from tenderness and inflammation. Fill a plastic, reclosable bag with crushed ice or use a bag of frozen peas and wrap in a towel. Lie down and place on the sore breast(s) for ten minutes.

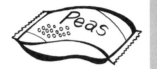

Note: Some women find alternating heat and cold, applying heat first for 30 minutes then cold for 10 minutes, helps minimize pain.

LIFESTYLE REMEDIES

Don't go braless. A well-fitting, supportive bra helps ease breast tenderness by immobilizing the breasts and eliminating the feeling of heaviness. If your breasts swell before your period, don't squeeze into your regular size. Buy the next size up.

Don't smoke.

Exercise regularly, eat a low-fat diet, and maintain an ideal weight. Body fat is the producer and storehouse of estrogen, the reproductive hormone often partially responsible for changes in the breasts. Being excessively overweight can predispose you to breast discomfort.

Don't use products made with ginseng. These can have steroidal effects similar to estrogen.

WHEN TO CALL THE DOCTOR

- Anytime you detect a new lump in your breast. A physician can determine if the lump is benign.
- If an existing lump increases in size or doesn't go away with menstruation
- If you feel a distinct lump, rather than a lumpy area
- If you think your birth control pills or hormone replacement therapies are aggravating your condition. Your doctor can recommend alternatives if these are part of your problem.
- If you experience a change in the size of one breast that's not related to your menstrual period or if your breast doesn't return to normal after menstruation

Flatulence
TAKING A PASS ON GAS

Who is the most glamorous person you know? Well, that person's not exempt from this particular problem. No one is. And it happens at the most awkward times, doesn't it? You feel that rumble way down deep in your belly, and it's traveling even lower. In the middle of very polite—and very quiet—company it gurgles inside, and you glance at the person next to you so no one will know that the undertone of the impending blast belongs to you.

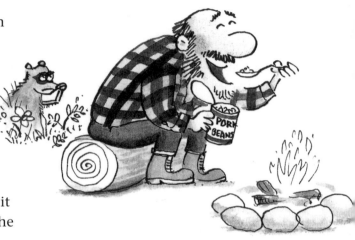

Well, gas happens. Called flatus, or flatulence when it finally does escape, it's normal. Its beginnings are in the foods we eat. We eat, therefore we pass gas. Why? Our stomach acids are breaking down last night's pasta primavera into elements that will either be absorbed into the body or eliminated. And that breakdown causes...you guessed it: Gas!

Bodily gas originates in the stomach and travels down to the intestines (unless it comes back up as a belch, see page 52). Its construction is pretty simple: carbon dioxide, hydrogen, nitrogen, and methane. Well, those gases make up about 99 percent of the gas we pass. The other 1 percent is divided among as many as 250 different gases, all of which occur naturally when carbohydrates are broken down. If you swallow air, you add oxygen to the mix.

Here are some other interesting flatus facts:

- Normal flatus production is 1 to 4 pints each day.
- There are at least 400 different kinds of bacteria living in your colon, waiting to mix and mingle with your food and give you gas.
- We pass gas, on average, 14 to 23 times each day.

Not all flatulence has an unpleasant odor, but some eye-watering "squeakers" can be enough to make you haul out the old gas mask. As bacteria in the gut munches on certain foods, it produces distinctly stinky gases.

Who's Prone

There are a few factors that make you more prone to passing gas. See if you're on the list:

- Anyone who dines regularly from the flatulogenic food list. See "Flatulogenic Foods," page 182.
- Those with certain stomach intestinal ailments, such as lactose intolerance or irritable bowel syndrome.
- Air-swallowers (See Belching, page 52)
- Those with gassy relatives. The tendency can be inherited.
- Anyone with food allergies that manifest in flatus after certain foods are eaten.

Gas is a side effect or symptom, not an illness in itself. And it's a symptom that can be treated several different ways with things you find in the kitchen.

DIETARY REMEDIES

Beano. Keep it sitting right next to that bag of dry beans to remind you it's a gas-busting enzyme that breaks down hard-to-digest disaccharides, thereby avoiding the formation of gas. Use this product as you eat the gassy foods, not afterward. It's available at groceries and pharmacies.

Caraway crackers. Caraway seeds and their oils are carminatives (they get rid of gas), but who wants to eat just the seeds? Caraway seed crackers and breads with caraway seeds are a tasty way to make your system gas-unfriendly.

SUGAR-FREE MISERY

Sorbitol, an artificial sweetener made of sugar alcohol that's used in many diet drinks and products, is often difficult to digest. Even a small amount, 10 grams, can cause bloating and gas. Double that and you may have cramping or diarrhea.

How do you know if you have sorbitol intolerance? That's easy. In mild cases, symptoms (normally gas) start 30 to 90 minutes after ingestion and go away after several hours. When diarrhea is present, it may take as long as 24 hours for sorbitol to clear the system. If symptoms last longer, call the doctor and explain that you've eaten something with sorbitol.

So, if you get gassy after you've consumed a sugar-free food or beverage, check the ingredients list. If sorbitol's there, chances are you can't handle it. And neither can your friends!

FLATULOGENIC FOODS

If you're plagued by gas, here are some foods that are definitely on the top of the flatus-maker list:

Beer
Bran
Broccoli
Brussels sprouts
Cabbage
Carbonated drinks
Cauliflower
Corn
Legumes (beans, lentils, dried peas)
Milk
Onions
Rutabaga

These are also gas-making culprits:

Apples
Apricots
Bananas
Carrots
Celery
Citrus fruits
Coffee
Cucumbers
Eggplant
Lettuce
Melon
Potatoes
Prunes
Radishes
Raisins
Soybeans
Spinach
Strawberries
Wheat products

Citrus fruits. Vitamin C in tablet form may cause gas, especially amounts in excess of 500 milligrams. So, reduce the dosage and replace the C with high-in-C fruits. Also try potatoes and sweet peppers, which are high in vitamin C.

Minimize milk consumption. Some people don't have enough of the enzyme lactase in their gut to digest lactose, the sugar in milk. If you are lactose intolerant, replace the milk in your diet with calcium-fortified orange juice or with calcium-fortified soy milk. Or try lactose-reduced milk, which is available at your grocer.

Pumpkin. It soothes the tummy, and best of all, it cuts down on flatulence. Try some baked, steamed, or broiled. Or make yourself a simple pumpkin soup.

Well-cooked beans. Beans that are undercooked are more likely to cause gas than beans that are well-cooked. To ensure that your beans are cooked thoroughly, pull out the pressure cooker and follow the manufacturer's advice for cooking beans. Or, cook them up to pressure for 30 minutes at 15 pounds per square inch on the gauge.

Yogurt with acidophilus. It alleviates digestive woes, including gas. But the yogurt must have live acidophilus, a bacteria that helps with digestion.

HERBAL REMEDIES

Cardamom seeds. These speed digestion. Add them to sautéed vegetables or to rice or lentils before cooking. You can also chew whole pods or steep pods in boiling water for several minutes to make a tea.

Cloves. They pep up digestion and are said to eliminate gas. Add 2 to 3 whole cloves to rice before cooking. Sprinkle on apples and pears when baking. Or steep 2 to 3 whole cloves in a cup of boiling water for ten minutes, sweeten to taste, and drink.

Coriander. This may help in the downward movement of foods being digested and can ease cramps, hiccups, bloating, and flatulence. Crush the seeds into powder and add to foods such as vegetable stir-fry. Its flavor really enhances curry and Middle Eastern dishes, too.

Fennel seeds. It's an acquired taste, but it may be one well worth acquiring if you're plagued by gas. Fennel's digestive powers are so good that in India fennel is customarily eaten after a meal to help digestion and freshen the breath. For gas, drink it as a tea by steeping ½ teaspoon seeds in 1 cup boiling water for ten minutes. Or, sprinkle them over those gassy vegetables during cooking or add to stir-fries. If you've acquired the taste, fennel also works well cooked into figs, apples, pears, and plums.

 Lemon. Stir 1 teaspoon lemon juice and ½ teaspoon baking soda into 1 cup cool water. Drink after meals.

Massage herbs. Add any of these to massage oil and rub over the abdomen to relieve gas: cardamom, clove, cinnamon, fennel, ginger. Warmed olive and sesame oils are wonderful for massages.

Rosemary. If you're eating a gassy food, sprinkle on a little rosemary to cut down the effect. You can do the same with sage and thyme, too.

Tea herbs. Steep and drink a tea made from any of these: aniseed, basil leaves, chamomile, cinnamon,

---

THINKING ABOUT GIVING THOSE BEANS THE BOOT?

Don't do it! Beans are loaded with cholesterol-lowering fiber and bone-saving calcium, and they have a hand in protecting against colon cancer and heart disease. So instead of bagging the beans, find out which ones cause you the most trouble and boot those out of your diet. Pintos, black beans, and Great Northerns are generally the biggest gas-makers. What's gassy for some, however, may not be gassy for others. It's all a matter of how your body digests them. Also see "De-Gas Those Beautiful Beans," page 184, for a great way to have your favorite beans without repercussions.

FASCINATING FACT

Flatus we expel is not too different from the air we breathe. Each time we suck in a lungful of air, we're getting:
Oxygen: 21%
Nitrogen: 78%
Hydrogen: less than 1%

DE-GAS THOSE BEAUTIFUL BEANS

If you love them but they don't love you back, there's a simple solution to eliminate most of the gas-causing effects.

1. Soak beans in water overnight.
2. Replace the water with fresh water and cook the beans for 30 minutes. Drain the water again.
3. Add fresh water and cook for another 30 minutes. Drain the water one more time.
4. Add fresh water and cook until done.

If you like the flavor of onion in those beans, skip the fresh onions. They share their gassy juices with everything that's in the bean pot. Instead, opt for dehydrated onions that will absorb the liquid already there instead of adding to it.

cloves, ginger, peppermint, sage. Steep about ½ teaspoon in 1 cup boiling water, then add honey or lemon to taste. Drink one to three times each day.

Turmeric. This may stop a gas problem altogether. Turmeric is one of the many flavorful and curative spices found in curry powder. You can add turmeric itself to rice or season a bland dish with curry powder, which contains turmeric. However you use it, it helps alleviate gas.

TOPICAL REMEDIES

Heating pad. The warmth of a heating pad placed on your abdomen can help alleviate discomfort.

Pressure. Apply pressure to your abdomen or lie facedown on the floor with a pillow bunched up under your abdomen to help relieve discomfort from gassiness.

Rock and roll. Sit on the floor with your knees drawn up to your chest and your arms wrapped around your legs, then rock back forth. The pressure and movement may provide relief.

LIFESTYLE REMEDIES

Cut back on carbonated beverages.

Don't sip drinks through a straw. You'll suck in air, which causes gas.

Don't stuff yourself when you eat. The more food in the gut, the more gas buildup.

Eat more slowly—you'll swallow less air.

Exercise. It stimulates digestion and the expulsion of gas. Do not exercise within two hours of eating, though. This can disrupt the normal digestive processes. A nice leisurely walk right after a meal is good, though.

Make a list. Write down the foods you eat. Include such information as the type of food, when you ate it, and how much you ate. Do you get gassy after gulping down cola? Or maybe it happens after eating ice cream? (See "Lactose Intolerance," page 289.) The truth about most gas is that you're likely causing it. Keeping a food diary is one of the easiest ways to pinpoint the cause.

Reduce the amount of fermented foods you eat. Cut back on cheese, soy sauce, and alcohol.

Stay calm. The digestive system is sensitive to emotional upset, stress, anxiety, and other strong emotions. When you're under stress, abdominal muscles tighten, causing painful spasms. This leads to gas, as well as swallowing air that can cause gas. (See "Belching," page 52.)

Try cutting back some on fiber, especially from legumes. Fiber is good for you, but increasing fiber intake too quickly can cause gas.

Wear loose clothing. Tight-fitting pants can compress the abdomen and cause pain.

MORE DO'S & DON'TS

- Try acupressure. Sit down and take off your shoes. Apply pressure to the sole of each foot, halfway above midline and below the ball, right in the middle, for about one minute. This is the stomach point in acupressure.
- Try over-the-counter aids. Activated charcoal products can help relieve gas. So do antigas medications. Check with your pharmacist to make sure they don't interact with medications you are already taking. If you have a condition in which salt intake can be detrimental, check with your doctor about taking any over-the-counter gas reliever.

WHEN TO CALL THE DOCTOR

- If you're experiencing sharp pain that starts near the naval and moves to the lower right side of the abdomen. Actually, call 9-1-1 for this one. It could be appendicitis.
- If you're experiencing pain in the upper right side of your abdomen
- If bloating and unexplained gas continues for more than three days
- If you're losing weight in addition to being unusually gassy
- If bowel movements smell worse than usual

Flu (Influenza)
SURVIVING THE SIEGE

The flu is a viral infection that strikes the entire body with a vengeance. Unlike the common cold, which causes a stuffy nose, sore throat, and sneezing, flu misery starts suddenly with chills and fever and spirals into more unpleasant symptoms that will take you out of commission. Flu's arsenal includes sore throat, dry cough, stuffy or runny nose, headache, nausea, vomiting, severe muscle aches and pains, weakness, backache, and loss of appetite. Some people even experience pain and stiffness in the joints.

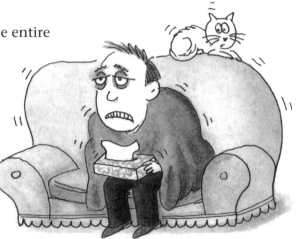

The worst of your symptoms will last about three to five days, but others, such as cough and fatigue, can linger for weeks. And a bout with the flu can deliver a double whammy if you develop a secondary infection, such as an ear or sinus infection or bronchitis. Even pneumonia can be a complication—and a potentially serious one—of influenza.

Flu viruses strike like clockwork in the United States. Every year they begin to show up in October and exit in April—although the 2009 outbreak of a new form of swine flu began in March–April, when flu is normal waning. As of June 2009, 21,940 cases had been reported worldwide, including 125 deaths. Peak flu season is typically December and January.

TAKE FLU SERIOUSLY
In the average year, influenza is associated with more than 36,000 deaths and 200,000 hospitalizations nationwide.

Flu is a highly contagious illness, spread by droplets from the respiratory tract of an infected person. These can be airborne, such as those released after a person coughs or sneezes, or they can be transferred via an infected person's hands.

Taking a yearly flu shot can help you ward off infection, and these are particularly recommended for senior citizens, people with compromised immune systems, or people with asthma. They won't give you 100 percent protection, but they will significantly increase your chances of avoiding it.

If you do get the flu, there are home remedies to help ease your suffering.

DIETARY REMEDIES

Broth. Canned broth, whether it's beef, chicken, or vegetable, will keep you hydrated and help liquefy any mucous secretions. Broth is easy to keep down, even when you have no appetite, and will provide at least some nutrients.

Honey. A hacking cough can keep you and every other household member up all night. Keep the peace with honey. Honey has long been used in traditional Chinese medicine for coughs. It's a simple enough recipe: Mix 1 tablespoon honey into 1 cup hot water, stir well, and enjoy. Honey acts as a natural expectorant, promoting the flow of mucus. Squeeze some lemon in if you want a little tartness.

Juice. Any flavor or kind will do. Just drink lots of juice both to keep yourself hydrated and to give yourself some extra vitamins.

Lemon. The lovely lemon may cause a puckered face if eaten raw, but in a hot beverage, lemons

MYTHS ABOUT THE DREADED FLU

Myth #1: The 24-hour flu.
Fact: There is no such thing as a 24-hour flu, although we wish it were so. The sudden onslaught of vomiting, diarrhea, and a general feeling of malaise that is intense for a few hours, but subsides after 24 hours, is indeed caused by a viral agent, but not the one that causes influenza. The correct term should be "the 24-hour attack of gastroenteritis," which is an infection that affects the gastrointestinal tract.
Myth #2: Going outside without a hat or catching a chill causes the flu.
Fact: Venturing outside ill-prepared for the elements may not be the brightest idea, but it doesn't directly cause the flu. Several scientific studies have shown that people exposed to cold temperatures for several hours fare no worse than those kept toasty warm. This myth grows from the observation that a severe chill is one of the first flu symptoms. Thus, people conclude that being chilled leads to the flu.

ALPHABET SOUP

Do you know your As, Bs, and Cs? These are the three strains of the flu virus:

Influenza A and B:
- Most responsible for illness
- Occur every winter
- Are the strains associated with hospitalization and deaths

Influenza C:
- Causes mild respiratory illness
- Doesn't strike in epidemic proportion
- Doesn't have a major health impact

will have you smiling. Hot lemonade has been used as a flu remedy since Roman times and is still highly regarded in the folk traditions of New England. Lemons, being highly acidic, help make mucous membranes distasteful to bacteria and viruses. Lemon oil, which gives the juice its fragrance, is like a wonder drug containing antibacterial, antiviral, antifungal, and anti-inflammatory constituents. The oil also acts as an expectorant. To make this flu-fighting fruit drink, place 1 chopped lemon—skin, pulp, and all—into 1 cup boiling water. While the lemon steeps for 5 minutes, inhale the steam. Strain, add honey (to taste), and enjoy. Drink hot lemonade three to four times per day throughout your illness.

Pepper. Pepper is an irritant, yet this annoying characteristic is a plus for those suffering from coughs with thick mucus. The irritating property of pepper stimulates circulation and the flow of mucus. Place 1 teaspoon black pepper into a cup and sweeten things up with the addition of 1 tablespoon honey. Fill with boiling water, let steep for 10 to 15 minutes, stir, and sip.

HERBAL REMEDIES

Lemon balm. For adults who can't catch their zzz's while coping with the flu, lemon balm acts as a mild sedative. It also contains antiviral compounds to help disinfect mucous membranes. To make this relaxing potion, place 1 teaspoon dried lemon balm in 1 cup boiling water. Cover and let steep for ten minutes. Strain, sweeten with honey (to taste), and drink as many as 4 cups per day. (Note: Lemon balm is also known as balm mint, bee balm, blue balm, garden balm, Melissa, and sweet balm.)

Mustard. This ancient remedy for the flu, chest colds, and bronchitis dates back to the ancient Romans, who early on understood the healing properties of mustard. Mustard is loaded with antimicrobial and anti-inflammatory properties, many of which can be inhaled through the vapors. Impress Grandma by making a mustard plaster with 1 tablespoon dry mustard and 2 to 4 tablespoons flour. Mix both with 1 egg white (optional) and warm water to form a paste. Next, find a clean handkerchief or square of muslin large enough to cover the upper chest. Smear the cloth the same way you'd smear mustard on a sandwich, then plop another cloth over it. Dab olive oil on the patient's skin and apply the mustard plaster to the upper chest. Check yourself or the patient every few minutes since mustard plaster can burn. Remove after a few minutes. Wash off any traces of mustard from the skin.

Peppermint. Running a fever of 102 degrees to 104 degrees Fahrenheit is common with the flu. A way to cool your hot head, via sweating, is with a cup of peppermint tea. As an added bonus, peppermint contains menthol, which works as a decongestant to help unstuff sinuses. And peppermint has antispasmodic properties to help that hack. To make this fever fighter, place ½ ounce peppermint leaves in a 1-quart jar of boiling water. Cover and let steep 20 minutes. Strain the liquid, add a little sugar if you'd like, and enjoy 2 to 3 cups per day.

Thyme. It's time to try thyme when the mucous membranes are stuffed, the head aches, and the body is hot with fever. Wonderfully fragrant, thyme delights the senses (if you can smell when sick) and works as a powerful expectorant and antiseptic, thanks to its constituent oil, thymol.

INFLUENZA, THE GRIM REAPER OF HISTORY

Throughout recent history there have been several noteworthy worldwide outbreaks of the flu, called pandemics, resulting in large numbers of deaths. The Centers for Disease Control and Prevention provides these alarming statistics:

- 1918–19: The Spanish flu caused the highest known influenza-related mortality. More than 500,000 deaths occurred in the United States, approximately 50 million or more worldwide.
- 1957–58: The Asian flu struck, resulting in 70,000 deaths in the United States.
- 1968–69: The Hong Kong flu caused 34,000 deaths in the United States.

WHEN TO CALL THE DOCTOR

- If flu symptoms are accompanied by a high fever that lasts more than three days
- If a cough persists, becomes worse, or is associated with chest pains and shortness of breath
- If the flu drags on and you don't get better
- If you have lung or heart disease, consult your physician at the first sign of flu. The elderly and the very young should also be taken to a doctor at the first sign of flu.

By cupping your hands around a mug of thyme tea and breathing in the steam, the thymol sets to work through your upper respiratory tract, loosening mucus and inhibiting bacteria from settling down to stay. Add 1 teaspoon dried thyme leaves to 1 cup boiling water. Let steep for five minutes while inhaling the steam. Strain the tea, sweeten with honey (to taste), and slowly sip.

Thyme and peppermint. Variety is the spice of life! Combine thyme and peppermint to make an herbal steam broth that will deliver healing aromas to your aching nose and throat. Combine 1½ quarts boiling water and 2 tablespoons each of dried thyme and peppermint in a large pot. Cover and steep for five minutes. Place the pot on a table and remove the lid. Lean in and cover both your head and the pot of steaming herbs with a large towel. Slowly breathe the herbal broth for 15 minutes.

Warning! Don't stick your nose too close to the broth or you'll risk a burn.

LIFESTYLE REMEDIES

Get plenty of rest. Okay, you may not need to be told this, at least when the flu first hits: Rest is essential to allow your body to fight the virus. So indulge yourself—you've got a good reason.

Drink lots of fluids. Water's good, as are teas, juice, and soups.

MORE DO'S AND DON'TS

- Don't give aspirin to anyone younger than age 18 because of the risk of Reye's syndrome, a potentially fatal illness that is linked with aspirin use and the flu in young people.

Food Poisoning
BEATING THE BUG

The company's annual 4th of July barbecue started out a huge success. The ribs were superb. The potato salad was excellent. Even Helen's famous coleslaw got rave reviews. But about the time the sun went down, people started sprinting in all directions, and they weren't running in the three-legged race. Most of them were headed for the nearest bathroom. Food poisoning claimed another round of victims.

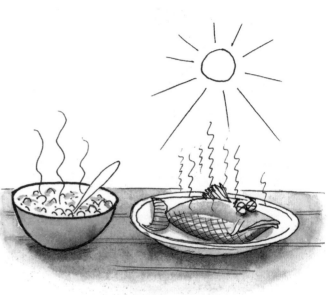

There are 76 million cases of food-borne illness every year, causing about 325,000 hospitalizations and 5,000 deaths, according to the Centers for Disease Control. Since the vast majority of food poisoning goes unreported, chalked up to the stomach flu or another bug, these estimates likely represent only a fraction of the number of actual cases. Even though the United States has strict guidelines when it comes to processing and handling food, there is always a risk of some food becoming contaminated. Food contamination has gotten more attention recently because of highly publicized outbreaks of *E. coli* found in hamburgers and fresh spinach, peanuts contaminated with salmonella, and vegetables and raw milk tainted with campylobacter. Ironically, though many cases of food poisoning do happen in restaurants, the most common place for foodborne illnesses to strike is your kitchen.

Spoiled Food Makes You Feel Rotten

The symptoms you have after eating a pork chop laden with bad bacteria can range from mild (a few stomach cramps) to severe (you spend a couple of days camped out on the bathroom floor). Many people describe food poisoning as akin to being hit by a

KEEPING BACTERIA AT BAY

Food that's very hot or very cold won't allow bacteria to grow. Here are the important numbers to know:

180°F: The ideal internal temperature to cook whole poultry.

165°F: The minimum internal temperature when cooking ground poultry.

160°F: The minimum internal temperature when cooking pork, ground beef, and ground veal.

145°F: The minimum internal temperature when cooking roasts, steaks, and chops of beef, veal, or lamb.

125°F: At this temperature, bacteria can survive and a few will grow.

140°F: Foods cooked and held at this temperature won't be free of bacteria, but bacteria will not be able to spread.

60°F: If risky food is left at this temperature for too long, bacteria will begin to take over.

40°F: The magic temperature at which potentially dangerous bacteria begin to grow.

32°F: Though most bacteria are halted at this temp, some bacteria will grow.

0°F: Bacteria don't die at this frigid temperature, but you can keep them from spreading.

very large truck. The most common symptoms are diarrhea, stomach pain, cramping, nausea, and vomiting.

Because most of the symptoms of food poisoning are similar to those of other illnesses, such as a stomach virus, people aren't always sure food is the problem. If you think you've got food poisoning but aren't sure, take note: Most people get sick about 4 to 48 hours after eating the suspect food. And if you got sick, chances are everyone else who ate a contaminated chop will be sick, too.

Foiling Food Poisoning

You've had some potato salad that's been sitting in the sun too long. Your stomach starts to cramp, and you make your first trip to the bathroom. Now what? There isn't really anything you can do to stop the symptoms of food poisoning once they start, and you shouldn't try. As awful as it is, the diarrhea and vomiting that happen when you contract a foodborne illness help your body get rid of the poison. Taking over-the-counter medications that halt the process can make you sicker. The best thing you can do is take care of yourself while you're sick. These remedies can at least make dealing with the symptoms more bearable and get you feeling better faster. There are also some home remedies that will help prevent food poisoning from visiting your house.

DIETARY REMEDIES

Bananas. As you spend more time embracing the porcelain

throne, your body is losing essential elements like potassium. Losing these vital nutrients can make that I've-been-hit-by-a-truck feeling worse. Once you've come to a lull in the bathroom visitations, usually after the first 24 hours, try eating a banana. It's easy on your stomach and can make you feel a bit better.

Chicken soup. Once you start feeling a bit better, start your stomach out with bland foods. Chicken soup is tasty and easy to digest.

Over-the-counter electrolyte solution. These products replace lost nutrients and help keep you hydrated.

 Sugar. Sugar helps your body hold onto fluid, and adding a spoonful of sugar to a glass of water or a cup of decaffeinated tea may be more palatable if you find sports drinks too sugary.

Sports drinks. Losing all that fluid means you're losing electrolytes (salts that keep your body functioning properly) and water. Replacing that fluid with a sports drink will help replace needed electrolytes, and the sugar in the drink will help your body better absorb the fluid it needs. If the sugar is too much for your tummy, tone the drink down by diluting it with water.

Water. You may not feel like having anything pass your lips, but you need to stay hydrated, especially when you are losing fluids from both ends. Start off with a few sips of this easy-to-swallow liquid and work your way up to more substantial stuff.

TOPICAL REMEDIES

Bleach. Scrubbing your counter with warm soapy water and bleach is one of your best defenses

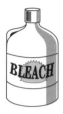

WHEN TO CALL THE DOCTOR

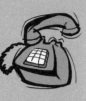

Food poisoning can be debilitating for a day or two, but you'll start feeling better after the poison leaves your system. Sometimes, though, food poisoning can be very dangerous. If you have any of these symptoms, see a doctor immediately:

- Diarrhea and vomiting that last more than 48 hours
- A fever of more than 101 degrees Fahrenheit
- Stomach cramps that keep getting worse
- Blood in your stool
- Dehydration
- Stiff neck, severe headache, and fever

   An important note: If the person poisoned is a young child, an elderly person, or someone with an impaired immune system (they're just getting over an illness or they have a more serious condition such as AIDS), see the doctor at the first sign of food poisoning.

against bacteria that tend to hover on countertops. It's a good idea to clean your cutting boards in a bleach and water solution: Try soaking them in a mixture of 2 teaspoons bleach to 1 quart water. Let the boards air dry.

Hot water bottle or heating pad. These can help ease your stomach cramps.

LIFESTYLE REMEDIES

Get lots of rest. Not that you'd feel like running a marathon or even attempting to go to the office, but take it easy at home. Stick to the bed or the couch, and let time do its magic.

Give your stomach and your intestines time to recuperate. Stay away from spicy, smoked, fried, or salty foods. Stay away from raw vegetables or rich pastries or candies, and don't drink alcohol.

Hand washing. Wash your hands thoroughly before and after handling food. You don't want to be like Typhoid Mary and pass your illness to everyone in the household.

Try not to use antidiarrheals or antinausea medications. When you've ingested bacteria-infected food, your body reacts with diarrhea and vomiting to help you get rid of it quickly. Don't interfere with that process if you can help it.

MORE DO'S AND DON'TS

- Be careful with pain medications. Prescription and over-the-counter pain medications, especially those containing aspirin or ibuprofen, may irritate the gastrointestinal tract and increase discomfort instead of relieving it. Acetaminophen is usually okay, but be sure to read the labels and product information before you use it.

- Tell your state health department about your woes. Telling your story may keep others from experiencing the same problems, especially if you experienced food poisoning after eating at a restaurant or other food establishment.
- Once you're sick, get someone else to go to the kitchen for you. You could be spreading more harmful bacteria and inviting others to share in your suffering.

BACTERIA'S BAD BOYS

There are somewhere around 100 bacteria that can cause food poisoning. But these are on the "Most Wanted" list:

- **Campylobacter jejuni.** A common cause of foodborne illness, this bacteria is found in raw and undercooked poultry and meat, unpasteurized milk, and untreated water. Cook food properly and clean hands and utensils to kill it.
- **Clostridium perfringens.** Known as the "buffet germ," this bacteria grows fastest in casseroles, stews, and gravies that are held at low or room temperature. Make sure hot foods are kept hot and cold foods cold.
- **Escherichia coli (E. Coli) 0157:H7.** This specific strain of *E. coli* can cause severe problems. Found mostly in raw or undercooked ground beef, unpasteurized milk, contaminated water, and minimally processed poultry. Kill this bacteria by cooking food properly.
- **Salmonella.** Found mostly in raw or undercooked meat, poultry, eggs, and fish, and in unpasteurized milk, salmonella is easy to get rid of. Cook foods thoroughly and drink only pasteurized milk.
- **Staphylococcus aureus.** Staph bacteria is found on people (skin, nose, throat) but is spread through contaminated foods. It can't be killed by cooking; avoid this one by keeping hands and kitchen utensils clean.
- **Vibrio vulnificus.** This bacteria is found in raw oysters; raw or undercooked mussels, clams, and whole scallops; and other shellfish.

Foot Discomfort
TLC FOR TOOTSIES

Overworked and taken for granted;
that's the lot of the lowly foot. But
feet are a marvelous work of nature
and an architectural wonder. Each one
of your feet is made up of 26 bones,
33 joints, and more than 100 tendons,
muscles, and ligaments. Together,
they comprise one-quarter of all the
bones in your body.

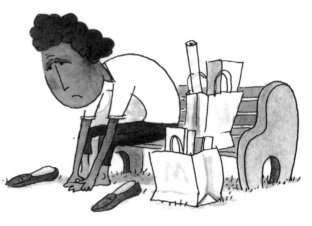

Every day, on average, moderately
active people take 7,500 to 10,000
steps. Highly active people take
12,500 steps a day or more. That adds up to four
hikes around the planet during a lifetime. And
each time a step is taken, the impact of hitting the
ground is about one and a half times your body
weight. No wonder, then, that most of us experience foot and ankle problems at some time.
Women have four times more foot problems than
men, mostly because of wearing high heels.

Here are some common problems that cause
foot pain, most often due to an overuse injury:

- Plantar fascitis. A heel injury affecting the
  area where the arch meets the heel. Plantar
  fascitis is marked by heel pain with first steps
  in the morning, possible swelling, and heel
  pain as you rest. It can usually be worked
  out with activity. What to do: Wear better
  shoes, or try orthopedic shoes prescribed
  by a podiatrist. Don't walk barefoot. Use ice

unless you have circulatory problems or are diabetic. Lose weight if you are overweight. Do foot stretches. Try heel cups in your shoes for shock absorption. If the pain is persistent, see a podiatrist.

- Heel spurs. A little outgrowth of the bone, a result of the bone's attempt to heal after repetitive stress and inflammation in the plantar fascia. What to do: If it causes foot pain, a simple surgery to shave the spur away may be required.
- Neuroma. A pinched nerve, causing pain between the third and fourth toes. It can feel like a tooth that needs a root canal. One of the most common causes is a poor shoe fit. What to do: Buy a shoe with a wider toe area.
- Tendinitis. An inflammatory process in the tendons, common in athletes. It can be a serious, painful, and persistent problem. What to do: Rest, ice, use anti-inflammatory drugs, and change exercise technique and shoe gear.
- Stress fracture. A crack in the bone usually resulting from repetitive pounding. Common to athletes. What to do: Limit weight bearing, and stick to low impact exercise. An orthotic device may be necessary to reduce pressure at the fracture site. Be sure to confirm and locate the stress fracture via X-ray for proper treatment.
- Ankle sprains. A ligament that is stretched or torn. It is the most common athletic injury, although it can occur when you simply step on an uneven surface. What to do: Ice, compression with an elastic bandage or splint to eliminate motion, and elevation to decrease

TOENAIL TIPS

- Soak your feet in equal parts vinegar and water to soften and clean the nail before you clip.
- Clip the toenail straight across with nail clippers. Leave enough nail so that there's a little white showing at the end of your nail.
- Remove rough edges with a nail file.
- For an ingrown toenail: Trim excess nail, then put cotton under the corner to separate it from the skin. Change cotton daily. If the area is red, apply hydrogen peroxide, then coat with an over-the-counter antibacterial cream. Cover with a bandage. Repeat daily.
- For a toe ache, soak in warm water.
- Call the doctor or podiatrist about that ingrown toenail if you experience severe pain or discharge around or under the nail, if you can't trim the nail yourself, or if you have diabetes and the ingrown nail becomes infected.

IF THE SHOE FITS
Shoe models change, even though their names may stay the same. Even if that last pair of shoes was the perfect fit, have a proper fitting each time you purchase new ones because they may not be quite the same.

swelling. Limit weight-bearing activities, and stay off feet for a few days. In cases of a severe sprain, your podiatrist may recommend a brace or surgery.

Here are a few more foot aches that aren't attributed to overuse. Instead, these are caused by simple everyday wear and tear, as well as poorly fit shoes.

- Black toenail. A hematoma (bruising) under the nail. What to do: Wear proper-fitting shoes that aren't too tight or too loose, clip toenails short so they won't rub against the shoe, soak foot in salt water.
- Bunions. A misaligned big toe joint in which the toe slants outward causing inflammation and swelling. The most common cause is tight-fitting shoes. What to do: Wear proper-fitting shoes and padding, and rest and soak the foot. Bunions must be treated by a podiatrist.
- Hammertoe. When a toe, usually the second, third, or fourth toe, bends up to look like a claw. It frequently is accompanied by calluses, and although the actual cause is a muscle imbalance, the underlying cause of that imbalance is usually an ill-fitting shoe that cramps the toes. What to do: Wear proper-fitting shoes and padding. Hammertoes must be treated by a podiatrist.
- Ingrown toenail. This happens when the side of your toenail cuts into your skin. The cause is usually a bad toenail clip job, but pressure from a bad shoe fit can cause it too. A mild ingrown nail can be removed with careful clipping, but if it is deep or painful, consider a trip to the podiatrist.

Bad Shoes, Good Shoes

Bad shoes are what many foot injuries have in common. Bad shoes, according to the American College of Foot and Ankle Surgeons, are to blame for the majority of all foot problems.

No matter what type of shoe you're wearing, a bad shoe is one that does not fit properly, has lost its shape, causes pain or rubbing, or is worn unevenly. Bad shoes cause foot and ankle problems, as well as leg and back problems.

To get a good fit for any type of shoe:

- Buy shoes at the end of the day, after work or exercise, when your feet are at their largest. If you buy shoes earlier in the day, they may be too tight.
- Measure both feet and fit your shoe to the largest one, since your feet aren't both the same size.
- Make sure you can wiggle your toes. If you can't, the fit is too tight. Also make sure the widest part of your foot is comfortable but secure.
- Walk around the store to see if the shoes are comfortable. Never buy shoes without first trying them on, and don't assume they will get comfortable with wear. If they don't feel good when you try them on, don't buy them.
- Try on shoes with the socks you plan to wear with them.
- When the shoe is on and you're standing up, make sure you can fit the width of your little finger between your heel and the back of the shoe—no more and no less.
- If your heel slides in the shoe as you walk, the shoe doesn't fit.

MASSAGE THAT PAIN AWAY

A foot massage feels wonderful, especially if you can get someone else to do it for you. Here's how.

- First, apply oil (olive oil from the pantry will work!) and condition the foot with medium-light strokes, using your thumbs and fingers.
- Starting with the ball of the foot, work across and down the entire foot, making small, circular motions with the thumbs.
- Use thumbs to make long, deep strokes along the arch, moving toward the toes.
- Gently squeeze, rotate, and pull each toe.
- End by cupping the foot between both hands and gently squeezing up and down the length of the foot.
- Sigh deeply, and say "ahhhh…"

FOODS THAT CAUSE FLUID RETENTION

Sometimes a simple dietary change is all it takes to get rid of those aching, swollen feet. Avoid these foods, which can make your feet puff up:

- Bacon and other cured meats. Curing is done with salt, which causes fluid retention.
- Lunch meats. These, too, have lots of salt.
- Canned foods. Salt is added to many canned foods, including vegetables. To reduce sodium in canned vegetables and beans, rinse before eating.

- Don't let anyone tell you the shoe will stretch. Good shoes fit properly when you buy them.
- No matter how much you're attached to your closet full of comfortable old shoes, toss them in the trash when they are worn out and get new ones.

Now that you know what that foot pain might be, as well as possible treatment options, here are a few home remedies to help heal those tired, aching dogs.

DIETARY REMEDIES

Asparagus. For swollen feet, look in the veggie drawer for that nice, fresh asparagus you bought. Steam and eat. Asparagus acts as a natural diuretic, which flushes the excess fluid out of your system.

Foods. For bloated, uncomfortable feet, here are some foods that can help balance your fluid levels: bananas, which are high in potassium that helps relieve fluid retention, and coffee or tea, both of which are diuretics. Also, poultry and fresh fish, both of which are low in sodium, and yogurt, which can reduce histamine-producing bacteria. Histamine causes fluid retention.

HERBAL REMEDIES

Cayenne pepper. To warm cold feet, sprinkle a

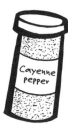

little cayenne pepper in your socks. Cayenne peppers have a chemical called capsaicin that warms, and it also relieves pain. However, this can be irritating to the skin after awhile, so carry some spare socks in case you need to change.

Cinnamon. Cure those cold feet with some hot cinnamon tea. Stir a gram of powdered cinnamon into a glass of hot water and steep for 15 minutes. Drink three times per day.

Cumin. For swollen feet, mix ¼ teaspoon each of cumin, coriander, and fennel in a cup of hot water, and drink two to three times per day.

Sage. Take a handful of sage leaves and rub them in your palm. (This is called bruising, and it releases the herb's curative chemicals.) Put them in a saucepan with ⅔ cup cider vinegar. Boil, then simmer for five minutes. After removing from the heat, soak a cloth in the solution and apply it to a sprain or sore foot, making it as hot as tolerable.

TOPICAL REMEDIES

Beans. Spread a few dried navy beans on the floor and practice picking them up with your toes. This is an exercise that will help keep your feet strong and flexible.

Carbonated water. Soaking your feet in sugarless carbonated water can be refreshing.

Epsom salts. For plain old tired feet, put 2 table-spoons Epsom salts into a basin of warm water. Soak for 15 minutes. Epsom salts can be drying, so moisturize your feet afterwards.

Ice. An ice pack will reduce the inflammation of tendinitis. You can use a bag of ice or a bag of frozen vegetables wrapped in a thin towel.

Olive oil. Use as a massage oil for tired feet. See "Massage that Pain Away," page 199.

Vinegar. To soothe tendinitis, sprains, strains, and general foot aches, alternate hot and cold vinegar wraps. First, heat equal amounts of vinegar and

DIABETES CAUTION
Foot problems can result in serious illness and even amputation for people with diabetes. To learn more about the care of diabetic feet, see page 137.

WHEN TO CALL THE DOCTOR

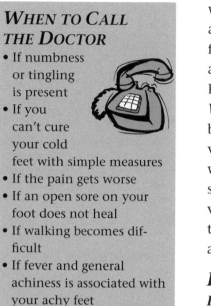

- If numbness or tingling is present
- If you can't cure your cold feet with simple measures
- If the pain gets worse
- If an open sore on your foot does not heal
- If walking becomes difficult
- If fever and general achiness is associated with your achy feet
- If the swelling does not diminish

water. Soak a towel in the mixture, wring it out, and wrap it around your foot. Leave it wrapped for five minutes. Then mix equal parts vinegar and cold water, and follow the same procedure. Repeat this entire sequence three times.

Water. Sometimes plain old water is the best cure of all. If you have varicose veins in your feet or ankles, this remedy will alleviate the ache and may even slow down the development of varicose veins. Dip your feet in hot water for 2 minutes, then in cold for 15 seconds. Repeat, and continue alternating hot and cold for 15 minutes.

LIFESTYLE REMEDIES

Don't stand too long, and don't stand on hard surfaces if you can avoid it. Foot pain is often muscle fatigue from standing. Take frequent breaks. Sit down and elevate your feet for ten minutes.

Don't ignore foot pain, tired legs, aching knees, lower-back problems, or sore hips. They could all be symptoms of serious conditions.

Maintain your ideal weight. The more weight you put on those puppies, the more they'll cause you pain.

Wear the right shoes. Choosing the right shoes is especially important when it comes to fitness footwear. Different sports and exercises have unique repetitive movements that require special support and cushioning. Spend the extra money to buy shoes that are specific for the activity you're doing, and replace sports shoes when cushioning starts to break down. The investment could save you and your feet a lot of pain, time, and money.

Foot Odor

STANCHING THE STENCH

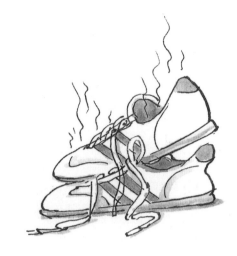

When you kick off your shoes, do you clear a room? That's one sure sign that your feet reek like week-old garbage. Your olfactory region may be blissfully unaware of the odors emitted from down below, but others' noses aren't so immune. Foot odor may leave you friendless, too, as the stink often (unfairly) implies bad hygiene to those who share your air.

Foot odor, known in the medical profession as *bromhidrosis,* can be traced to bacteria that find your moist and warm feet, socks, and shoes the perfect place to breed and multiply. Thousands of sweat glands on the soles of the feet produce perspiration composed of water, sodium chloride, fat, minerals, and various acids that are the end products of your body's metabolism. In the presence of certain bacteria (namely those found in dark, damp shoes), these sweaty secretions break down, generating the stench that turns people green.

Foot odor is only a temporary curse and can easily be cured. Kick off your shoes without worry after trying some of these refreshing remedies.

TOPICAL REMEDIES

Activated charcoal. Dust some activated charcoal in your shoes. It's an effective (but messy) odor absorbent. Or you can purchase inexpensive foot pads that contain it.

Baking soda. Don't just let those shoes sit there without odor support! Bring on the baking soda! Deodorize shoes by sprinkling 1 or 2 teaspoons baking soda inside to absorb moisture and hide odors. For added fragrance, combine 3 tablespoons baking soda with 3 tablespoons ground, dried sage leaves. Combine the sage and baking soda and place into an airtight glass jar. After removing your shoes for the

OUT-OF-THIS-WORLD ODOR

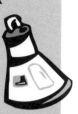

No stinky shoes make it into space. NASA employs a "master sniffer," who spends his days smelling all sorts of stuff. His olfactory region determines whether odors generated by a certain object would be too offensive to astronauts. Everything is tested, including footwear. Sound silly? Don't laugh. In the early '70s, two Soviet cosmonauts aborted a mission aboard the Salyut Space Station due to an overwhelming stench.

SLOSHING AROUND IN SWEAT

Each foot has more than 250,000 sweat glands and produces as much as ½ pint of sweat daily.

PEE-U

An unorthodox home remedy that we can't recommend, but many swear by, is to pee on your feet. That's right...miss deliberately. This begs the question: If foot odor is viewed as unhygienic, than what do you call this remedy?

day, sprinkle 1 tablespoon of the mixture into each shoe. Shake and leave overnight. The following day, keep the sage-soda in the shoes. In the evening remove excess sage-soda mix, and replace it with a fresh supply. Repeat nightly.

Another way to use baking soda is in a foot bath. Add 2 tablespoons baking soda to a bowl of warm water. Soak feet every night for a month.

Black tea. Soak tootsies in black tea. Tannic acid, a component of tea, is thought to have astringent properties that prevent feet from perspiring. To make a foot-tea soak, brew 5 bags black tea in 1 quart boiling water. Let cool, add ice cubes (during summertime), and soak in this "iced tea for the toes" bath for 20 to 30 minutes.

Cornstarch. A less fancy solution to keeping shoes deodorized and dry is to sprinkle the inside with 1 to 2 teaspoons cornstarch.

Ginger. Mash a 1- or 2-inch piece of ginger into a pulp, put it into a handkerchief or piece of gauze, and soak it in some hot water for a 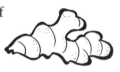 few minutes. Rub the ginger liquid onto each foot nightly after taking a shower. Try for two weeks.

Radish. You can't squeeze blood from a turnip, but you can squeeze an antistink solution from a radish. Using a juicemaker, juice about two dozen radishes, add ¼ teaspoon glycerine, and pour in a squirt or spray-top bottle. Spritz on toes to reduce foot odor.

 Salt. Add table salt or Epsom salts to water for a foot soak. Pour a few teaspoons of salt into a tub of warm water. Soak for ten minutes.

Vinegar. Soak your feet several times a week in an apple cider or plain vinegar bath. Mix ⅓ cup vinegar into a bowl of warm water. Soak for 10 to 15 minutes.

Water. Alternate footbaths of hot and cold water to help reduce blood flow to your feet and reduce perspiration. After the hot foot bath, shock those toes by dipping them into a second foot bath containing cool water, ice cubes, and 1 to 2 teaspoons lemon juice (if available). Rub your feet with alcohol following the bath. Try this treatment once per day, especially in warmer months.

LIFESTYLE REMEDIES

Give your feet a rest...from your shoes, that is. The secret to keeping your favorite pair of shoes in first place is to let them air out at least 24 hours between wearings. If not, the sweat buildup keeps them moist and makes bacteria happy.

Watch what you eat. Strong, pungent foods such as garlic, onions, scallions, peppers, and curry spices can cause foot odor. The odoriferous products in each pass through the bloodstream and concentrate in the perspiration.

Go barefoot or wear sandals when possible.

Wear moisture-wicking socks. Look for such fabrics as orlon, polypropylene, and brand-name patented fabrics like CoolMax. If possible, change socks at least twice a day.

MORE DO'S AND DON'TS

- Don't wear solid rubber or synthetically lined shoes. Neither lets your feet breathe easily, allowing odor-producing bacteria to grow.
- Once a month, toss those tennis shoes into the washing machine. Let them air dry.
- When the shoe fits, wear it. When it starts to stink, throw it out with the garbage.

WHEN TO CALL THE DOCTOR

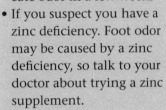

- If home remedies and frequent washings of feet and socks have failed to eradicate odor in a few weeks
- If you suspect you have a zinc deficiency. Foot odor may be caused by a zinc deficiency, so talk to your doctor about trying a zinc supplement.

THE TEN-TOED SAHARA

The average temperature inside the shoe is 110 degrees Fahrenheit.

A BIT ABOUT BAKING SODA

Baking soda, aka sodium bicarbonate, is a mild base that can neutralize acidic environments (in this case, smelly shoes and feet). The white powder works by balancing the pH, bringing acidic and basic odors back to a neutral, odorless state.

Gallbladder Problems
AVERTING AN ATTACK

Unless you've had problems with your gallbladder, you probably don't know much about it. Be thankful. If you do know the specifics of your gallbladder, you're probably one of the estimated 25 million Americans who have gallstones. One-quarter of those with gallstones require treatment to relieve symptoms such as discomfort and pain in the upper abdomen, indigestion, nausea, and intolerance of fatty foods. A gallbladder attack, which occurs when a gallstone gets stuck in the bile duct, can double you over in pain for hours and leave you wishing something, anything, could make you feel better.

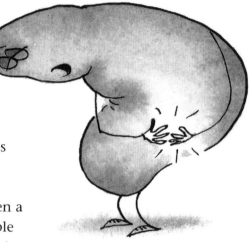

Casting Stones

The gallbladder is a little pear-shaped pouch tucked behind the lobes of the liver. Its main job is to store up the cholesterol-rich bile that's secreted by the liver. Bile helps your body digest fatty foods. When that piece of prime rib reaches the intestines, they send a message up to the gallbladder to send some bile their way. Once the bile saturates your steak, it becomes more digestible and easily makes its way through the rest of the digestive process.

At least that's the way things should work. But the reality is that many people, especially older people and women, will have some gallbladder trouble. The majority of the time that trouble is in the form of gallstones. Gallstones form when

GOOD-BYE GALLBLADDER

Every year, 500,000 people have their gallbladder removed.

the bile contains excessive amounts of cholesterol. When there isn't enough bile to saturate the cholesterol, the cholesterol begins to crystallize, and you get a gallstone. These tough bits can be as tiny as a grain of sand or as large as a golf ball. You may not even know you have gallstones unless you happen to have an ultrasound or X-ray of your tummy. But the 25 percent of the time that gallstones do cause problems, it's excruciatingly painful.

Gallstones become a problem when they get pushed out of the gallbladder and into the tube that connects the liver and the small intestine. The tube gets blocked, and you get 20 minutes to 4 hours of indescribable agony. Pain usually radiates from your upper right abdominal area to your lower right chest, and it can even leave your shoulder and back in agony. Gallstones typically fall back into the gallbladder or make their way through the duct, leaving you feeling better. After you have an attack, you'll probably be sore and wonder what in the world happened.

Sometimes, though, the gallstones can get stuck in the bile duct. Symptoms of a stuck gallstone include chills, vomiting, abdominal cramping, and possibly jaundice in addition to the pain described above.

Who's at Risk?

Pregnancy, obesity, diabetes, liver disease, a sedentary lifestyle, a high-fat diet, and certain forms of anemia can all increase the risk of gallstones. People who are overweight and lose and gain weight repeatedly are more susceptible to gallstones, as are women who have had two or more children. Lack of exercise is a significant contributor to the development of gallstones. In

SURVIVING WITHOUT A GALLBLADDER

Believe it or not, you actually can get along just fine without your gallbladder. Instead of being stored in the gallbladder, bile flows directly from the liver into the small intestine. Diarrhea may be a side effect; chronic diarrhea affects about 1 percent of those who have had their gallbladder removed. And you may have higher blood cholesterol levels. You may also risk stomach upset if you eat too much fat at one time. But aside from that, life will continue as normal—that is, minus the chronic pain from gallbladder attacks.

ETHNICITY AND GALLSTONES

Gallstones are most common in fair-skinned people of Northern European descent, Hispanic people, and Native Americans. They are least common among Asian and African American people.

LAY OFF THE LIVER

"Liver flush" is a popular, but unsafe, folk remedy for gallstones. Folk healers recommend drinking 1 cup olive oil with the juice of 2 lemons for breakfast several days in a row. Some people swear this remedy helped them pass their gallstones. The problem with "liver flush" is it's more likely to block the liver duct that leads to the small intestine than it is to get rid of gallstones. Some experts believe drinking so much olive oil may actually increase the cholesterol in the gallbladder, making you *more* at risk for developing gallstones. So if you've got gallstones, skip this home remedy. It may do more harm than good.

fact, according to the Nurses' Health Study, inactivity can actually account for more than half of the risk of developing gallstones. Women are twice as likely as men to develop gallstones, although the reasons are unclear. And people older than 60 years of age have a greater risk of gallstones.

Other risk factors include a family history of gallstones and taking hormones, such as birth control pills or estrogen.

Take heart. There are some specific things you can find in your home to help you avoid a gallstone attack and even prevent gallstones from forming in the first place. What you eat has a great effect on whether or not you develop gallstones. And research is finding that certain foods can help you avert a painful attack or, better yet, avoid gallstones altogether.

DIETARY REMEDIES

Alcohol. Moderate alcohol intake appears to reduce gallstone attacks. But don't go overboard. The study didn't find that drinking more than half a glass would offer any more protection.

Coffee. Studies have found that drinking a couple of cups of java a day can prevent gallstones. One study discovered that men who drank 2 to 3 cups of regular coffee per day cut their risk of developing gallstones by 40 percent. Four cups per day reduced the risk by 45 percent. Researchers are not sure what it is about coffee that helps reduce the risk of forming gallstones, but the effect was the same whether it was cheap, store-bought instant coffee or high-priced espresso. It might be the caffeine; however, teas and soft drinks containing caffeine did not produce the same effect—and neither did decaffeinated coffee.

High-fiber cereal. People who eat a sugary, high-fat diet probably will have more problems with their gallstones. But adding in some fiber-rich foods and avoiding the sugary snacks and fatty foods can help you keep your gallbladder healthy. Grabbing some cereal in the morning will also get something in your tummy. Studies have shown that going for long periods without eating, such as skipping breakfast, can make you more prone to getting a gallstone.

Lentils. An interesting study found that women who ate loads of lentils, nuts, beans, peas, lima beans, and oranges were more resistant to gallbladder attacks than women who didn't eat much of the stuff.

Nuts. Scientific studies in 2004 showed that men and women who ate five or more ounces of nuts a week had a lower risk of developing gallstones. Both peanuts and other nuts had the same protective qualities.

Red bell pepper. Getting loads of vitamin C in your diet can help you avoid gallstones, and one red bell pepper has 95 mg of the helpful vitamin—more than the 90 mg a day the government recommends for adult men and 75 mg daily for adult women who are not pregnant or breastfeeding. A recent study found that people who had more vitamin C in their blood were less likely to get the painful stones.

SHOCKING THOSE STONES: THE WAVE OF THE FUTURE

Until recently, most people who had recurring painful bouts with gallstones had one choice—get rid of the gallbladder. But there's a new procedure that may allow people to get rid of their gallstones without losing any body parts. The procedure is based on the same shock-wave theory that demolishes kidney stones. This time, though, the shock waves are more specific, delivered directly to the gallstones. It is an invasive procedure. The doctor inserts a tube into the gallbladder via a small puncture hole, and the electric shock is delivered directly to the gallstones. Then the fragments of the stones are scooped up and removed from the body. The whole process takes about an hour and leaves you on R & R for a few days. Compared to the major surgery required to remove your gallbladder, this procedure is a breeze.

Salmon. Research is finding that omega-3 fatty acids, found in fatty fish such as salmon, may help prevent gallstones.

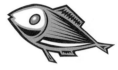

Vegetables. Eating your veggies is a good way to ward off gallstones. One study found that vegetarian women were only half as likely to have gallstones as their carnivorous counterparts. Researchers aren't sure exactly how vegetables counteract gallstones, but they believe vegetables help reduce the amount of cholesterol in bile.

LIFESTYLE REMEDIES

Exercise! Staying active can cut your risk of developing gallstones in half.

Lose some weight. Being overweight, even as little as 10 pounds, can double your risk of getting gallstones.

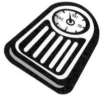

Diet sensibly. If you are overweight, plan on shedding pounds slowly. Losing weight too fast can increase your chances of developing gallstones.

Reduce your saturated fat intake. Too much fat in the diet increases your risk of gallstones. But don't cut back too drastically. You need some fat to give the gallbladder the message to empty bile. If you're trying to lose weight, don't go below 20 percent calories from fat.

Eat a low-fat, low-cholesterol, high-fiber diet. Multiple studies show this is your best bet for a healthy body and a healthy gallbladder.

Genital Herpes
COUNTERACTING RECURRENCES

Genital herpes is a sexually
transmitted disease (STD)
caused by the herpes simplex
virus type 1 (HSV-1) and
type 2 (HSV-2). The type 1 virus
is the same one that causes cold
sores on the mouth, face, and
lips (see Cold Sores, page 91),
although it can also cause sores
on the genitals. The type 2
virus, however, most often causes
sores on the genitals.

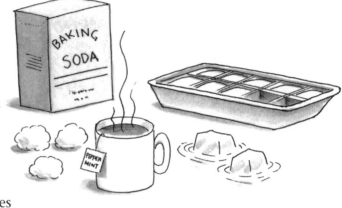

How You Get Genital Herpes

Herpes can spread to the genitals from a cold sore
if hand washing and other hygiene precautions
are not taken. Or, it can be spread though oral or
genital sexual contact. And be warned: The virus
does not have to be in an active state—that is,
blisters do not have to be present—for a partner
to become infected. The virus can also be passed
during the preactive state, when there is itching
or tingling in the area in which the sores generally appear. Sometimes, the virus can be passed
along before the infected person is even aware
that the virus is being shed. What's more, saliva
also carries the virus!

Symptoms

The first episode usually starts within a couple
weeks of exposure, and the initial onset can be

pretty bad, including an initial round and then a second round of painful sores, flulike symptoms, fever, and swollen glands. Sometimes the symptoms are mild, however, and appear as little more than insect bites or a rash.

Once you have genital herpes, you have it for life. Luckily, it spends most of its life, and yours, dormant. But like cold sores, genital herpes recurs, often as many as four or five times per year. Check the cold sore triggers list (page 92) to see some of the reasons why these demons return.

There are a few home remedies that can help you through an episode, however.

DIETARY REMEDIES

Food. Eat well to boost your immune system. For some immune-boosting foods, see pages 299-301.

HERBAL REMEDIES

Peppermint Tea. A nice cup of peppermint tea may help reduce pain and fever.

Tea. Place a cold wet tea bag right on the sores. Tannic acid can soothe genital tissues. Throw away the tea bag afterward.

TOPICAL REMEDIES

Baking soda. Using a cotton ball, pat baking soda on the sores to dry them out and decrease itching. Just be careful not to double dip: You don't want to contaminate the unused baking soda.

Cornstarch. This also can help dry out the sores and help alleviate itching. Use a cotton ball that's been dipped in cornstarch and dust it onto the sores.

Ice. To reduce pain and itching, apply ice to the sores. Fill a plastic bag with crushed ice or use a bag of frozen peas. Wrap the bag in material the thickness of a sheet. Apply for 10 or 15 minutes, and repeat several times per day. Be careful about the time because prolonged exposure to ice can cause tissue damage.

Milk. For pain relief and to promote healing, soak cotton balls in milk and apply to the area.

LIFESTYLE REMEDIES

Don't depend on a condom to protect you or your partner. They help, but they may not cover the entire area. Viral shedding may also occur in the infected area, making the spread of the disease to a sexual partner easy, even if protection is used. Be sure to use a latex or vinyl condom between outbreaks.

Don't wear tight-fitting pants or underwear.
Shower, don't soak in the tub. Shedding virus can escape into the water.

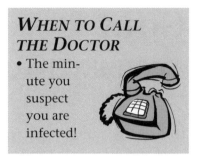

WHEN TO CALL THE DOCTOR
- The minute you suspect you are infected!

Gout
AVOIDING EXCESS

The word gout may make you think of kings and medieval history. But gout isn't a disease of the past. It's very much with us today. That's because gout is an inflammatory joint disease and a form of arthritis, not some mysterious illness of the rich and powerful.

Gout, which occurs in about five percent of people with arthritis, results from the buildup of uric acid in the blood. Uric acid is the result of the breakdown of waste substances, called purines, in the body. Usually it is dissolved in the blood, processed by the kidneys, and passed out of the body in the urine. But in some people there is an excess amount of uric acid—too much for the kidneys to eliminate quickly. When there is too much uric acid in the blood, it crystallizes and collects in the joint spaces, causing gout. Occasionally, these deposits become so large that they push against the skin in lumpy patches, called tophi, that are visible.

A gout attack usually lasts five to ten days, and the most common area under siege is the big toe. In fact, 80 percent of people with gout will be affected in the big toe at some time.

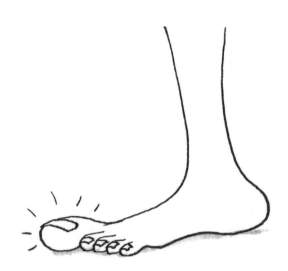

Gout in the big toe can become so painful that even a bedsheet draped over it will cause intolerable pain. Besides the big toe, gout may also develop in the ankles, heels, knees, wrists, fingers, and elbows.

Who Gets Gout?
Though anyone can get gout, it's primarily a man's disease. Women have the good fortune of being more efficient in the way they excrete uric acid. And children rarely get it.

Other risk factors include:
- Age. Men older than 70 are at greatest risk.
- Being postmenopausal. A woman's risk increases after menopause.

- Family history of gout. Twenty percent have family members with gout.
- Overweight. Excessive eating steps up the production of uric acid.
- Eating too many foods with purines, such as organ meats (liver, kidney, brains, sweetbreads), sardines, anchovies, meat extracts, dried peas, lentils, and legumes.
- An enzyme defect that prevents the breakdown of uric acid.
- Heavy alcohol use.
- Exposure to environmental lead.
- Using certain medications, including diuretics, salicylates (aspirin), and levodopa.
- Taking niacin, a vitamin that's also called nicotinic acid.

Gout symptoms come on quickly the first time, often overnight. You may also experience joint swelling and shiny red or purple skin around the joint. If you're already predisposed to gout, you can trigger an episode by

- Drinking too much alcohol
- Overeating, especially purine foods
- Having surgery
- Experiencing a sudden severe illness or trauma
- Going on a crash diet
- Injuring a joint
- Having chemotherapy
- Being under stress. The link isn't the stress itself, but the comfort eating or drinking that may accompany it.

If you have gout, professional medical treatment is required. There are several prescription medications that are very effective at eliminating excess uric acid. Untreated, gout may progress to

GOOD FOODS, BAD FOODS

Diet plays an important role in gout prevention. Here are some foods that will help to keep gout under control:

- Whole-grain cereals and whole-wheat bread. These are loaded with zinc that may be depleted during a gout attack.
- Breakfast cereals and breads fortified with folic acid. These can slow the production of uric acid.
- Bread, pasta, low-fat milk and dairy products, eggs, lettuce, tomatoes. These are low-purine foods.
- Citrus fruits. They have vitamin C that may assist the kidneys in ridding the body of uric acid.

And if you have gout and don't want it to come back, avoid these foods:

- Asparagus, spinach, cauliflower, mushrooms. They have purines.
- Shrimp and crabs. They also contain purines.
- Alcohol. It increases uric acid production in foods. That means beer, too!
- Dried fruit and fruit sugar. If you eat it, do so in moderation. The fructose in it produces uric acid.

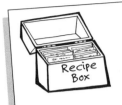

EASY CHERRY SOUP DESSERT

1 pound cherries, pitted
water
1 teaspoon cinnamon
1–2 tablespoons cornstarch
honey or apple juice concentrate
whipped cream

Put the cherries in a saucepan, cover with water, add 1 teaspoon cinnamon. Simmer until cherries are tender. To thicken the mixture, combine 1 to 2 tablespoons of the cooled cherry mixture with 1 to 2 tablespoons cornstarch. Add the cooled mix to the hot soup and stir in. Sweeten to taste with honey or apple juice concentrate. Chill. Top with whipped cream and serve.

Serves 4

GOUT FACTS

- It's not contagious, it doesn't spread from joint to joint, and there is no cure.
- Three million people in the United States had gout in 2005; 6.1 million adults have ever had gout.
- 62 percent of those who have a first gout attack will experience a second attack within a year.
- 95 percent of those with gout experience a second attack within five years.

serious joint damage and disability. Also, excess uric acid can cause kidney stones. There are several home remedies that, along with medication, can help alleviate the pain and symptoms.

DIETARY REMEDIES

Apple preserves. This may neutralize the acid that causes gout. Peel, core, and slice some apples. Simmer in a little water for three hours or more, until they turn thick, brown, and sweet. Refrigerate. Use as you would any preserve.

Cherries. These may remove toxins from the body, clean the kidneys, and even help give you a rosy complexion. Because of their cleansing power, they're at the top of the gout-relief list. Anything cherry works, including cherry pie, cherry juice, and cherry jam. See the Recipe Box, above, for an easy cherry remedy.

Water. To get rid of uric acid, you must keep your body flushed out. Drink at least 2 quarts of water per day—more, if you can manage it.

HERBAL REMEDIES

Mustard powder. Make a mustard plaster and apply to the achy joint. Mix 1 part mustard powder (or crushed mustard seeds) to 1 part whole-wheat flour and add enough water to form a thick paste. Slather petroleum jelly or 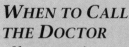 vegetable shortening on the affected area. Spread a thick coat of mustard paste on a piece of gauze or cloth, then apply over the greased-up area. Tape down and leave in place for several hours or overnight.

Thyme. Add 1 to 2 teaspoons to a cup of boiling water. Sweeten, if desired, and drink as a tea.

LIFESTYLE REMEDIES

Avoid foods that are high in purine. These include turkey, organ meats, herring, anchovies, meat gravies, beer, and red wine.

Elevate and immobilize the joint. This reduces pain and helps prevent joint damage.

Keep your toes warm. Gout seems to rear up more often when it's chilly.

Lose weight. Uric acid levels increase as weight increases.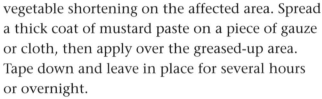

Stay hydrated. Heat and humidity increase the risk of a gout attack, so be sure to drink extra fluids.

Take fish oil supplements to ease inflammation.
Take ibuprofen, not aspirin, for pain and swelling.
Wear shoes with plenty of room for your big toe.

MORE DO'S & DON'TS

- Don't ice or heat the achy area.
- Don't take nonprescription diuretics. They can keep you from properly excreting uric acid.

WHEN TO CALL THE DOCTOR

- If you experience any of the symptoms described on page 215
- If, with your gout attack, you experience fever or other unusual physical symptoms
- If you notice any joint deformity
- If the pain is unmanageable with over-the-counter remedies

Hangovers
MORNING-AFTER MISERY

Well, you partied from sundown to sunup, and now you're paying the price. You've got the pounding headache, the queasiness, the dizziness, the sensitivity to light and sound, the muscle aches, and the irritability that comes from overconsumption of alcoholic beverages. How quickly last night's fun turns into next morning's nightmare when you have a hangover!

Why Such Suffering?

Although we don't like to think of it as such, especially when we're having such a good time, alcohol is actually a drug. It's a depressant, and when taken in excess, it fills your body with toxins. Your body reacts as it would to any drug overdose: It tries to metabolize and get rid of the offending substances.

Researchers aren't sure what in the alcohol causes a hangover. But they do know that the debilitating symptoms you experience are a result of the body's inability to get rid of the toxins quickly enough, and they build up in your bloodstream.

Your body's attempts to flush out the alcohol puts a strain on the liver, which madly draws on the body's water reserves to get the job done. Since alcohol is a major diuretic, causing you to urinate more frequently, you lose more water than your body takes in with the beverage. As strange as it may sound, the more alcohol you drink, the more vital fluids you lose. The considerable water loss associated with drinking alcohol increases the liver's burden to get a hold of water anywhere it can. It will take water from the brain and from other vital organs. The resulting dehydration is what's behind many of the worst symptoms of a hangover.

The process of metabolizing the alcohol and excreting large quantities of water also robs the body of glucose and other vital nutrients. Being malnourished further contributes to the unpleasant hangover symptoms.

In addition to dehydration, fatigue is also behind some of your hangover pain. Excessive drinking and late nights usually go hand-in-hand. But more than that, alcohol interferes with a normal sleep pattern, robbing you of the dream state, which is essential to feeling rested. You may pass out on the floor and sleep for hours, but it won't be the kind of sleep that will allow you to restart your engine in the morning. Lack of proper rest contributes to the malaise a hangover brings.

Prevention

The best way to prevent a hangover is, of course, drinking in moderation or abstaining from alcohol. Keeping yourself well-hydrated and well-nourished when you're drinking can also go a long way toward minimizing the morning-after symptoms. Try drinking a glass of water or other noncaffeinated beverage for each alcoholic beverage you drink. And don't drink on an empty stomach. Food helps slow the absorption of alcohol, giving your body time to metabolize it

FACTS ABOUT HANGOVERS

According to the Alka-Seltzer Morning Relief Hangover Survey of 900 Americans aged 21 or older:

- The average number of drinks that cause a hangover is 3.2.
- About 1 in 10 people older than age 21 get hangovers after 1 or 2 drinks.
- 55 percent of Americans of legal drinking age consume alcoholic beverages at least once a week.

PICK YOUR POISON CAREFULLY

If you do drink, know that your beverage choice may determine your hangover fate. Keep these recommendations in mind when seated at the bar.

- Mixing different types of alcohol makes for a difficult recovery.
- Darker-colored liquors (such as bourbon or rum) will give you worse hangovers than light-colored liquors (gin or vodka). Darker liquors contain more impurities called congeners, which are by-products of fermentation.
- Red wine can cause a worse hangover because of an amino acid it contains called tyramine.

- Carbonation in drinks speeds up the absorption of alcohol.
- Don't choose quantity over quality. Cheap liquors make you sicker quicker.
- Tropical drinks with creams and sugars (such as piña coladas) mask the taste of alcohol, sing a siren song to your sweet tooth, and make you want "just one more."

and decreasing the chances of a hangover.

The best cure for a hangover: time. Of course, people ignore the prevention and don't have "time" for the cure. So, here are some remedies to ease the suffering for those who have had one drink too many.

DIETARY REMEDIES

Bananas. Bananas are your best friend! While you were drunk and peeing like a racehorse, lots of potassium drained from your body. Eating a banana bursting with potassium will give you some giddy-up and go. All you have to do is peel and eat.

Honey and Lemon. The classic hot toddy (nonalcoholic, of course) is honey, lemon, and hot water. Easy to swallow, this beverage replenishes fluids and sugars lost to a hangover. It is vital, however, to use honey instead of white sugar. Honey contains fructose, which competes for the metabolism of alcohol. Some healthy competition is needed, since it prevents the rapid change in alcohol levels that results in headaches. Plain sugar contains sucrose, which isn't absorbed as quickly. To make a toddy, boil 1 cup water and mix in honey and lemon juice to taste. Enjoy a toddy several times per day.

Juice. Juice, especially freshly squeezed orange juice, will help raise your blood sugar levels and help ease some of your hangover symptoms. However, if your stomach is upset, skip acidic juices such as orange juice and stick with apple juice instead.

Rice, Soup, or Toast. Food is probably the last thing you want to look at while recovering, but you do need some substance for 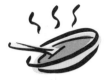 energy. Stay with clear liquids until you can tolerate something solid. Then start off slowly with mild, easy-to-digest foods such as plain toast, rice, or clear soup.

Sports drinks. These are a good way to replace fluids as well as electrolytes and glucose.

Water. Next to time, drinking water is the best cure for a hangover. Dehydration does a doozy on your body and causes much of the discomfort associated with a hangover. Stick to water, be it tap, bottled, or carbonated. Drink more than 8 glasses per day while recovering.

HERBAL REMEDIES

Gingerroot. Ginger has long been used to treat nausea and seasickness. And, since having a hangover is much like being seasick, this easy remedy works wonders. If you're really green, the best bet is to drink ginger ale. (No preparation required, but be sure to choose a brand that actually contains ginger!) If you can remain vertical for 10 minutes, brew some ginger tea. Cut 10 to 12 slices of fresh ginger root and combine with 4 cups water. Boil for 10 minutes. Strain and add the juice of 1 orange, the juice of ½ lemon, and ½ cup honey. Drink to your relief.

TOPICAL REMEDIES

Ice. Put an ice compress on your aching head. Place crushed ice in a plastic bag, wrap in a dry towel,

WHEN TO CALL THE DOCTOR
- If a person passes out from too much alcohol
- If you are severely dehydrated
- If symptoms don't improve after a few days' rest
- If drinking in excess becomes a habit. Seek professional help.

HANGOVER CURE MYTHS

Myth #1: A strong cuppa joe cures a hangover.

If only it were as easy as stopping off at Starbucks! Coffee does little, if anything, to help you sober up and may, in fact, work against you. Like alcohol, coffee is a diuretic and can further dehydrate your system. Moreover, the acidic nature of coffee can sour a sensitive stomach. What coffee can do is ease your aching headache by constricting blood vessels, but it does so at a price. Instead of brewing a cuppa, it's a better (and easier) idea to take two nonaspirin pain relievers, especially acetaminophen. Aspirin can aggravate the stomach.

Myth #2: Slurp a raw egg and sober up.

You really have to be drunk to handle this unappetizing cure. Besides the strong possibility of vomiting, you risk salmonella poisoning if you down an uncooked egg. Another cure, equally repulsive, is the Prairie Oyster concoction: 1 egg yolk, a dash of Worcestershire sauce, a dash of ketchup, ½ ounce port, a celery stick, salt and pepper. That's one drink that makes even the sober shudder.

Myth #3: A morning-after drink will cure a hangover.

Along the lines of the "hair-of-the-dog-that-bit-you" philosophy, drinking a glass of what you drank the night before (or any other alcohol for that matter) won't help. A morning-after drink only recreates the problem and worsens symptoms.

Myth #4: Down a big, all-American breakfast for a quick cure.

Greasy bacon, runny eggs, and fried potatoes will send you running to the toilet faster than you can say "hangover cure." Your poor stomach, already irritated by alcohol, isn't prepared for this hard-to-digest, fatty trio. Give the tummy a break and stick to toast, perhaps with a little marmalade on top.

and apply it to where it hurts. Or just rinse a washcloth under cold water, place it on your forehead, and rest.

LIFESTYLE REMEDIES

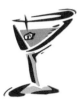 ***Drink to the night.*** If you can remember one thing while intoxicated, remember this: Guzzle plenty of water before going to bed. It will help nip dehydration, and you'll feel much better in the morning.

Never drink and drive.

Rest. Pull the shades down, unplug the telephone, and go to sleep.

Stick to 1 drink (or less) per hour, and sip it slowly. One hour is about the time it takes for the average adult body to process an alcoholic beverage. One drink is a 5-ounce glass of wine, a 12-ounce beer, or 1.5 ounce of hard liquor.

Take a multivitamin with B vitamins. This will replace those lost during your night of carousing.

Try Pepto-Bismol. Or take an antacid to relieve queasiness and settle your stomach.

Headaches
THWARTING THE THROBBING

The day starts with screaming kids, continues slowly onward with stop 'n' go traffic, and ends on a sour note with an angry boss. By this point, you are ready to chop your head off in order to relieve the pounding pain.

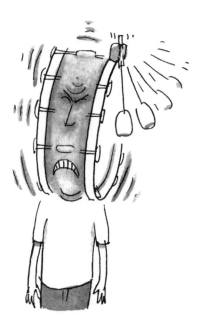

You can take a little comfort in knowing that almost everyone has had such a day...and such a headache. Yet some people fare worse than others do. An estimated 45 million Americans get chronic, recurring headaches, and as many as 25 million of those suffer from painful, debilitating migraines.

The Three Kinds of Headaches

Although there are nearly two dozen types of headaches, they all fall into three basic categories: tension, vascular, and organic.

Tension headaches, the most common of the trio, cause a dull, nonthrobbing pain, usually accompanied by tightness in the scalp or neck. Triggers range from depression to everyday stresses.

Vascular headaches are more intense, severe, throbbing, and piercing: They take first prize for pain. Cluster and migraine headaches fall into this category. Triggers for cluster headaches are unknown, although excessive smoking and alcohol consumption can ignite them. Migraines are thought to be caused by heredity, diet, stress, menstruation, and environmental factors such as cigarette smoke.

Less common are organic headaches, in which pain becomes increasingly worse and is accompanied by other symptoms, such as vomiting, coordination problems, visual disturbances, or speech or personality changes. Triggers include tumors, infections, or diseases of the brain, eyes, ears, and nose.

HERBAL REMEDY

If you suffer from recurring headaches, you might want to plant a little feverfew in your herb garden (or grow the herb in a windowsill pot). This lovely, easy-to-nurture herb has long been used as a headache remedy, especially for migraines. Feverfew causes blood vessels to dilate and inhibits the secretion of substances that cause pain and inflammation (such as histamine and serotonin) through the substance parthenolide.

You have two choices when it comes to taking feverfew: eating it raw or drinking it in a tea. If you prefer the au naturel way, chew on 2 to 3 of the bitter-tasting leaves each time you have a headache. (Don't exceed 4 leaves a day.) Feverfew may cause mouth irritation. Should this occur, place a leaf in a salad or sandwich. To make a tea, place 1 tablespoon dried feverfew into 1 cup boiling water. Steep for ten minutes, strain, and sip.

If you are prone to the usual tension headache, there are a variety of remedies that can help your throbbing head.

DIETARY REMEDIES

Avoid trigger foods. Some headache sufferers find their pain is set off by certain foods, such as aged cheese, processed meats, food additives, alcohol, very cold foods, MSG, or salty foods.

Peach juice. Drinking peach juice or apricot nectar may help alleviate the nausea that sometimes accompanies a bad headache. It is a well-tolerated drink for those suffering from nausea.

HERBAL REMEDIES

Peppermint. A dab of peppermint oil rubbed on the temples can ease a tension headache. Don't try this with children or if you have sensitive skin as the oil can have a burning effect.

Cloves and other spices. A blend of scented herbs eases tension headaches. Do you have dried marjoram, rosemary, and mint? They work well together. And if you have dried lavender and rose petals, they make wonderful additions to the mix. Put 4 tablespoons of each (or whichever you have) into a cloth sachet bag. Add 1 tablespoon cloves. Close the sachet bag, and whenever you have a headache or feel one coming on, hold the bag to your nose and inhale deeply until you feel it subsiding. A clean handkerchief works fine, too. You can also apply this bundle of herbs to your head when you rest.

Rosemary. Rosemary is a well-recognized folk cure in the United States, China, and Europe for easing pain. One of its constituents, rosmarinic acid, is an anti-inflammatory similar to aspirin and ibuprofen. Since rosmarinic acid is also an important constituent in sage, the two herbs are often combined to make a pain-relieving tea. Place 1 teaspoon crushed rosemary leaves and 1 teaspoon crushed sage leaves in a cup. Fill with boiling water. Cover to prevent the volatile oils from escaping, and steep until the tea reaches room temperature. Take ½-cup doses two to three times per day. You don't have to mix the two herbs to benefit from rosmarinic acid, however. If you only have one, make a tea of it alone.

TOPICAL REMEDIES

Alternating cold and heat. Some find relief when they alternate heat and cold for 10 minutes each.

Ice. For some, a washcloth dipped in ice-cold water and placed over the pain site helps relieve a headache. (For others, it aggravates it.) An ice compress  can work well, too. Place a handful of crushed ice cubes into a zipper-type plastic bag, and cover it with a dry washcloth. (A bag of frozen vegetables is a good substitute.) Apply where needed. Whatever method you use, try to apply the compress as soon as possible after the headache develops. Relief typically starts within 20 minutes of use.

Hot water. If snow is falling and the last thing you want on your head is an ice pack, turn to heat for soothing relief. Dip a washcloth into hot but not scalding water. Squeeze out and apply over your eyes or on the pain site. Leave the compress on for 30 minutes, rewarming as necessary.

LIFESTYLE REMEDIES

Check for tension. Many people unconsciously clench their jaw muscles, grip the steering wheel tightly, furrow their brows, or make fists when

PLEASURE AND PAIN

Ice cream, that summertime delight, can truly make you scream—or at least writhe in agony. Eating ice cream can cause an ice-cream headache, and anyone who has eaten an icy treat too fast knows the pain well. What sparks this headache is a change in mouth temperature. As the icy dessert touches the top of your mouth (or back of your throat), it causes a nerve reaction that swells blood vessels in the head. The result: an intense, shooting pain that lasts for 30 to 60 seconds. The cure: Spend more time licking your ice cream 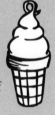 cone and less time gulping it down— and keep icy cold foods to the side of your mouth.

FASCINATING FACT

Onions to the rescue! The onion seemed to be the cure-all for many ailments back in the Middle Ages. Not only was it used to battle headaches, but the onion supposedly cured snakebites and hair loss.

WHEN TO CALL THE DOCTOR

- If you get daily headaches
- If you get headaches after intense coughing or sneezing
- If you have pain in the ear or eyes
- If you experience nausea or vomiting
- If you experience vision changes
- If you have hallucinations
- If you experience sensitivity to light and sound
- If you have weakness or dizziness
- If you experience loss of consciousness
- If you have a severe, debilitating headache

they're tense. All of these can lead to a headache. If you notice you're tense, force yourself to breathe slowly and deeply.

Don't smoke. Aside from the fact that it's unhealthful, smoking can give you a headache or make one worse.

Get regular exercise. When you exer-

cise, you release the physical and emotional tension that can trigger headaches. And aerobic exercise—the kind that gets your heart pumping, such as walking, jogging, and dancing—helps boost the body's production of endorphins, which are naturally occurring pain-relieving substances.

Rise and retire at the same time every day. That means seven days a week! Getting up and going to bed at the same time gives you a stable body rhythm. Oversleeping actually causes body chemistry changes that set off migraines and other kinds of headaches.

MORE DO'S AND DON'TS

- Lie down. Sometimes the best headache treatment is to go to bed and sleep. For some headaches, sleep interrupts the pain cycle.
- Keep it dark. Bright light, whether it's sunlight or the glare of a computer screen, can bring on a headache or make one you already have worse. If you're sensitive to light, wear sunglasses outdoors and adjust your blinds so that intense light doesn't hit your eyes. If you've already got a headache, darken the room where you're resting.

Heartburn
PUTTING OUT THE FIRE

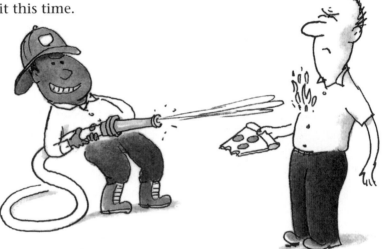

Boy, oh boy, did you do it this time. You added that heaping second helping to all the platter pickings you couldn't resist, and what do you have? Indigestion (an incomplete or imperfect digestion), that's what. And it may be accompanied by pain, nausea, vomiting, heartburn, gas, and belching. All this because you couldn't resist temptation. But don't worry. It happens to everybody, and it goes away.

So, now that you've eaten until you're about ready to burst, what's next? The couch, maybe? Stretch out, let your digestive system do its thing, take a nap?

Wrong! The worst thing you can do after a binge is to lie down. That can cause heartburn, also known as acid indigestion. Whatever you call it, it's the feeling you get when digestive acid escapes your stomach and irritates the esophagus, the tube that leads from your throat to your stomach. After you eat, heartburn can also fire up when you bend forward, exercise, and strain muscles.

Why Acid Backs Up

Occasionally the acid keeps on coming until you have a mouthful of something bitter and acidy. You may have some pain in your gut, too, or in your chest. Along with that acid may come a belch, one that may bring even more of that stomach acid with it.

The purpose of stomach acid is to break down the foods we eat so our body can digest them. Our stomachs have a protective lining that shields it

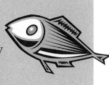
from those acids, but the esophagus does not have that protection. Normally that's not a problem, because after we swallow food, it passes down the esophagus, through a sphincter, and into the stomach. The sphincter then closes.

Occasionally, though, the muscles of that sphincter are weakened and it doesn't close properly or it doesn't close all the way. Scarring from an ulcer or frequent episodes of acid reflux (when the acid comes back up), stomach pressure from overeating, obesity, and pregnancy can all cause this glitch in the lower esophageal sphincter (LES). And when the LES gets a glitch and allows the gastric acid to splash out of the stomach, you get heartburn.

Generally, heartburn isn't serious. In fact, small amounts of reflux are normal and most people don't even notice it because the swallowing we do causes saliva to wash the acids right back down into the stomach where they belong. When the stomach starts shooting back amounts that are larger than normal, especially on a regular basis or over a prolonged period of time, that's when the real trouble begins, and simple heartburn can turn into esophageal inflammation or bleeding.

WHO'S PRONE TO HEARTBURN?

Just about anybody. According to the National Digestive Diseases Clearinghouse, 15 million adults suffer from heartburn daily and about 50 million Americans get gastroesophageal reflux and heartburn at least once a month.

There are several prescription medicines available for the treatment of long-term or serious heartburn or acid reflux, and over-the-counter remedies are available at your pharmacy too.

There are also several remedies right in your own home that can fight the fire of heartburn.

DIETARY REMEDIES

Almonds. Chewing 6 or 8 blanched almonds when you have heartburn may relieve the symptoms. Chew them well, though, to avoid swallowing air and causing yourself more discomfort.

Apples. They cool the burn of stomach acid. Eat them fresh, with the skin still on, or cook them for desserts.

Baking soda. Take ½ teaspoon in ½ glass water. Check the information on the box about antacid use before using this remedy, however. *Warning!* If you're on a salt-restricted diet, do not use baking soda. It's loaded with sodium. And do not use it if you're experiencing nausea, stomachache, gas, cramps, or stomach distention from overeating.

Buttermilk. This is an acid-reliever, but don't confuse it with regular milk, which can be an acid-maker, especially if you are bothered by lactose intolerance.

Cabbage. Like apples, this is a natural fire extinguisher for stomach burn. For the best relief, put the cabbage through a juicer, then drink it.

Cream of tartar. For an acid neutralizer, mix ½ teaspoon with ½ teaspoon baking soda in a glass of water. Take 1 teaspoon of the solution as needed.

Brown rice. Plain or with a little sweetening, rice can help relieve discomfort. Rice is a complex carbohydrate and is a bland food, which is less likely to increase acidity or relax the sphincter muscle.

OLD WIVES' TALE (OR NOT?)

Cabbage's ability to heal the digestive system has been known for 450 years, since 1557 when a Dutch doctor by the name of Drodens recorded the benefits of cabbage, especially in juice form. Taken a step further, there are many hearty Germans who swear by the internal healing properties of sauerkraut juice. If you have a taste for it, you may be able to find it in your grocery store. If not, look for it in a specialty market.

GUMMY FACTS

Gum-chewers are notorious air-swallowers. And air-swallowers are prone to indigestion. So if you're a gum-chewer who gets frequent indigestion, skip the gum for awhile to see if there's a connection.

If you are already suffering with a bout of heartburn, however, chewing sugarless gum can bring relief. It increases the flow of saliva, which washes down the acid. Skip the mint flavors and don't chew too much because that can lead to air-swallowing.

Fruit juices. Skip juices from citrus fruits, but try these stomach-cooling juices for heartburn relief: papaya, mango, guava, pear.

Papaya. Eat it straight to reap the benefit of its indigestion-fighting enzyme papain. Or drink 1 cup papaya juice combined with 1 teaspoon sugar and 2 pinches cardamom to relieve acid. *Warning!* Pregnant women should not eat papayas; they're a source of natural estrogen that can cause miscarriage.

Potato. Mix ½ cup raw potato juice with ½ cup water, and drink after meals. To make raw potato juice, simply put a peeled raw potato through a juicer or blender.

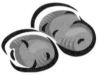

Soda crackers. This is an old folk cure that actually works. Soda crackers (preferably unsalted) are bland, they digest easily, and they absorb stomach acid. They also contain bicarbonate of soda and cream of tartar, which neutralize the acid. Tip: You know that package of soda crackers they always give you at the restaurant that you leave on the table? From now on, take them with you. These come in handy when you're plagued by heartburn and can't seek immediate relief.

Water. Drink water in between meals, not with meals. If you drink fluids with meals, you increase the volume of stomach contents, which makes it easier for heartburn to happen.

Yogurt. Make sure it has live cultures in it. Because of the helpful and digestive-friendly microorganisms in yogurt, it may sooth the acid-forming imbalances that can lead to heartburn. Choose low-fat or nonfat yogurt, as fat can aggravate heartburn.

HERBAL REMEDIES

Aloe vera gel. Mix 2 tablespoons aloe vera gel with a pinch of baking soda for quick heartburn relief.

Cardamom. This old-time digestive aid may help relieve the burn of acid indigestion. Add it to baked goodies such as sweet rolls or fruit cake, or sprinkle, with a pinch of cinnamon, on toast. It works well in cooked cereals, too.

Chicory. This herb is an acquired taste and is found most commonly in coffee. It can neutralize acid indigestion. Brew up a little tea with 3 tablespoons chicory root and 1 quart boiling water. Let it cool completely, then drink a cup whenever necessary.

Cinnamon. This is a traditional remedy for acid relief. Brew a cup of cinnamon tea from a cinnamon stick. Or try a commercial brand, but check the label. Cinnamon tea often has black tea in it, which is a cause of heartburn, so make sure the brand you buy doesn't contain black tea. For another acid-busting treat, make cinnamon toast.

Ginger. A tea from this root can soothe a burning belly. Add 1½ teaspoons gingerroot to

WHEN TO CALL THE DOCTOR

- If you've tried home remedies or over-the-counter medications and they're not working. Your heartburn could be a symptom of another ailment, such as an ulcer, gallbladder disease, or hiatal hernia.
- If heartburn happens on a prolonged or regular basis, even if home treatments are working.
- Call 9-1-1 or go to the nearest emergency room if you're experiencing chest pain that spreads into your arm, jaw, or shoulder, especially when accompanied by any of these symptoms: sweating, nausea, dizziness, shortness of breath, fainting. This could be a heart attack.

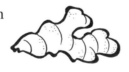

SAGE TEA

2½ cups boiling water
¼ cup fresh sage leaves
1 teaspoon sugar or honey
juice of ½ lemon

Combine ingredients and steep for 20 minutes. Strain and drink warm. The best relief comes from small, frequent doses.

CONSIDER YOUR OVER-THE-COUNTER ANTACID CHOICES

Choosing an over-
the-counter (OTC)
antacid is not always
as simple as grabbing the first box
or bottle you come to on the shelf.
Antacids come with their own
unique qualities as well as risks. If
a simple OTC is your choice, talk
with your doctor or pharmacist
about which is best for you. People
with high blood pressure, for
instance, should NOT take over-
the-counter antacids without first
checking with the doctor.

Ask your pharmacist about possible interactions with other drugs
you're taking. Most pharmacies
have readily available printouts
about drug interactions that are free
for the asking. In the meantime,
here are some common antacid
ingredients and their possible side-
effects.

- Aluminum hydroxide. Can cause
  constipation. Because there may
  be a link between Alzheimer's
  disease and aluminum, antacids
  with aluminum hydroxide are not
  recommended for people with, or
  who are at risk for, AD.
- Magnesium salts. May cause
  diarrhea. However, choosing an
  antacid containing both aluminum hydroxide and magnesium
  salts may balance out the consti-
  pation/diarrhea side effects.
- An antacid with alginic acid may
  prevent reflux.

1 cup water; simmer for ten minutes. Drink
as needed.

Sage. For a tea that can relieve stomach
weakness that allows acid to be released
back into the esophagus, see the Recipe
Box on the previous page.

Warning! If you are pregnant, talk with
your doctor before taking herbal remedies
for heartburn.

LIFESTYLE REMEDIES

Avoid foods that often trigger heartburn.
These include spicy or high-fat foods,
alcohol, chocolate, carbonated beverages,
and caffeinated drinks.

Don't eat right before bedtime. Give your
stomach a two- or three-hour break before
you sleep. And if you're plagued by the
burn at night, sleep with your head elevated on pillows.

Eat smaller meals. The more food in your
belly, the more likely that bulk will push
stomach acid right back up.

Eat slowly, chew thoroughly. Sometimes
heartburn will flare because the food is
simply too large to get through the digestive tract and it, along with the acids, is
forced back up.

Lose weight. All that baggage pushing in
on the abdomen increases pressure on the
stomach, which causes heartburn.

Keep a food diary. This can tell you which
foods or food combinations cause that
heartburn.

Let the gravity be with you. Stay upright
so the gastric contents are forced to stay

down. In other words, don't head for the couch after you eat. If you must snooze, try the recliner, but don't recline too steeply.

Quit smoking. Smoking can make heartburn worse.

Stay in shape. Heartburn hates people who are fit. Just don't exercise strenuously for a couple hours after a meal. Instead, go for a nice leisurely walk. This will help keep the stomach acid in its place.

MORE DO'S & DON'TS

- Loosen your belt. Tight clothing and belts can create enough pressure to cause heartburn.

THE USUAL SUSPECTS

Here's the food list that's commonly associated with heartburn. Cut back on these, or cut them out altogether, and see what happens:

Fried and fatty foods, pies, cakes, cookies, butter, margarine, oils, cream: These may weaken your lower esophageal sphincter (LES). Also, fatty foods take longer to digest, meaning the gastric juices are working overtime and have more opportunity to cause a backup.

Peppermint in any form*: It relaxes the stomach muscle and valve, allowing the release of acids back up into the esophagus.

Caffeinated beverages, such as coffee, tea, cola: Caffeine causes extra acid production.

Chocolate: It contains methylxanthines, a second cousin to caffeine, and can weaken the stomach valve.

Fruit and vegetable juices, especially tomato and citrus juice: They can irritate the throat and cause pain if heartburn has already caused irritation. Pineapple juice has an especially potent punch.

Garlic and onions: May weaken the LES.

Spicy, pickled, or fermented foods: These are heartburn-makers, too.

Alcohol: It causes the LES to relax.

Smoking and certain drugs such as aspirin, ibuprofen, and some antibiotics: These also relax the LES, causing acid reflux.

*Warning! Peppermint is often prescribed for other symptoms of indigestion but should never be used when heartburn is present.

Heart Disease
TENDING YOUR TICKER

The heart is an amazing structure, tough yet fragile. It's a muscle, and its network of arteries and veins transport blood through your body, nourishing organs and tissues. When the heart is working as it should, you barely notice it. But when your heart starts acting strangely, you have cause to worry. Thankfully, you live in a day when heart disease can be treated very successfully, and in some cases, the condition can even be reversed.

Heart Trouble

Heart disease is any condition that keeps your heart from functioning at its best or causes a deterioration of the heart's arteries and vessels. Coronary heart disease (CHD), also known as coronary artery disease, is the most common form of heart disease, affecting 16.8 million people in America and is the single leading cause of death.

If you are diagnosed with CHD, it means you have atherosclerosis, or hardening of the arteries. Arteries become hard when plaque accumulates on artery walls. This plaque develops gradually as an overabundance of low-density lipoprotein (LDL) cholesterol (the bad stuff) makes itself at home in your arteries. The plaque builds and narrows the artery walls, making it more and more difficult for blood to pass through the heart and increasing the opportunity for a blood clot to form. If the heart doesn't get enough blood, it can cause chest pain (angina) or a heart attack.

Not treating coronary heart disease can also lead to congestive heart failure (CHF). CHF happens when your heart isn't strong enough to pump blood throughout the body—it fails to meet the body's need for oxygen. This often causes congestion in the lungs and a variety of other problems for your heart and the rest of your body.

Honing In on Heart Disease

There are many risk factors for heart disease, some you can do something about, and some you can't. A family history of heart disease puts you at much greater risk for developing it yourself. While you can't do anything about your genes, there are a number of risk factors that you can control. These are the ones you can do something about:

- High levels of low-density lipoprotein (LDL) cholesterol (the bad stuff), and low levels of high-density lipoprotein (the good stuff) (See High Cholesterol, page 254).
- High levels of triglycerides. Triglyceride levels increase when you eat too many fatty foods or when you eat too much—excess calories are made into triglycerides and stored as fat in cells. Having an abundance of triglycerides has been linked to coronary heart disease.
- High blood pressure (see High Blood Pressure, page 248)
- Smoking
- Lack of regular exercise
- A high fat diet
- Being overweight or obese
- Diabetes (see Diabetes, page 131)
- Ongoing stress or depression

THE HEART OF A WOMAN

Heart disease isn't a subject that comes up much in discussions of women's health. But nearly twice as many women die of heart disease, stroke, and other cardio-vascular disease each year as from all kinds of cancer combined, including breast cancer. Each year, 1 out of every 2 women who die do so from heart disease or stroke, but only 1 in 35 will die of breast cancer. It seems heart disease needs a little more attention by the gentler gender. Estrogen helps reduce the risk of coronary heart disease (CHD), which is why younger women are less prone to heart attacks than men. But after menopause, when estrogen levels drop, women are on equal footing with men in their risk for getting CHD.

How to Know If You Have Heart Disease

Many people who have heart disease don't even know it until something serious happens. That's why it's a good idea to see your doctor for a regular checkup and to have your cholesterol and triglyceride levels and your blood pressure checked and monitored. If you experience any of these symptoms, schedule a checkup as soon as you can.

- Chest pain (angina). If you feel like you have an elephant sitting on your chest after climbing the stairs, your body could be giving you a warning signal.
- Shortness of breath. This is especially noticeable after a game of one-on-one with your daughter or an intense meeting with your boss.
- Nausea or stomach upset. This could be more than the guacamole you ate at dinner, especially if you have recurrent bouts of tummy trouble.
- Sweating. Even when you haven't been exercising.
- Feeling weak or tired.

DIETARY REMEDIES

Bran. Bran cereal is a high-fiber food that will help keep your cholesterol levels in check. Other high fiber foods in your cupboard include barley; oats; whole grains such as brown rice and lentils; and beans, such as kidney beans and black beans.

Broccoli. Calcium is another heart-healthy nutrient, and milk isn't the only calcium-rich food. In fact, there are lots of nondairy foods that are rich in calcium, such as kale, salmon, figs, pinto beans, and okra. One cup of broccoli can supply you with 90 mg of calcium.

Chicken. Three ounces of chicken will give you one-third of your daily requirement for vitamin B6, a necessary nutrient for maintaining heart health.

Dark Chocolate. Now you've got an excuse to indulge (a little) in chocolate—as long as it's dark chocolate. Research shows 6.7 grams (0.23 ounces) per day can significantly reduce the arterial inflammation that leads to cardiovascular disease.

Olive oil. The American Heart Association and the American Dietetic Association recommend getting most of your fat from monounsaturated sources. Olive oil is a prime candidate. Try using it instead of other vegetable oils when sautéing your veggies.

 Nuts. The amount of evidence supporting the beneficial effects of nuts on heart health convinced the U.S. Food and Drug Administration (FDA) to approve a qualified health claim for certain nuts in 2003. Producers of almonds, walnuts, pecans, hazelnuts, pistachios, and peanuts can now say on their package labels and ads that "scientific evidence suggests, but does not prove, that eating 1.5 ounces per day of most nuts, as part of a diet low in saturated fat and cholesterol, may reduce the risk of heart disease."

Peanut butter. Eat 2 tablespoons of this comforting food and you can get one-third of your daily intake of vitamin E. Because vitamin E is a fat-soluble vitamin (other antioxidant vitamins are water soluble), it is found more abundantly in fattier foods like vegetable oils and nuts. If you're watching your weight, don't go overboard on the peanut butter because it is high in calories.

HEARTWARMING NEWS
The number of deaths from heart attack declined 19 percent between 1995 and 2005.

Pecans. These tasty nuts are full of magnesium, another heart-friendly nutrient. One ounce of pecans sprinkled over a spinach salad can give you one-third of your recommended daily allowance of this vital mineral.

Salmon. Adding fatty fish to your diet is a good idea if you're at risk for heart disease. Three ounces of salmon meets your daily requirement for vitamin B_{12}, a vitamin 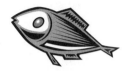 that helps keep your heart healthy, and it's a good source of omega-3 fatty acids, which have been proven to lower triglycerides and reduce blood clots that could potentially block arteries in the heart.

Spinach. Make yourself a salad using spinach instead of the usual iceberg lettuce and get a good start on meeting your folic acid needs (½ cup has 130 mcg of folic acid). Along with the other B vitamins, B_6 and B_{12}, folic acid can help prevent heart disease.

 Strawberries. Oranges aren't the only fruit loaded with vitamin C. You can fill up on 45 milligrams of the heart-healthy vitamin with ½ cup of summer's sweet berry. Vitamin C is an antioxidant vital to maintaining a happy heart. Strawberries are also a good source of fiber and potassium, both important to heart health.

Sweet potatoes. With double your daily requirements for vitamin A, a heart-protecting nutrient, sweet potatoes are a smart choice for fending off heart disease.

Tea. Both black tea and green tea are good for your heart, but you do need to drink quite a lot. A reduced risk of heart disease and stroke has been linked with drinking 3 cups of black tea in one study and 6 cups of black tea in another. And a Japanese study reported in the Journal of the American Medical Association in 2006 showed a 26 percent decrease in cardiovascular disease risk in people who drank more than 5 cups of green tea per day.

Whole-wheat bread. Slather some peanut butter on a slice of whole-wheat bread and you've got a snack that's good to your heart. One slice of whole-wheat bread has 11 mcg of selenium, an antioxidant mineral that works with vitamin E to protect your heart.

Wine. Research is finding that drinking a glass of alcohol a day may help in the battle against heart disease. Health experts are quick to note that alcohol in moderate amounts is helpful. They  define moderate as one glass a day for women and two glasses of alcohol a day for men—although women who are at high risk for breast cancer should avoid alcohol because even small amounts raise your risk of developing the disease. What's in one drink? Twelve ounces of beer, five ounces of wine, or 1.5 ounces of hard liquor.

Herbal Remedies

 Garlic. Chock full of antioxidants, garlic seems to be able to decrease plaque buildup, reduce the incidence of chest pain, and keep the heart generally healthy. It is also a mild anticoagulant, helping to thin the blood. The advantages may take some time: One study found that it took a

When to Call the Doctor

- If you have any symptoms in "How To Know If You Have Heart Disease," page 236. However, if you have any of the following symptoms, go to the nearest emergency room or call 9-1-1 immediately:
- Painful pressure or squeezing in the chest that lasts for a few minutes or goes away and returns
- Pain that radiates to the shoulders, neck, or arms
- Lightheadedness, fainting, sweating, nausea, or shortness of breath along with chest pain.

couple of years of eating garlic daily to get its heart-healthy benefits.

LIFESTYLE REMEDIES

Coenzyme Q-10. This nutrient, found in fatty fish, is not classified as a vitamin or a mineral. But studies have found that it is necessary for heart health. Coenzyme Q-10 re-energizes heart cells, especially in people who have already been diagnosed with heart failure. It blocks the process that creates plaque buildup in the arteries and helps lower blood pressure. It has been used to treat congestive heart failure in Japan for decades. Talk to your doctor before trying the supplement.

Don't be a smoke stack. People who smoke are twice as likely to have a heart attack.

Eat healthy. The American Heart Association (AHA) suggests getting 25 to 35 percent of your calories from fat. Less than 7 percent should be the saturated kind and less than 1 percent should be *trans* fat. You should get no more than 300 mg of cholesterol per day.

Get moving. Your heart is a muscle, and if you don't exercise it, it will get weaker.

Pass on the salt. A low-sodium diet can help control high blood pressure, a risk factor for heart disease. Healthy people should eat no more than 2,300 mg of sodium per day. Some people—African Americans, middle-age and older adults, and people with high blood pressure—should keep their sodium intake under 1,500 mg daily, according to the AHA.

Watch your weight. Even 10 to 20 pounds of extra weight for a person of average height increases the risk of death, especially for people between the ages of 30 and 64.

Hemorrhoids
DEALING WITH DISCOMFORT

Hemorrhoids are a sore subject, and millions of people suffer from them. Also known as "piles," hemorrhoids are swollen, stretched out veins that line the anal canal and lower rectum. Internal hemorrhoids may either bulge into the anal canal or protrude out through the anus (these are called prolapsed). External hemorrhoids occur under the surface of the skin near the anal opening. Both types hurt, burn, itch, irritate, and bleed.

About half of Americans will develop hemorrhoids before age 50. Most cases are caused by constipation or physical strain during a bowel movement. Other causes include heredity, age, constipation from a low fiber diet, obesity, improper use of laxatives, pregnancy, anal intercourse, prolonged sitting, and prolonged standing.

Fortunately, most hemorrhoids respond well to home treatments and changes in the diet, so you can keep this sore point under wraps.

DIETARY REMEDIES
Oranges. Vitamin C plays a role in strengthening and toning blood vessels, so eat lots of vitamin C-rich fruits and vegetables.

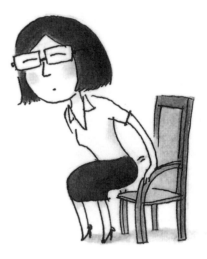

Prunes. Prunes have a laxative effect and help soften stools. Try to eat 1 to 3 per day.

Water. Think of water as the plumber of the digestive tract, without the $85-an-hour fee. Water keeps the digestive process moving along without block-ups—one of the main causes of hemorrhoids. Drink a minimum of 8 large glasses of water and other fluids, such as juice, per day and eat plenty of water-loaded fruits and vegetables.

TOPICAL REMEDIES
Ice. This remedy will wake you up and soothe hemorrhoid pain. Break ice into

THE HEALING BENEFITS OF WITCH HAZEL

Witch hazel has long been used as a soothing, cooling astringent for hemorrhoid pain, itching, and bleeding. It has anti-inflammatory properties and, when applied to hemorrhoids, tightens up the tissues and stanches bleeding. A dab of witch hazel applied to the outer rectum with a cotton ball (after dry wiping) is one of the best and easiest remedies available for external hemorrhoids. Give your hemorrhoids a cool treat by keeping a bottle of witch hazel refrigerated. You can also make a compress soaked in witch hazel and leave it on your bottom while resting.

small cubes (easier for the ice to shape itself around certain regions), and place it in a plastic, reclosable bag. Cover with a thick paper towel and  sit on it! The ice numbs the region and reduces blood flow to those distended veins.

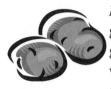 **Potato.** A poultice made from grated potato works as an astringent and soothes pain. Take 2 washed potatoes, cut them into small chunks, and put them into a blender. Process until the potatoes are in liquid form. Add a few teaspoons water if they look dry. Spread the mashed taters into a thin gauze bandage or clean handkerchief, fold in half, and apply to the hemorrhoids for five to ten minutes.

Warning! Some folk remedies have you place raw potato pieces in places that don't see the light of day. Don't use potatoes or any other food as a suppository without first talking to your doctor.

Vinegar. Applying a dab of apple cider or plain vinegar to hemorrhoids stops itching and burning. The vinegar has astringent properties that help shrink swollen blood vessels. After dry wiping, dip a cottonball in vinegar and apply.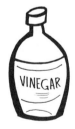

HERBAL REMEDIES

Aloe vera. The anti-inflammatory constituents in the aloe vera plant help reduce the irritation of hemorrhoids. Break off a piece of the leaf and apply only the clear gel to the hemorrhoids.

Chamomile. German folk medicine uses chamomile to treat hemorrhoids. It contains strong anti-inflammatory substances that may reduce the pain or itching associated with hemorrhoids. Combine 1 ounce dried chamomile with 2 quarts boiling water to make a tea. Let steep until warm. 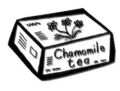 Pour the tea into a tub deep enough to sit in and soak for 15 minutes. If possible, bathe two to three times per day for acute hemorrhoids. Or, you can make the tea and apply it to the hemorrhoids with a cotton ball after having a bowel movement. Do not use chamomile if you have pollen allergies.

Witch Hazel. Put some on a cotton ball and apply to the anal area. Witch hazel is an astringent that can help relieve itching and pain and reduce swelling of hemorrhoids.

LIFESTYLE REMEDIES

Get off the pot. Avoid straining during a bowel movement. Don't sit on the throne if you're not doing business.

Exercise. Regular aerobic exercise helps the digestive system work more efficiently.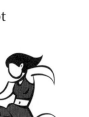

Easy does it. After a bowel movement, don't vigorously clean yourself with dry toilet paper. Buy premoistened wipes designed for anal care or, after gently wiping with toilet paper, apply the witch hazel or the vinegar remedy (mentioned previously) to clean yourself.

Soak in the tub. A bath does much to soothe inflamed tissues and ease pain. Take a sitz bath three to four times per day for 30 minutes at a time. If you don't have time, try a mini-soak. Apply a washcloth moistened with warm water to the hemorrhoids for a few minutes a few times per day.

WHEN TO CALL THE DOCTOR
- If you have rectal bleeding. Although rectal bleeding is associated with hemorrhoids, it can also be a warning sign of colon and rectal cancer.
- If you are pregnant and develop hemorrhoids
- If you are in pain

Hiccups
INTERRUPTING THE PATTERN

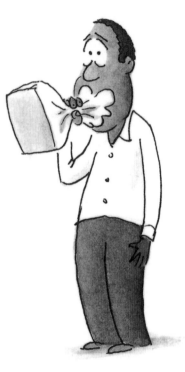

Even before you were born, you got the hiccups. Just ask your mom. And those strange muscle spasms will continue to come over you for the rest of your days. Everyone gets hiccups, but thankfully most people only deal with a case of them three to five times a year. Most bouts with the hiccups are pretty short-lived, lasting at most a few hours. Hiccups can be somewhat embarrassing, though. Imagine hiccuping through a first date or, worse, making a sales presentation you've worked on for months and letting out a loud "hic" right as you move in for the kill.

How You Hiccup

Having a little biological background on hiccups may not cure your case, but it can ease your mind about what's going on in your body. A hiccup starts as your diaphragm (the muscle that separates your lungs and heart from your stomach and intestines) has an involuntary spasm. As the diaphragm involuntarily contracts, it causes your glottis, the flap of skin that covers the windpipe, to close. The breath you started to take can't get through, and you make that loud "hic" noise in response to the blocked breath. The reflex of the diaphragm and glottis is similar to the one you get when the doctor taps on your knee.

One of the physiological reasons experts give for hiccups is an irritation of the nerve that leads from the brain to the abdominal area. Aggravating this nerve starts a chain reaction that touches off

> ### HOW MANY HICCUPS CAN A HICCUP HIC?
> Most people have between 4 and 12 hiccups per minute. In more severe cases, you may hiccup as many as 100 times in one minute. That's one hiccup every 0.6 seconds.

the nerve that activates the diaphragm. But what sets the nerve off in the first place?

Why Hiccups Happen

You get the hiccups for all sorts of reasons. Digestive disturbances, such as eating too fast, eating too much, eating an irritating food, or eating hot and cold foods together, are frequent triggers. Alcohol and fizzy drinks have been blamed for hiccups, and some experts believe they can be caused by emotional stress. But sometimes they occur for no reason. You may be sitting quietly reading a book, when all of a sudden, "hic!" There's no one reason why you get hiccups, and there's no one way to get rid of them!

Halting Your Hiccups

Hiccups are one problem that literally everyone and their grandmother has a cure for. But the truth is, there's not much scientific basis to most home remedies, and what works once may not work again. Most cures involve interrupting your breathing pattern, causing you to take a deep breath or an irregular breath (such as breathing while you swallow). But when you've got the hiccups, you will try almost anything to get rid of them. So any or all of these home cures may be worth a shot.

DIETARY REMEDIES

Honey. Try swallowing a tablespoon of honey. This overwhelms the mouth with a sweet flavor and may short-circuit the irritated nerve.

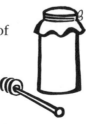

Ice. Drink a glass of ice water—a cold drink is believed to shock the system. Or simply apply a piece of ice to the back of the

THE SECRET'S IN THE SWALLOW

Many remedies for hiccups are designed to get you to do one thing—swallow. Gulping down a drink seems to disrupt the diaphragm function that keeps you hiccuping. Some folk remedies say that swallowing nine times quickly does the trick, while others say five or seven times. No matter, it's the quick swallow action that seems to make the remedy so effective. Drinking a glass of plain old water should suffice, but folk-medicine healers believe one of these items may be worth a swallow: dill seeds, peanut butter, sugar, lemonade, strong coffee, water, crushed ice, or cold carbonated water.

GYPSY HICCUP CURE

This herbal tea is believed to have sedative and antispasmodic properties, which could bring you some relief, especially if your hiccups seem to return often.

Take a handful each of dried valerian root, blackberry leaf, fennel seeds, chamomile flowers, peppermint leaf, and sage leaf.

Crush the herbs and mix well in a bowl.

Place 2 tablespoons of the herbs in a 1-pint jar. Fill the jar with boiling water and cover. Allow to steep for 10 to 15 minutes and strain.

Drink 1 cup warm tea three times per day for as long as ten days.

neck. This may shock your body and cause you to take a deep breath.

Lemon. Lemons are believed to overwhelm irritated nerves with a sour taste. This may divert the nerves' attention and get rid of your hiccups.

Pineapple juice. Some think the acidic content of the juice helps stop the hiccups.

Sugar. Experts give a thumbs-up to this remedy. Simply place a spoonful of sugar in your mouth, toward the back of the tongue where tastes are detected. This will enhance the sweet overload you're delivering.

Water. Bartenders swear by this hiccup-relieving trick—quickly downing a glass of water with a spoon in it. The swallowing is probably the reason the hiccups go away, but the spoon seems to take the person's mind off their hiccups. And some people believe gargling with water relieves the hiccups.

HERBAL REMEDIES

Dill seed. Swallowing a teaspoon of dill seeds is an old folk remedy that may work for you. No one is sure if it's an ingredient in the dill seeds that helps or if simply swallowing the seeds is what does the trick.

TOPICAL REMEDIES

Cotton swab. Tickling the roof of your mouth with a cotton swab, or your finger, may help cure your hiccups.

Paper bag. Breathing into a paper bag will increase the amount of carbon dioxide in your body. Since your body takes that as a signal of suffocation, your respiratory system urges the body to take deeper breaths. Those deeper breaths may stop the diaphragm spasm. This method is a favorite in hospitals.

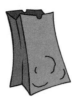

Stick 'em up. Putting your hands over your head may help you breathe a bit deeper and lessen the tension on the diaphragm.

Stick it in your ear. Putting your fingers in your ears seems to have some scientific merit in curing hiccups. It works by rerouting the action of the irritated nerve that sparks hiccups. Just be careful not to stick those fingers in too far and cause damage to your inner ear.

Stick out your tongue. Or pull on your tongue. These actions stimulate the glottis and may help keep it open (a closed glottis causes that hiccuping sound)—averting your hiccups. Pulling on your tongue also may stimulate your diaphragm and stop its annoying spasms.

Suck it in. Holding your breath works in much the same way that breathing into a paper bag does. It overwhelms your body with carbon dioxide and causes deeper breathing.

MORE DO'S AND DON'TS

- Take an antacid. A couple of antacid tablets may help quiet suspect digestive nerves.
- Get scared. Having someone sneak up on you may shock your body and change your breathing, relieving that "hic!"

WHEN TO CALL THE DOCTOR

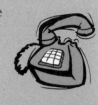

- If you have hiccups that last for more than 24 hours. There are certain diseases and infections that can be signaled by a lasting case of the hiccups.
- If you keep having regular bouts with hiccups

High Blood Pressure
REVERSING THE TREND

Sometimes what you don't know *can* hurt you. Such is the case with high blood pressure, or hypertension. Although one in three adults has high blood pressure, according to the American Heart Association (AHA), about 20 percent of them don't know they have it.

That's because high blood pressure often has no symptoms. It's not as if you feel the pressure of your blood coursing through your circulatory system. When the heart beats, it pumps blood to the arteries, creating pressure within them. That pressure can be normal or it can be excessive. High blood pressure is defined as a persistently elevated pressure of blood within the arteries.

Over time, the excessive force exerted against the arteries damages and scars them. It can also damage organs, such as the heart, kidneys, and brain. High blood pressure can lead to strokes, blindness, kidney failure, and heart failure.

In 90 to 95 percent of all cases, the cause of high blood pressure isn't known. In such cases, when there is no underlying cause, the disease is known as primary, or essential, hypertension. Sometimes the high blood pressure is caused by another disease, such as an endocrine disorder. In such cases, the disease is called secondary hypertension.

> **FASCINATING FACT**
> High blood pressure killed 57,356 Americans in 2005. From 1995 to 2005, there was a 25 percent increase in the death rate from high blood pressure.

Who's at Risk?

Although no one knows the exact cause of hypertension, there are specific factors that put you at risk of developing it. These include:

- Age. The older you are, the greater the likelihood of developing hypertension.
- Weight. The heavier you are, the greater your risk of hypertension.
- Race. African Americans are more prone to developing high blood pressure—and at an earlier age—than Caucasians and Asian Americans.
- Heredity. If high blood pressure runs in your family, you have an increased chance of developing it.
- Alcohol use. Heavy drinking increases blood pressure.
- Sodium consumption. Too much salt in your diet will do you in if you're sodium sensitive.
- A sedentary lifestyle. Couch potatoes are at an increased risk for hypertension.
- Pregnancy. Some expectant mothers experience elevated blood pressure.
- Oral contraceptives. Some women who take birth control pills develop hypertension, especially if other risk factors are also present.

What to Look For

Hypertension is known as "the silent killer" because it has few or no obvious symptoms. The symptoms that it does present are shared by other diseases and conditions. But if you have any of these symptoms, be sure to have your blood pressure checked to rule out high blood pressure:

- Frequent or severe headaches
- Unexplained fatigue

TASTY, NOT SALTY

Americans nearly preserve themselves with salt. The average American consumes between 3,000 and 6,000 mg of sodium each day. (The maximum intake suggested is 2,300 mg, which is about the amount in a level teaspoon of salt.) A diet high in salt, or sodium chloride, is directly linked to high blood pressure in salt-sensitive individuals, so start on the road to lower blood pressure by waving bye-bye to the saltshaker. There are several salt-free substitutes you can purchase, or you can make your own salt-free substitute that will spice up your meals without compromising your health.

- Dizziness
- Flushing of the face
- Ringing in the ears
- Thumping in the chest
- Frequent nosebleeds

Diagnosis

Finding out whether you have high blood pressure is simple. You just need to have your blood pressure checked by a doctor, nurse, or other health professional. Often you can even find blood pressure check booths at your local mall or at the pharmacy. The blood pressure test is simple, quick, and painless, but the results can save your life.

A blood pressure reading is given in two numbers, one over the other. The higher (systolic) number represents the pressure while the heart is beating, indicating how hard your heart has to beat to get that blood moving. The lower (diastolic) number represents the pressure when the heart is resting between beats.

Blood pressure of less than 120 (systolic) over 80 (diastolic) is considered a normal reading for adults, according to the AHA. A reading equal to 120 to 139 over 80 to 89 is considered prehypertension, and a reading greater than 140 over 90 is considered hypertension (high). Blood pressure higher than 120/80 should be watched carefully.

The key to controlling high blood pressure is knowing you have it. Under the guidance of a physician, you can battle hypertension through diet, exercise, lifestyle changes, and medication, if necessary. The home holds several blood pressure helpers.

DIETARY REMEDIES

Bananas. Potassium-rich bananas have been proved to help reduce blood pressure. The average person needs several servings of potassium-rich fruits and vegetables each day.

If bananas aren't your favorite fruit, try dried apricots, raisins, currants, orange juice, spinach, boiled potatoes with skin, baked sweet potatoes, cantaloupe, and winter squash, as well as fish and low-fat dairy foods.

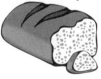

Breads. Be good to your blood with a bit more "B," as in the B vitamin folate. Swimming around the blood is a substance called homocysteine, which at high levels is thought to reduce the stretching ability of the arteries. If the arteries are stiff as a board, the heart pumps extra hard to move the blood around. Folate helps reduce the levels of homocysteine, in turn helping arteries become pliable. You'll find folate in fortified breads and cereals, asparagus, brussels sprouts, and beans.

Broccoli. This vegetable is high in fiber, and a high fiber diet is known to help reduce blood pressure. So indulge in this and other fruits and vegetables that are high in fiber.

Celery. Because it contains high levels of 3-N-butylphthalide, a phytochemical that helps lower blood pressure, celery is in a class by itself. This phytochemical is not found in most other vegetables. Celery may also reduce stress hormones that constrict blood vessels, so it may be most effective in those whose high blood pressure is the result of mental stress.

SALT WEARS MANY DISGUISES

Sodium chloride isn't the only name for salt. Labels that list soda or sodium also contain salt.

- Monosodium glutamate (MSG) is a popular flavor enhancer in restaurant cooking and in packaged and canned foods and seasoning mixes.
- Baking soda (sodium bicarbonate or bicarbonate of soda) and baking power are often used to leaven breads and cakes.
- Disodium phosphate is found in some quick-cooking cereals and processed cheeses.
- Sodium alginate is used by some manufacturers to make ice cream smooth.
- Sodium benzoate is used as a preservative in many condiments.
- Sodium hydroxide is used to soften and loosen skins of ripe olives and certain fruits and vegetables.
- Sodium nitrate is used to cure meats and sausages.
- Sodium propionate helps inhibit the growth of mold in baked goods.
- Sodium sulfite is used to bleach foods that will then be colored or glazed. It's also used as a preservative in some dried fruits.

Cocoa and chocolate. A 2007 review of 10 studies of chocolate's effects on blood pressure indicated that flavonoid-rich cocoa and chocolate can be part of a blood-pressure-lowering diet as long as the total calorie count of the diet stays the same. On average, chocolate products lowered systolic pressure by 4 to 5 points and diastolic pressure by to 2 to 3 points—enough to lower heart-disease risk by 10 percent and stroke risk by 20 percent.

Milk. The calcium in milk does more than build strong bones; it plays a modest role in preventing high blood pressure. Be sure to drink skim milk or eat low-fat yogurt. Leafy green vegetables also provide calcium.

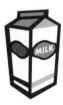

Polyunsaturated oils. Switching to polyunsaturated oils, such as canola, mustard seed, or safflower, can make a big difference in your blood pressure readings. Switching to them will also reduce your blood cholesterol level.

HERBAL REMEDIES

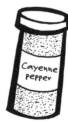

Cayenne pepper. This fiery spice is a popular home treatment for mild elevated blood pressure. Cayenne pepper allows smooth blood flow by preventing platelets from clumping together and accumulating in the blood. Add a dash of cayenne to a salad or salt-free soups.

LIFESTYLE REMEDIES

Avoid strength training exercise, such as weight lifting, unless you first consult with your doctor. This kind of exercise can be dangerous for people with hypertension.

Do aerobic exercise. Aerobic exercise that elevates your pulse and sustains the elevation for at least

20 minutes will help reduce your blood pressure if you do it several times a week. It will also help you lose weight, which will help lower your blood pressure. Check with your doctor before starting an exercise program if you've been sedentary.

Lose the saltshaker. Although there is some debate about salt's role in high blood pressure, most experts agree that cutting back on salt intake can reduce blood pressure.

Quit smoking. Smoking causes blood pressure to rise, and it increases your risk of stroke.

Skip processed foods. They're loaded with sodium (salt) and high in saturated (read: artery-clogging) fat. Read labels, as it's not always obvious which foods contain the most sodium and saturated fat.

Vitamin C. An antioxidant, vitamin C helps prevent free radicals from damaging artery walls, and it may help lower high blood pressure. Take a supplement or eat foods rich in vitamin C.

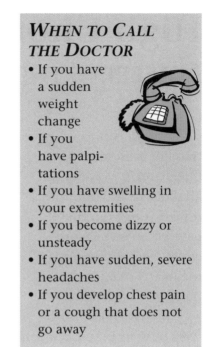

WHEN TO CALL THE DOCTOR

- If you have a sudden weight change
- If you have palpitations
- If you have swelling in your extremities
- If you become dizzy or unsteady
- If you have sudden, severe headaches
- If you develop chest pain or a cough that does not go away

AN HERBAL REMEDY

Lemon balm relaxes blood vessels, helping to reduce blood pressure. There are two ways to enjoy balm's benefits: as a tea on cold days and as a sorbet on hot ones. To make the tea, use a handful of crushed fresh leaves per teapot of boiling water. Let steep for ten minutes, strain, and enjoy.

For a cool sensation, try lemon balm sorbet:

  2 large apples, peeled and chopped
  Leaves from 6 lemon balm sprigs
  2 cups water
  1 cup honey
  Juice of 2 lemons

Puree apples and lemon balm in a blender or food processor. Transfer puree to a saucepan, add water and honey. Simmer over low heat until thick and bubbly. Strain. Add lemon juice, stir briskly, and cook. Place mixture in an ice cream maker and freeze. If you don't have an ice-cream maker, freeze as usual and then blend the mixture just before serving. Enjoy as a dessert or between courses.

High Cholesterol
LOWERING THE NUMBERS

Cholesterol is that waxy, soft stuff that floats around in your bloodstream as well as in all the cells in your body. It takes a bad rap these days because the word cholesterol strikes fear in the hearts of even the healthiest of people.

Having some cholesterol in your blood is normal, and it's even healthy because cholesterol is used in the formation of cell membranes, tissues, and essential hormones. So, in proper amounts, cholesterol is good. In excessive amounts, though, it can clog the arteries and cause coronary disease, heart attack, or stroke.

Cholesterol comes from two sources: the foods you eat and your very own liver. And the truth of the matter is, your liver can produce all the cholesterol your body will ever need. This means that what you get in your food isn't necessary. Some people get rid of extra cholesterol easily through normal bodily waste mechanisms, but others hang on to it because their bodies just aren't as efficient in removing it, which puts them at risk.

So, what makes people prone to high blood cholesterol?

- Family history
- Eating too many foods high in saturated fats
- Diabetes
- Kidney and liver disorders
- Alcoholism
- Obesity
- Smoking
- Stress

Good and Bad Cholesterol?

There are two kinds of cholesterol, and yes, one's good and one's bad. Cholesterol can't get around on its own, so it hitches a ride from lipoproteins to get to the body's cells. Problem is, there are two different rigs picking it up: One is called HDL, or high-density lipoprotein, the other is called LDL, or low-density lipoprotein. HDL is the good ride; it travels away from your arteries. LDL is the bad ride; it heads straight to your arteries. Bottom line: You want more HDL and less LDL.

High cholesterol can be cured two ways: by medication and by diet. There are numerous effective drugs on the market that will make drastic reductions in cholesterol levels, but they all come with side effects and require frequent blood tests to monitor for possible problems. But there are home remedies that may work on their own or along with conventional treatment. Whatever your cure, it must come with advice from your doctor since your heart is at risk.

DIETARY REMEDIES

Almonds. Studies indicate that snacking on almonds regularly for as few as three weeks may decrease LDL by as much as 10 percent.

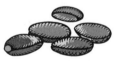

Honey. Add 1 teaspoon honey to 1 cup hot water in the morning, and you may rid your system of excess fat and cholesterol, according to Ayurvedic medicine. Add 1 teaspoon lime juice or 10 drops cider vinegar to give that drink a more powerful cholesterol-fighting punch.

Apples. Apples are high in pectin, which can lower cholesterol levels.

Artichokes. These veggies can actually lower cholesterol levels. Early studies pointed to their beneficial cholesterol-busting

---

CHOLESTEROL COUNTER

- The average American male gets 337 mg cholesterol per day from the food he eats.
- The average American female gets 217 mg cholesterol per day from the food she eats.
- The American Heart Association recommends limiting cholesterol from food to no more than 300 mg. For people with coronary disease, that recommendation drops to less than 200 mg of cholesterol per day.

FASCINATING FACT

Every one-percent reduction in cholesterol levels produces a two-percent reduction in heart disease risk.

FASCINATING FACT

- 20 percent of all Americans have high blood cholesterol.
- 33 percent have borderline high levels.

FASCINATING FACT
The egg yolk has 213 milligrams of cholesterol, but the white has 0. In recipes that call for an egg, cut out the cholesterol by using 2 egg whites in place of 1 whole egg.

FASCINATING FACT
• 42 to 50 percent of all Americans have total blood cholesterol levels of more than 200 mg/dL
• 12 to 18 percent have total cholesterol levels of more than 240 mg/dL

properties, but recent studies have shown that artichokes may be even more effective than they were first thought to be.

Beets. Full of carotenoids and flavonoids, beets help lower—and may even prevent—the formation of LDL, the bad cholesterol. Choose fresh beets, rather than canned.

Carrots. Full of pectin, they're as good as apples in lowering cholesterol levels.

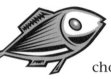

Fish. Although fish doesn't lower cholesterol, choosing it over beef will help you cut your cholesterol intake. Fish are also a rich source of omega-3 fatty acids, which are unsaturated fats that have been shown to protect the heart. Fatty fish have the most omega-3s, so choose mackerel, lake trout, herring, sardines, albacore tuna, and salmon. The American Heart Association recommends eating fish twice per week.

Oats. In any pure form, oats are a traditional cholesterol buster. Eating oatmeal, along with a low fat diet, may reduce cholesterol levels.

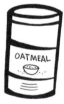

Olive oil. It protects your heart by lowering LDL, raising HDL, and preventing your blood from forming clots.

Pears. These are high in soluble fiber, which helps regulate cholesterol levels.

Rhubarb. Yep, this is a cholesterol-buster. Consume it after a meal that's heavy in fats. You can cook it in a double boiler, with a little honey or maple syrup for added sweetness, until done. Add cardamom or vanilla if you like.

Rice. The oil that comes from the bran of rice is known to lower cholesterol. And brown rice is particularly high in fiber, which is essential in a cholesterol-lowering diet. One cup provides 11 percent of the daily fiber requirement.

Walnuts. A cholesterol-lowering diet that includes walnuts eaten at least four times per week may lower LDL by as much as 16 percent. And studies indicate that those who munch on these nuts regularly cut their risk of death by heart attack in half when compared to non-walnut munchers.

Yogurt. Eating 1 cup plain yogurt with active cultures per day may reduce LDL by four percent or more and total cholesterol by at least 3 percent. Some scientists believe that eating yogurt regularly may even reduce the overall risk of heart disease by as much as 10 percent.

HERBAL REMEDIES

Chicory. Studies indicate that chicory root may have a significant role in lowering cholesterol. Shave a root, brew it into a tea, and drink 1 to 2 cups every day to reap the benefits.

Garlic. Studies show that garlic may not only reduce LDL but raise HDL and decrease the amount of fat in your blood. Add some fresh garlic regularly to your cooking to keep your heart healthy.

Turmeric. This may lower blood cholesterol. Added to eggplant, you may reap twice the cholesterol-fighting benefit. Mix ¾ teaspoon turmeric with 2 tablespoons cooked, mashed eggplant and 1½ tablespoons boiling water.

FAT FACT

The more liquid the margarine (tub or squeeze bottle), the less hydrogenated it is and the less trans fat it contains. Trans fatty acids raise total blood cholesterol levels, so the less of them you eat, the better off you will be.

WHEN TO CALL THE DOCTOR

Call 9-1-1 for:

- Crushing chest pain, possibly accompanied by nausea, vomiting, shortness of breath, sweating, weakness
- Dull chest pain or a feeling of tightness or heavy pressure
- Pain that starts in the chest, possibly radiating to the arms and jaw
- Symptoms of stroke: loss of speech, balance problems, sudden weakness or paralysis on one side of the body, sudden vision problems, numbness in your extremities

Call the doctor for:

- Weakness or pain in the buttocks, legs, or feet during exertion
- Cold feet that never get warm
- Leg or foot sores that won't heal
- Discolored skin on legs and feet
- Sharp, sudden leg or foot pain during rest

Spread it on whole wheat bread and eat after a meal heavy in fats.

LIFESTYLE REMEDIES

Avoid trans fats. Partially hydrogenated vegetable oil contains trans fatty acids, which increase the cholesterol-raising properties of fat. Trans fats are found in processed baked goods and snack foods, margarines, and many other foods.

Bulk up. Whole grains are high in fiber. Stick to complex carbohydrates, too, because they fill you up faster and leave you feeling satisfied. Try eating more fruits, veggies, pasta, rice.

Exercise. Regular exercise can boost HDL.

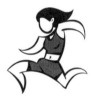

Read the food labels. They list the cholesterol content, so keep your cholesterol goal in mind—less than 300 mg per day.

Eat small meals. Instead of three big meals a day, go for five or six small meals. The body deals with cholesterol intake more efficiently when it comes in small amounts.

MORE DO'S & DON'TS

- Don't grease those pans. Use a nonstick olive oil spray or buy an inexpensive oil mister in a kitchenwares store and make your own spray.
- Change the way you cook. Don't fry your foods, because that requires added fat. Instead, broil or steam what you're cooking.

Hives
CATCHING THE CULPRIT

You decide to make two special batches of birthday brownies for your office—one with nuts and one without because one of your coworkers has a nut allergy. But to save on dishwashing, you bake both batches in the same pan. Big mistake! About an hour after eating your nut-free brownies, red spots begin radiating up the arm and neck of your nut-sensitive coworker. The essence of walnuts left in the unwashed baking pan was enough to spark a mild reaction. You remind yourself to fix cheesecake next time there's a birthday bash.

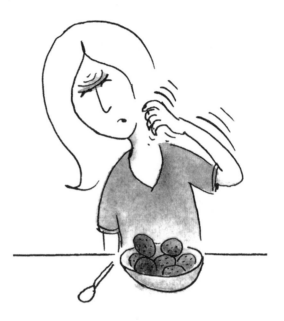

Hives, Histamine, and You

When you eat a food that you're allergic to, your body reacts by producing histamine. Histamine can do all sorts of things in the body in response to an allergen, such as making your eyes water or your tongue or throat swell. In the case of hives, histamine causes blood vessels to leak blood plasma into the skin. This blood leakage comes to the surface, causing inflammation and itching, and, lucky you, you've got a case of hives.

Hives, whose technical name is urticaria, can be as tiny as a dot or as big as a dinner plate. They have very defined edges and are usually irregularly shaped. If you've ever had hives, you know that though the swelling can be uncomfortable, it's the itching that drives you bonkers. The good news is hives usually run their course in a couple of hours. Sometimes, though, they can last as long as a couple of days. If they last longer than that, you should contact your doctor.

Those Annoying Allergens

Because hives are an allergic reaction, your best bet in preventing future

FASCINATING FACT
Hives are usually worse at night.

flare-ups is finding the source of the problem. You'll need to do a little detective work to figure out what caused your itchy bumps. If you can't put your finger on the culprit, you're not alone: About 50 percent of the time the trigger is unde-termined. To help your investigation along, here's a look at the primary causes of hives. Perhaps you'll be lucky and discover the source of your itchy bumps below:

- *Foods.* Certain foods are more likely to cause a heaping helping of hives. Strawberries are a problem for many people because they promote the production of histamine in the body. Other well-known hive producers are nuts, chocolate, fish, shellfish, soy, wheat, tomatoes, eggs, fresh berries, and dairy prod-ucts. If you're going to have an itchy reac-tion to food, it will probably happen within 30 minutes of eating it.
- *Food additives.* Food colorings, flavorings, preservatives, and emulsifiers or stabilizers in some foods can cause a hive outbreak. If you think food additives might be the reason your skin's so red, look for ingredients such as salicylates, sulfites, and polysorbate on the label of any processed foods you've eaten.
- *Medications.* Penicillin and aspirin are the two most common drug offenders. Penicillin and other antibiotics are the number one cause of drug-related hives.
- *Heat.* Getting too hot by spending too much time outside on a summer day or by exercis-ing are two causes of heat-induced hives. Sometimes known as "prickly heat," these heat-related hives calm down as your body temperature returns to normal.

- **Cold.** Sticking your arm in ice-cold water may cause cold-induced hives. These hives happen when you're exposed to cold objects or water, or even when you step outside on a cold, blustery day. Like heat-related hives, your oversize chill bumps will disappear once your body temperature normalizes.
- **Insect bites or stings.** Components of insect venom are allergenic. Some people have a systemic (bodywide) reaction to these components that produces hives.
- **Infections.** Bacterial, viral, and yeast infections can cause an outbreak of hives. Fever is also related to hive production.
- **Everyday objects.** Sometimes hives simply happen from pressure on the skin; from contact with everyday objects such as furniture, towels, watchbands, or bedsheets; or from wearing clothing that's too tight.
- **Stress.** Many people find that stress triggers an episode of hives.
- **Diseases.** Hives can be a symptom of thyroid disease, hepatitis, lupus, and even some cancers. That's why you shouldn't ignore a lingering case of the hives.

What Are Your Chances of Bumping Into Hives?

If you've never had a run-in with the itchy inflammation, you've got a 10 to 20 percent chance that you'll end up with it at sometime in your life. Young adults are most likely to get hives. Children and adults are at the same risk for getting the itchy red patches, but from different sources. Kids seem to get hives from food allergies or infections, while adults tend to break out in hives in reaction to a medication.

Whether or not you can uncover the source of your hives, there are some home remedies that can help relieve your symptoms while you're investigating.

HERBAL REMEDIES

Basil. The Chinese believe bathing in basil tea is a good antidote for hives. Put 1 ounce dried basil in a 1-quart jar and fill the jar with boiling water. Let cool to room temperature and use it as a wash.

Herbal tea. De-stress yourself by relaxing with a soothing cup of herbal tea.

TOPICAL REMEDIES

 Baking soda. Add ½ to 1 cup baking soda to a warm bath to soothe your itching.

Cotton gloves or oven mitts. Put these on your hands to keep you from scratching. Tape them at the wrist, and you'll be less tempted to remove them to start scratching. If you wear the gloves to bed at night, you won't do damage if you scratch your itches unconsciously.

Hydrocortisone. An over-the-counter, one percent topical cortisone preparation may help. Follow the directions on the package.

Ice. An ice pack helps shrink blood vessels, which alleviates swelling. Put the compress, wrapped in a thin towel, on your skin five minutes at a time, three or four times per day.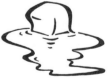

Oatmeal. Add 1 to 2 cups finely ground oatmeal to a warm bath (not hot or you might have breakfast for the next month in your tub) to ease your itches.

Milk. Calm your hives with a milk compress. Wet a cloth with cold milk and put it on your skin for 10 to 15 minutes.

LIFESTYLE REMEDIES

Calm down. Emotional stress has been known to spark a case of hives. But even if stress isn't the cause, worrying about your hives can make the pain and itching worse. Relax: Your hives will disappear shortly.

Get loose. Wearing clothes or shoes that are too tight can induce a case of hives. Try loosening up waistbands, bra straps, or any other clothing that is snug.

MORE DO'S AND DON'TS

- An over-the-counter antihistamine can keep your hives from spreading and can lessen the severity of itching and swelling. Remember that most antihistamines make you very, very sleepy. If you're planning on driving, take one of the newer nondrowsy antihistamine products.
- Ignore the itch. Sure that's easier said than done, but scratching can increase swelling and may cause your hives to spread.
- Leave the lotions alone. Nonprescription anti-itch lotions can cause an allergic reaction, making your itching more irritating.

WHEN TO CALL THE DOCTOR

Most hives run their course within a couple of days. However, if you have any of the following symptoms, head to your doctor's office or the closest emergency room:

- Significant swelling around your face and throat
- Nausea or dizziness
- Difficulty breathing
- Fever
- Weight loss
- Fatigue and lethargy
- Hives that come and go for six weeks or more

Incontinence
CHECKING THE FLOW

Laughter is the best medicine, unless, of course, it causes you to wet your pants. Then it's no laughing matter. The leaking of urine that occurs when laughing, exercising, coughing, sneezing, or lifting heavy objects is called incontinence and varies by degree. Whether it is a small leak or a major plumbing disaster, incontinence is an embarrassing problem to an estimated 12 to 20 million Americans, the majority of them women.

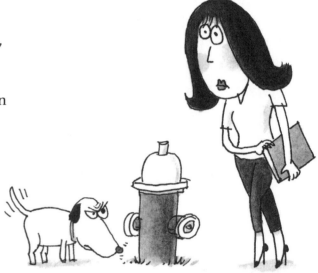

What Causes the Leak?
The causes of incontinence may be as minor as an infection triggered by a cold, bladder irritation, constipation, or the use of certain medications. In women, incontinence is often the result of sagging pelvic-floor muscles. These muscles at the bottom of the pelvis support the lower internal organs and help them maintain their shape and proper function. Childbirth and certain types of surgery, such as a hysterectomy, can cause these muscles to weaken, allowing urine to squeeze out at inappropriate times.

There are four main types of incontinence. They are:

Stress incontinence. This type occurs from rigorous or spontaneous activity such as jumping, running, coughing, laughing, or sneezing.

Urge incontinence. This type is marked by a sudden need to urinate. The person loses urine as soon as there is a strong need to use the toilet. Often the bathroom is one step too far away. This is most common in older adults.

Mixed incontinence. This is a mix of stress and urge incontinence and is most common in older women.

Overflow incontinence. This is a full bladder that starts leaking. In men, it can occur when the prostate is enlarged.

Other factors: Decreased mobility, medications, and cognitive impairment (particularly from Alzheimer's disease) can contribute to incontinence.

Fortunately, most types of incontinence can be solved, especially by doing pelvic-floor exercises and vaginal weight training recommended by your doctor. In extreme cases, medication or surgery may be recommended. In addition, there are several home remedies to help you remain dry and free from embarrassment.

DIETARY REMEDIES

Juice. Grape, cranberry, cherry, and apple juices are not irritating to the bladder and may help control the odor of your urine. They may also help diminish urinary tract infections.

Water. Drink to your bladder! Cozy on up to the sink and down a glass of water. Sounds strange, considering the bladder is leaking, but being well hydrated actually helps. If you cut back on fluid intake, you may become dehydrated, resulting in constipation. This, in turn, irritates nerves that may trigger the bladder to let loose. Schedule water consumption so you can regulate the fullness of your bladder. Stick to the recommended eight 8-ounce glasses of water each day.

TOPICAL REMEDIES

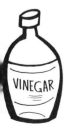

Vinegar. A person prone to leakage is also at risk for developing irritated skin from the wetness. Always clean damp areas with plain soap and water, followed by a rinse of diluted vinegar to disinfect and control odors. For a quick clean-up, keep a bottle of diluted vinegar and cotton balls close to the toilet.

THE EVER-EXPANDING BLADDER

The normal bladder holds about 2 cups of fluid. Normal bladder function is considered to be urinating every two to five hours during the day (7 to 9 times per day) and 0 to 1 times at night younger than 65 years old and 1 to 2 times per night if you're older than 65.

HOW TO CURE URINE STAINS

Urine accidents on clothing should be cleaned immediately. First rinse the clothing with warm water. Then mix 3 tablespoons white vinegar and 1 teaspoon liquid soap. Apply the mixture to the stained area, and leave it on for 15 minutes. Rinse the clothing well and dry.

WHEN TO CALL THE DOCTOR

- If you experience frequent leakage
- If leakage comes on suddenly after an injury
- If you are at high risk for developing diabetes

IRRITATING FOODS

Cleanse your refrigerator (and kitchen) of foods that irritate the bladder lining. Experts aren't sure why certain foods rub the bladder the wrong way, in turn causing leakage, but it is worth trying to eliminate a few suspects. Decrease your intake of the following and note any improvements:

- Hot spices and sauces
- Tomato-based foods
- Sugars
- Chocolate
- Coffee
- Carbonated sodas (except seltzer)
- Alcohol
- Grapefruit juice and tomato juice

LIFESTYLE REMEDIES

Empty your bladder. This is especially important before a long trip or watching long movies.

Go, then go again. Empty your bladder before you leave home, whether or not you feel the need. After voiding, stand up and then sit down again. Lean forward, which will compress the abdomen and put pressure on the bladder, helping to empty it completely.

Strengthen pelvic-floor muscles. Be diligent about doing strengthening exercises recommended by your doctor.

Maintain your normal weight. Adding more pounds puts more pressure on the pelvic-floor muscles, causing them to sag or weaken.

Stop smoking. Nicotine irritates the bladder, and a smoker's hack only heightens problems for the person susceptible to leakage while coughing.

Wear clothing that is easy to take off.

FEELING PLUGGED UP?

Constipation, while uncomfortable, can also aggravate incontinence. Be sure to get enough fiber by eating plenty of fresh fruits and vegetables. One fiber-rich recipe recommended by the National Association for Continence is an easy-to-make snack.

¼ cup prune juice
1 cup each applesauce and oat bran
Spices as desired, such as cinnamon and nutmeg

Combine the prune juice, applesauce, and oat bran. Store the mixture in your refrigerator. Begin by taking 2 tablespoons every day, followed by a large glass of water or juice. After seven to ten days, increase to 3 tablespoons. You should start noticing improvements in two weeks.

Insomnia/Sleep Disorders
RECLAIMING YOUR REST

The house is completely quiet. The kids are in bed. Your hubby is sawing logs. But you are staring at the ceiling listening to the fan hum. You've tried everything: counting sheep, counting dots on the ceiling, reading *War and Peace,* watching old sitcoms. Nothing is working, so you resign yourself to another dreary day of being a poster child for the walking dead.

Two-thirds of adults have some sort of trouble sleeping, according to the National Sleep Foundation. There are more than 20 common sleep disorders that plague men and women, from sleep apnea to restless legs syndrome. The number one sleep problem for men and women is insomnia. One-third of Americans have insomnia occasionally, and 10 to 15 percent deal with sleeplessness almost every night. This wouldn't be such an unsettling statistic if lack of sleep was no big deal, but your body and mind need to shut down for a while at the end of the day.

Insufferable Insomnia

Insomnia can be classified in one of three ways—trouble falling asleep (called sleep-onset insomnia), trouble staying asleep (called sleep-maintenance insomnia), or waking up feeling groggy and sleepy after what should have been a

WHEN YOUR LEGS WANT TO DO SOME WALKING...BUT YOU WANT TO SLEEP

Restless legs syndrome is a frustrating condition. The name of the problem explains it all. When you finally get into bed, your legs decide it's time to get up and move. The symptoms of restless legs syndrome have been described as tingling, crawling, or prickling sensations that peak during times of inactivity, such as when you're trying to go to sleep. Walking, massaging your legs, or taking a hot shower can help relieve the problem for a bit, but it'll come back, leaving you with a sleep-deprived night. Restless legs syndrome has been connected with a deficiency in iron and folic acid. The problem worsens with age and is more frequently diagnosed in people older than 65. It can be treated with prescription medicines.

full night's sleep. Most episodes of insomnia last anywhere from a couple of nights to a few weeks. There are myriad causes, including stress, anxiety, depression, disease, pain, medications, or simply not creating a relaxing sleep routine.

There's no magic number when it comes to how many hours you should sleep. Some people get by just fine on a few hours, while others need more than eight. You will know if you're not getting enough sleep because you'll wake up exhausted and feel sleepy most of the day.

Suffering Through Sleepless Nights

Women are twice as likely to experience insomnia than men. Half of all adults older than 65 are affected by insomnia. Having problems in your marriage makes you more likely to have insomnia, as do hormonal changes such as those that occur during menopause, menstruation, and pregnancy. Stress, mourning, certain medications, and other factors also play a part.

Insomnia's Ill Effects

Insomnia can have a significant impact on your health and well-being. If you don't get enough sleep, you're setting yourself up for some serious problems. People with insomnia are

- More likely to be diagnosed with depression.
- More likely to have a serious illness, including heart disease.
- More likely to have an accident on the job, at home, or on the road.
- More likely to miss work and accomplish less on the job than well-rested coworkers.

DIETARY REMEDIES

Cookies. Yes, that comforting nighttime snack of milk and cookies may be just what the doctor ordered to get you back in bed. Sugary foods eaten about 30 minutes before bedtime can actually act as a sedative, and you can wake up without the morning fuzziness that accompanies sleeping pills. Be careful to eat only a few cookies, though; eating too much sugar can keep the sandman at bay.

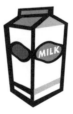

Honey. Folk remedies often advise people with sleeping difficulty to eat a little honey. It has the same sedative effect as sugar and may get you to bed more quickly. Try adding 1 tablespoon honey to some decaffeinated herbal tea or even to your warm milk for a relaxing presleep drink.

Milk. Drinking a glass of milk, especially a glass of warm milk, before bedtime is an age-old treatment for sleeping troubles. There is some debate, however, about what it is in milk—if anything—that helps cause slumber. Some scientists believe it's the presence of tryptophan, a chemical that helps the brain ease into sleep mode, that does the trick. Others believe it may be another ingredient, a soothing group of opiatelike chemicals called casomorphins. Whatever the reason, milk seems to help some people hit the sack more easily. And warm milk seems to be more effective at relaxing body and mind. Other foods high on the tryptophan scale

SELLING SLEEP

Over-the-counter (OTC) sleep aids seem to be everywhere these days. They can be helpful for occasional sleeplessness, but you must be sure to use them properly. Many OTC sleep aids contain antihistamines, which are medications typically used to clear up stuffy noses. A side effect of antihistamines is that they can make you sleepy, which is why they are included in sleep aids. Just because these medications are available over the counter doesn't mean they're safe. They can have side effects, and adverse reactions do occur. Here are some safety recommendations if you decide to go the OTC route:

- Don't combine OTC sleep aids with alcohol or other prescription or nonprescription drugs containing sedatives.
- Be cautious if you are older and want to take an OTC sleep aid. Slower metabolism could mean the effect lasts longer than you want it to.
- Certain medical conditions may not mix well with a sedative. If you have breathing problems, glaucoma, chronic bronchitis, or an enlarged prostate, or if you're pregnant or nursing, skip the OTC sleep helpers.
- Use OTC sleep aids only occasionally. If you find yourself relying on them on a regular basis, talk with your doctor. You may have an underlying health condition that is causing insomnia.

WATER CREATES SLEEP WAVES

Folk remedies for insomnia often include hydrotherapy. Depending on the person and how their body reacts, ice, cold water, hot water, steam, or water infused with special minerals may bring on a restful sleep. Cool water can increase circulation. Cold water can stop blood flow to an area, but when the blood rushes back to warm the area, it creates a sedating effect. Hot water can draw blood to an area, creating a relaxing feeling. Try these hydrotherapy sleep solutions to see if any of them work for you:

- Soak a cloth in cold water and place it on the back of the neck. Then cover with a warm towel. Keep it in place for 15 minutes.
- Soak a cloth in hot water and place it on the spine for 20 to 30 minutes before you go to bed.
- Soak your feet in hot water for 15 minutes before bed.
- Soak in a hot tub for as much as an hour before bed.
- Fill a tub with cool water until it reaches just above your belly button. Rest your feet on the edge of the tub so it covers only your hips and stomach. Soak for up to two minutes before going to bed.
- Add 1 ounce valerian, hops, chamomile, or lavender to a pot and cover with 1 quart boiling water. Strain the fragrant water and add it to your bath. Or simply add a couple drops of essential oil to your bathwater.

are cottage cheese, cashews, chicken, turkey, soybeans, and tuna.

Toast. High carbohydrate, low-protein bedtime snacks can make sleeping easier. Carbohydrate-rich foods tend to be easy on the tummy and can ease the brain into blissful slumber.

DIETARY SUPPLEMENT REMEDIES

5-HTP. Some experts believe a tryptophan deficiency can cause problems with sleep. Made from tryptophan, 5-HTP helps the body make serotonin. Low levels of serotonin are often a factor in sleepless nights. Taking a 5-HTP supplement may be a benefit if your body has low levels of tryptophan. How do you know if you're low? Low levels of tryptophan are most common in people who are depressed. If your insomnia is associated with depression, it might be a good question to ask your doctor. In one study, 100 mg of the supplement was enough to make sleep longer and better.

Melatonin. Melatonin is the timekeeper of the body. It's a hormone that regulates your biological clock. As you get older you make less melatonin, which experts believe is probably why older folks have more trouble sleeping. Research is suggesting that taking a melatonin supplement can help with some kinds of sleep problems. Ask your doctor about taking 1 to 3 mg of melatonin 1½ to 2 hours before bedtime.

HERBAL REMEDIES

Chamomile. Chamomile tea is one of the most popular sleep-inducing drinks on the market. It's been used in folk medicine for years and is best used for sleep problems due to upset stomach. To brew your own chamomile tea: Put 1 heaping tablespoon chamomile flowers in a cup. Add boiling water, cover, and let steep for ten minutes.

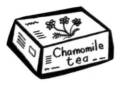

Dill seed. Though scientists haven't proved its worth, this herb is often used as a folk cure for

THE BEDROOM RULER

Louis XIV could be remembered as the king of beds. He loved staying in bed so much that he often held court in his bedroom. He also owned 413 beds, most of which were very spacious and very ornate.

DREAM A LITTLE DREAM

Everyone dreams three, four, even five times a night. Dreams are so intriguing that some people have made a career out of analyzing them. Books about what dreams mean are best-sellers, even though there's no way to determine their accuracy. Some people remember every detail of their dreams, and some don't remember them at all.

Whether you dream about a date with a movie star or your upcoming business meeting, most dreams fall into four categories:

- Lucid dreams. These dreams are usually pretty entertaining. In the dream, you have complete control over the situation. You can move from the mountains to the beach, get rid of the blonde your movie star is eyeing, or create a candlelit dinner in a garden. It's all up to you.
- Recurrent dreams. Every so often you have a dream that you're trapped in the trunk of a car and can't move. Dreams that you have over and over again may have some psychological—or even physiological—basis. For instance, when you are in a certain stage of deep sleep, your body becomes paralyzed. That may be why you have an unconscious feeling that you can't move.
- Nightmares. You lost your little girl in the aisles of the grocery store. You found her safe and sound, but that night you have a horrible dream that she was kidnapped. Nightmares are often horrifying dreams that reveal issues you didn't know were bothering you.
- Night terrors. Kids are most susceptible to night terrors. Your little boy wakes up everyone in the house with his screaming. Once you get to him, he can't remember what scared him so much. If your child has night terrors, be cautious; they can often go hand-in-hand with sleepwalking, which potentially could be dangerous.

insomnia in China. Its essential oil has many sedative-producing properties.

Lavender. The scent of lavender is so calming that in one study it was actually as potent as a tranquilizer. In Germany, where herbs are prescribed for medical conditions, doctors often give lavender for insomnia. You can find lavender essential oil at natural food stores.

Valerian. United States physicians listed this potent herb as a sedative until the late 19th century. Studies have found that it's as effective as Valium in coaxing sleep in some people, but it can act as a stimulant in others. Use cautiously. These days valerian is often combined with another herb, such as hops, to avoid any overstimulating effects.

Other herbs that might help you catch some ZZZs. Catnip, cinnamon, clove, hops, juniper, passionflower, peppermint, pine, sage, and skullcap. The best way to get the most relaxing effect from most of these herbs is to drink them in warm teas. Drink ½ cup an hour before bedtime and a second dose right before you hit the sack.

TOPICAL REMEDIES

Epsom salts. Naturopathic practitioners recommend this remedy for sleepless nights. Add 1 to 2 cups Epsom salts to a hot bath and soak for about 15 to 20 minutes before hitting the hay.

LIFESTYLE REMEDIES

Avoid alcohol. Yes, alcohol is a sedative, but the effects soon wear off and you'll end up tossing and turning.

Create bedtime bliss. Make your bedroom as dark, quiet, and peaceful as you can, and reserve the bed for sleep and sex only.

Cut the caffeine.
By its nature,
caffeine stimulates
your brain. When
you're trying to snooze, it can
cause problems. Having a
couple of cups of coffee or a
soda early in the day is fine,
but switch to decaf after lunch,
and if that doesn't work, try
eliminating it completely.

Get physical. Exercise helps
you sleep better, but watch the
timing. Exercising too close to
bedtime can make you too
keyed up to rest.

Maintain a relaxing routine.
Try to do the same relaxing
things before turning in, such
as taking a hot bath or reading
a book. This will prepare your
brain for sleep.

Nix the nap. People who have
trouble falling asleep or staying
asleep shouldn't try to sleep
during the day. It usually adds
to the problem. If you simply
must have some rest, don't nap
longer than 30 minutes early
in the afternoon.

Don't try too hard. If the
sandman doesn't come within
30 minutes of hitting the sack,
get up and do something
relaxing like reading. Try again
when you're feeling tired.

PAY ATTENTION TO APNEA

Your husband is having a Fred Flintstone moment. His snoring is so loud you keep waiting for the neighbors to complain. Just when you're about to elbow him into more peaceful slumber, you hear a gap in the noise. For a scary few seconds you notice he's not breathing at all. Your sweetie may have sleep apnea, a sleep disorder that affects more than 12 million Americans.

Sleep apnea literally takes your breath away. It's a condition in which there is prolonged lack of breathing or irregular breathing during sleep. People with sleep apnea stop breathing for 10 to 30 seconds at a time up to 400 times per night.

The National Sleep Foundation divides sleep apnea into three categories: obstructive apnea, central apnea, and mixed apnea. Obstructive apnea happens when the back of the throat relaxes so much that it blocks the upper airway. Breathing stops for a few seconds, and catching that breath causes you to wake up (though you probably wouldn't remember waking up). This is the most common apnea and is the kind associated with obnoxious snoring. Central apnea happens when the diaphragm and chest muscles stop working. Again, you wake to catch a breath, but you probably wouldn't remember it either. You have mixed apnea if you experience both central and obstructive apnea during the night at different times.

Middle-aged men and people who are overweight are more likely to suffer from sleep apnea. If left untreated, the condition can cause sleepiness during the day because of the constant awakening during the night. Sleep apnea can also cause high blood pressure and increase the risk of heart attack and stroke.

Not everyone who snores has sleep apnea, but if you think you or your spouse might have it, see your doctor immediately.

Irritable Bowel Syndrome
CONQUERING CRAMPING

Does this sound familiar? You're enjoying a nice meal at a nice restaurant, feeling pretty good. Coffee and dessert come and you're lingering over pleasant conversation, then all of a sudden wham! You've got a belly cramp, a gut gurgle that registers a 3.5 on the Richter scale. Suddenly you're off to find the nearest facility. There was no warning, no nothing. It just hit, and now your evening is on hold, changed, or canceled until you see how this latest attack resolves itself.

Irritable Bowel Syndrome (IBS) is a real condition, with real symptoms. (A decade ago it was one of those things doctors thought was just "in your head.") But it's a mysterious one to medical experts, who still don't know what it is or what exactly causes it. What they do know is that it's common—about 15 percent of all adults are afflicted with it sometime in their lives—and that it is a malfunction of the digestive tract.

Symptoms of irritable bowel syndrome include:

- diarrhea or constipation, or alternate bouts of each
- abdominal pain or cramping
- gas and bloating
- nausea, especially after eating
- headache
- fatigue
- depression or anxiety
- mucus-covered stools
- the urge to have another bowel movement after you've just had one

What We Know

Irritable bowel syndrome is also called spastic colon. It's an apt name that describes the abnormal digestive function that's typical of IBS. Normally, food is pushed through the intestine by synchronized muscle contractions. They are all dancing the same dance. But then something happens and one of those dancers steps out of the chorus line, does its own dance, and messes up everybody else's rhythm. As a result, the food that's being passed down that chorus line is suddenly disrupted in its travel.

Why does the muscle contraction become unsynchronized? No one knows for sure. Stress and poor diet are at the top of the suspected culprit list, since the majority of people with IBS seem either to be stressed-out or to have poor dietary habits. But that's only a guess. The other triggers most likely to cause it are: food intolerance, abdominal operations, medications, and hormonal changes during menstruation.

IBS is frustrating and inconvenient, but it's not serious, even though it does stand shoulder to shoulder with the common cold as a major reason for people to miss work. The good news is, IBS doesn't lead to other more serious intestinal conditions, and it can be treated with medications that relieve the symptoms. However, treatment isn't always easy, since the cause isn't known.

Regardless of the source of the problem, it does seem that there are some remedies for IBS symptoms right in your own home.

DIETARY REMEDIES

Cabbage. Juice of the cabbage soothes the symptoms of intestinal ills (although in some people it can cause gas). To turn this veggie into juice, simply wash and put through a juicer or blender. If these are not available to you, cook the cabbage in a very small amount of water—just enough to keep it from scorching or burning—until very mushy. Then pulverize with a fork or mixer.

Carrots. These little gems help prevent the symptoms of IBS as well as regulate diarrhea and

FASCINATING FACT

- One-third of all people who have IBS claim that stress exacerbates the problem.
- Half of all people who have digestive complaints have IBS.
- More women than men have IBS, and they are especially prone to symptoms around the time of their menstrual period.

NO-NO FOODS

You may have your own personal list of foods that cause your IBS flare-ups, but many people find these foods trouble them:

- Dairy products
- Cereals, especially wheat cereals
- Red kidney beans
- Lentils
- Peas
- Apples
- Grapes
- Raisins
- Brussels sprouts
- Broccoli
- Cauliflower
- Preserved, processed, or cured meats

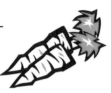

constipation. Eat them raw, by themselves or in salads, or cooked—steamed and tossed with a little melted butter and brown sugar for a sweet treat. Or put raw carrots through the juicer, adding a little pure apricot nectar to make it a juicier mix. Any way you eat a carrot is fine, just don't overcook them.

Lettuce. You can eat it raw to relieve symptoms of IBS, but it's especially helpful if lightly steamed. And when you're picking out your lettuce, go for the darker varieties. The darker the color, the more nutrients it contains.

Oat bran. Increasing fiber is a cure for almost every intestinal ill, and oat bran is especially good for IBS because it's mild and usually colon-friendly. So use some every day: a bowl of oatmeal, oat bran bread, oatmeal cookies. Don't expect immediate results, however. It may take as long as a month to get any IBS relief.

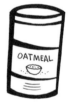

Pears. Fresh, ripe, sweet pears are a nutritious fruit that also help relieve the symptoms of IBS. Buy them when they're still hard and let them ripen at room temperature for a few days. Pure pear juice and dried pears are also helpful in treating this intestinal woe.

Yogurt. Yogurt with active cultures will supply your digestive tract with the helpful kind of bacteria, which can ease IBS symptoms. You can also try mixing 1 cup yogurt with ½ teaspoon psyllium husks (or psyllium bulk you can buy in any pharmacy) and eating the mixture one hour after meals.

HERBAL REMEDIES

Fennel seeds. These may relieve bloating and the intestinal spasms associated with IBS. Steep the seeds into a tea by adding 2 to 3 teaspoons crushed fennel seeds to 1 cup boiling water. Steep for 10 to 15 minutes. Drink up to 2 cups per day. Or add them to veggies such as carrots or cabbage, both of which soothe IBS symptoms. You can also sprinkle the seeds on salads or roast them and snack on them after a meal to reduce IBS symptoms and freshen your breath. To roast, spritz a baking sheet with olive oil, then cover with fennel seeds. Bake at 325 degrees Fahrenheit for 10 to 15 minutes. *Warning!* Do not take fennel if you are allergic to celery.

Flaxseed. Make a tea using 1 teaspoon flaxseed per cup of water, and drink at bedtime for relief of symptoms. Flaxseed can act as a laxative, so avoid it if you have diarrhea.

Peppermint. Steeped into a relaxing tea, this can relieve intestinal spasms. Use 1 heaping teaspoon dried peppermint, and steep in 1 cup boiling water for ten minutes. Drink as often as necessary.

TOPICAL REMEDIES

Heat. For cramping, try a hot bath or apply a hot compress or a heating pad to your abdomen.

LIFESTYLE REMEDIES

Avoid stress. Relax during meals. Give yourself enough time to complete your tasks. Get up a few minutes early to avoid the morning rush. Spend a few minutes working on progressive relaxation.

Drink between meals, not with meals. Drinking when you eat dilutes digestive juices and frustrates digestion.

TRAVELED LATELY?

If you recently traveled to an area where water is untreated, or went camping and drank fresh water from a mountain spring, those IBS symptoms you suddenly started experiencing might not be IBS at all. Instead, you could be suffering from a parasite that was having a swim in the water you drank. Parasitic illnesses such as amoebiasis and giardiasis, as well as other bacterial woes, can cause nausea, diarrhea, cramping, and fatigue. So if you've sipped from the untreated source and are now experiencing some of these symptoms, call your doctor and mention the possible link.

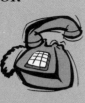
Eat slowly. Some people with IBS find their symptoms flare up when they bolt their food.

Exercise moderately. This will make the entire digestive system work better, but don't overdo it. In people with IBS, strenuous exercise can lead to symptoms.

Get enough fiber. It helps maintain good bowel function. You need about 35 grams a day. Chances are you're only getting about half of what you need.

Keep a food diary. Track the foods that seem to trigger the attacks. Eliminate a specific food for a couple of weeks to see if that makes a difference. If it does, you may have isolated the cause. If not, choose another food you've eaten around the time of an attack and eliminate it. This is called an exclusion diet, and if what you're eating is a trigger for IBS, this is the best way to find out what it is. Also make note of anxiety or stress you're feeling and what you think is causing it. If you notice that your attacks seem to come during stressful events, you may need to consider ways to eliminate them.

Limit alcohol and caffeine. They irritate your stomach lining, which can lead to IBS symptoms.

Nix the tobacco. It can cause stomach cramps.

Skip the gassy foods. For a list of gassy foods, see page 182. And try to eliminate air swallowing. The more gas you introduce into your intestine, the more likely a flare-up of IBS.

MORE DO'S & DON'TS

- Don't use the artificial sweetener called sorbitol. It can cause bowel problems, including constipation.

Itching
SOOTHING WITHOUT SCRATCHING

To scratch or not to scratch, that is the question. When confronted with an itch, most of us tend to throw self-discipline out the door and scratch to our skin's content. Although that may prove momentarily satisfying, scratching excessively can injure your skin. And if you break the skin, you leave yourself open to infection.

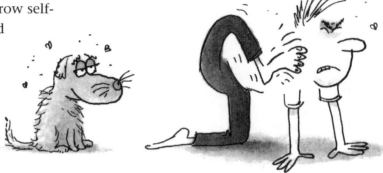

Itching, medically known as pruritus, is caused by stimuli bugging some part of our skin. There are a lot of places to bother on the body, too. The average adult has 20 square feet (2 square meters) of skin, all open to the world of irritants. When something bothers our skin, an itch is a built-in defense mechanism that alerts the body that someone is knocking. We respond to an itch with a scratch, as most people want to remove the problem. But the scratching can also set you up for the "itch-scratch" cycle, where one leads to the other endlessly.

An itch can range from a mild nuisance to a disrupting, damaging, and sleep-depriving fiasco. Itches happen for many reasons, including allergic reactions; sunburns; insect bites; poison ivy; reactions to chemicals, soaps, and detergents; medication; dry weather; skin infections; and even aging. More serious itches, such as those caused by psoriasis or other diseases, are not covered here.

Scratching isn't the only solution to an itch. The cupboards hold a few more.

TOPICAL REMEDIES
Baking soda. Baking soda battles itches of all kinds. For widespread or hard-to-reach itches, soak in a

SCRATCHING HIS WAY TO JAIL

Scratching nether regions in public is not only bad manners in American society, it could get you arrested. As reported in a dermatology journal, "Curtis," a 36-year-old machinist, emerged from his job site covered in irritating fiberglass dust. He ventured to the store but, while standing in line, was overwhelmed by an itch in his groin. He submitted and scratched away in relief. Somebody noticed and called the police, who arrested him for "lewd and indecent behavior." Charges were dropped, but not before he spent a night in the slammer...itching, presumably.

baking soda bath. Add 1 cup baking soda to a tub of warm water. Soak for 30 to 60 minutes and air dry. Localized itches can be treated with a baking soda paste. Mix 3 parts baking soda and 1 part water. Apply to the itch, but do not use if the skin is broken.

 Lemon. Many American folk remedy recipes call for using a lemon to treat itchy skin—and rightly so. The aromatic substances in a lemon contain anesthetic and anti-inflammatory properties, which may help reduce itching. Squeeze undiluted lemon juice on itchy skin and let dry.

Oatmeal. Add 1 to 2 cups finely ground oatmeal to a warm—but not hot—bath to ease your itches.

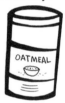

HERBAL REMEDIES

Aloe vera. The same constituents that reduce blistering and inflammation in burns also reduce itching. Snap off a leaf, slice it down the middle, and rub only the gel on the itch.

Basil. Like cloves, basil contains high amounts of eugenol, a topical anesthetic. Place ½ ounce dried basil leaves in a 1-pint jar of boiling water. Keep it covered to prevent the escape of the aromatic eugenol from the tea. Allow to cool. Dip a clean cloth into the tea and apply to itchy skin as often as necessary.

Cloves and juniper berries. Native Americans of the Paiute, Shoshone, and Cherokee tribes knew how to stop an itch in its tracks. They used juniper berries. (No need to run out in the wilderness to gather berries. They are available in some grocery stores.) These berries contain anti-inflammatory substances. When combined with cloves, which contain eugenol to numb nerve endings, the result is no more itch. To make a salve of both spices, melt 3 ounces of unsalted butter in a saucepan. In a separate pan, melt a lump of beeswax—about the amount of 2 tablespoons. When the beeswax has melted, combine with butter and stir well. Add 5 tablespoons ground juniper berries and 3 teaspoons ground cloves to the mixture and stir. Allow to cool and apply to itchy skin. *Note:* It is best to grind the spices at home because the volatile substances are preserved better in whole berries and cloves.

Mint. If you're saving that basil for spaghetti sauce, try a mint tea rinse instead. Chinese folk medicine values mint as a treatment for itchy skin and hives. Mint contains significant amounts of menthol, which has anesthetic and anti-inflammatory properties when applied topically. In general, mint also contains high amounts of the anti-inflammatory rosmarinic acid, which is readily absorbed into the skin. To make a mint tea rinse, place 1 ounce dried mint leaves in 1 pint boiling water. Cover and allow to cool. Strain, dip a clean cloth in the tea, and apply to the itchy area when necessary.

Thyme. If you're saving that mint for a glass of lemonade, there is one more spice on the rack that makes a good anti-itch rinse: thyme. This fragrant herb contains large amounts of the volatile constituent thymol, which has anesthetic and anti-inflammatory properties. In other words, it numbs that darn itch while reducing inflammation caused by all your scratching. To make a thyme rinse, place ½ ounce dried thyme leaves in a 1-pint jar of boiling water. Cover and allow to cool. Strain and dip a clean cloth into the tea,

SCRATCH THAT SUPERSTITION!

- If your nose itches, someone will kiss you or you'll shake hands with a fool.
- If your right palm itches, you'll soon be getting money.
- If your left palm itches, you'll soon be paying money.
- If your right ear itches, someone is speaking ill of you.
- If your left ear itches, a loved one is talking about you.
- If the bottom of your feet itch, you will go on a long journey.

WHEN TO CALL THE DOCTOR

- If the itching is severe and lasts more than 24 hours

- If the skin is broken, blistered, or damaged by scratching
- If you are experiencing other symptoms with the itch, such as difficulty breathing, nausea, faintness, etc.

then apply to affected areas. Note: In Chinese folk medicine, dandelion root, easily plucked from most yards, is added to this rinse. If in season, place 1 ounce dried dandelion root and ½ ounce dried thyme leaves into 1 quart boiling water and proceed as directed.

MORE DO'S AND DON'TS

- Try not to scratch!
- Wear gloves, if need be, to keep yourself from opening your skin by scratching with your nails.

ITCHES IN NETHER REGIONS

Some types of itches are just not socially acceptable, especially when it comes to those around the derriere. Pruritis ani is the medical term for an "itchy bottom," and it's one itch that isn't discussed in polite company.

For those who silently suffer this unspeakable condition, the itching is often unbearable and no relief is available if you're in a public setting. The causes of an itchy bottom are many:

- Tight clothing and underwear
- An allergic reaction to perfumed or rough toilet paper
- Offending condiments such as hot sauces and acidic foods such as tomatoes, citrus drinks, coffee, and alcohol
- Pinworm infestation
- Infections by viruses, yeast, or bacteria.

For the less-serious causes, there are some cures that can be used in the privacy of your home.

- Be free. If you want to make your own petri dish, wear tight-fitting underwear! With no air flow, combined with moist, warm conditions, your underwear and skin become a science experiment with itchy results. Throw out any snug underwear. Men should switch to boxer shorts too.
- Splurge on softness. Plush, soft toilet paper may provide some relief to your itchy bottom. It costs more, but the "end" result is probably worth a few extra pennies. If you're really willing to splurge, purchase alcohol-free, pre-moistened wipes designed for anal care.
- Back it up with soap. During the day, plenty of unpleasant things, such as sweat and fecal material, can gather down below and cause irritation and itch. Clean your rectal area every night with warm water and non-irritating, fragrance-free soap. Let yourself air dry, and apply witch hazel or vinegar as needed.

SCRATCHING ON THE PLAYING FIELD

Watch a baseball game (or other sports event) for ten minutes and you'll soon spot some player (usually of the male species) scratching his privates. He may be adjusting his snug-fitting underwear or protective cup, but more likely he's relieving his jock itch.

Jock itch is typically caused by a fungus infection but can also result from a bacterial infection or an allergic reaction to clothing, chemicals, or medications. Symptoms are redness, scaliness in the groin and thigh, and that all-too-noticeable itch.

The itch's namesake, the jockstrap (or athletic supporter), is often the villain behind all the scratching. After a workout, this protective device is usually carelessly thrown back into a dark, dank locker without being laundered or aired out. This cycle of wearing without washing makes the athletic supporter the perfect playground for fungi and bacteria.

Women aren't immune to jock itch, despite not wearing athletic supporters. Under similar conditions, women's sports bras, cycling pants, and protective padding can sport fungi growth.

To make sure jock itch doesn't become a major-league problem, try to use some of the following home remedies before and after exercise.

TOPICAL REMEDIES

Cornstarch. Before a game, dust some cornstarch on the groin area to keep it dry and reduce friction from underwear elastic, athletic supporters, or other sporting gear.

Soap and water. Simple soap can help prevent jock itch. Shower after a workout using antibacterial soap. Afterward, dab the groin area with a vinegar solution made from 2 tablespoons white vinegar and 1 pint cool water. Let yourself air dry. (Don't apply vinegar to broken skin.)

Vinegar and baking soda. After each workout or game, wash the athletic supporter (or other close-to-the-body clothing) in warm water with mild, non-irritating detergents. A cup of vinegar or ½ cup baking soda added to detergent freshens laundry and helps detergents work more efficiently.

LIFESTYLE REMEDIES

Wash athletic supporters immediately after use. If you can't wash the athletic supporter, at least air it out. Never leave it in a locker or gym bag!

Don't hang out in workout clothes. After exercising, shower, dry off completely, and change into clean and comfortable clothing.

Hang loose. Tight-fitting underwear can ruin the day. Wear boxers during the day, and sleep in the nude or in loose-fitting pajamas at night.

WHEN TO CALL THE DOCTOR

• If home remedies don't work and the jock itch becomes unbearable.

• If you suspect that an allergic reaction to a substance or medication is causing the itch.

Kidney Stones
CLEARING THE PATH

In one episode of a famous sitcom, one of the characters is in labor with triplets. As she screams during a contraction, her (male) friend doubles over in pain. Thinking he's having sympathy pains, he shouts, "I didn't know I cared so much!"

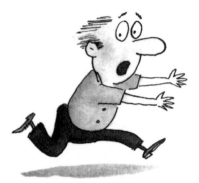

Alas, he soon discovers his agony isn't because he's such a sympathetic guy. He has a kidney stone.

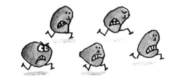

The rest of the show examines the parallels between having a baby and passing a stone, a comparison many kidney-stone sufferers would echo. And since four out of five people who get kidney stones are men, there are many husbands gaining new respect for their spouses. (And many wives of kidney-stone sufferers believing that justice has finally been served!)

The Stone Source

Each about the size of your fist, your kidneys are located in your back, just below your rib cage. The main function of kidneys is to get rid of extra waste and fluid, clear impurities from the blood, and keep your blood pressure under control. The majority of kidney stones form when there's not enough fluid passing through the kidneys. Certain minerals, namely calcium, magnesium, and phosphate, along with oxalate, a substance found in some foods, begin to crystallize on the sides of the kidneys. When the stones break loose, these little calcified pebbles make a path through your ureter, the tube that connects your kidneys with your bladder. The majority of kidney stones are small—90 percent are less than five millimeters, about the size of a tiny pea—and usually pass without notice. Occasionally, however, kidney stones can grow quite large, some even as big as golf balls. As these grainy, rough rounds pass through your ureter, you experience the legendary anguish of passing a stone.

What causes stones? Scientists don't know for sure. But there are some factors that put you at greater risk. These include:

- Inadequate fluid intake
- Lack of exercise
- Heredity. If your mom or dad battled the stones, you probably will, too.
- Frequent urinary tract infections
- A high-protein diet
- Some diuretics
- Taking calcium-based antacids
- Some metabolic disorders, such as hyperparathyroidism
- Gout
- Excessive intake of vitamin D

Stone Stats

The National Kidney Foundation estimates that one million Americans are treated for kidney stones each year. This doesn't account for the brave souls who pass stones without visiting a doctor. The majority of those with kidney stones will be men, although the number of women with kidney stones is increasing. Experts blame that growing statistic on high protein diets. Too much animal protein in the diet can spark kidney stone formation. Most people have their first

WHEN YOU'VE GOT TO GO

The average adult can hold as much as 24 ounces in the bladder, which is equivalent to three glasses of water. Most people feel the urge to go when their bladder contains between 10 and 16 ounces of fluid.

THE YOUNGEST STONE

Joshua Price, of Jacksonville, TX, holds the distinction of being the youngest person to ever have a kidney stone removed. A couple of months shy of seven years old, Joshua had a stone removed from his left kidney on October 5, 1993. A painful claim to fame, but Joshua's story now resides in the *Guinness Book of World Records*.

attack between ages 20 and 40. And if you have one attack, odds are you'll have another. Fifty percent of people who have kidney stones will have another attack within five years.

If you've ever had a kidney stone, there's some good news. Turns out even those at higher risk for kidney stones can prevent another attack simply by watching what they eat. Here are some suggestions for staying free of kidney stones.

DIETARY REMEDIES

Bran flakes. Fiber helps get rid of calcium and oxalate in your urine, which cuts the risk of kidney stones. A bowl of bran flakes can give you 8 mg of fiber.

Carrots. Vitamin A is an essential ingredient for healthy kidneys. One carrot can give you twice your daily requirements for this kidney-friendly nutrient.

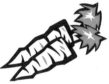

Chicken. The B vitamins, specifically vitamin B_6, are well-known stone fighters. Vitamin B_6 keeps the body from building up excess oxalate. Too much oxalate is a major factor in kidney stone formation. But don't eat too much, since high-protein diets can contribute to kidney stones. Three ounces of chicken provide more than one-third of your daily needs.

Lemonade. Drink a glass of lemonade a day. It can be homemade from real lemons, from frozen concentrate, or a ready-made liquid. Just don't use a powdered mix. Lemonade increases the levels of citrate in your urine, which helps to prevent kidney stone formation.

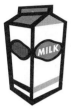

Milk. Although calcium is one of the major minerals in kidney stones, recent evidence shows that not getting enough calcium can actually increase the chances of getting a stone. The reason: Dietary calcium binds with oxalates so they can't be absorbed from the intestine and excreted by the kidney to form stones. One study found that men who ate the most calcium reduced their chance of developing kidney stones by 34 percent compared with those who ate the least amount of calcium. Research has also found that women who have a high intake of calcium are less likely to develop kidney stones than women whose calcium intake is lower. How much is enough? Meeting your recommended daily allowance, which for most adults is between 1,000 and 1,200 mg per day, the amount in about three glasses of milk, should do the trick.

Tea. Both women and men can benefit from drinking tea. In the Nurses' Health Study, there was an 8 percent decrease in the risk of kidney stones for every 8 ounces of tea the women drank daily. And a Harvard study of men found that there was a 14 percent decrease in kidney stone development for every 8 ounces of tea they drank daily. People with oxalate kidney stones should avoid black tea, because of it high oxalate content.

Water. Hippocrates was the first to recognize the benefits of drinking water for averting kidney stones. Most modern-day docs recommend drinking about a gallon of water per day if you're at risk for kidney stones. And drinking fluids at night is more beneficial.

ROLL THOSE STONES AWAY

Too much oxalate- or calcium-rich food may be to blame for some kidney stones. If you're at risk for kidney stones, check with your doctor about cutting back on these foods:

Apples
Beer
Berries
Broccoli
Cheese
Chocolate
Cocoa
Coffee
Grapes
Ice cream
Milk
Oranges
Peanuts and peanut butter
Rhubarb
Spinach
Swiss chard
Yogurt

WHEN TO CALL THE DOCTOR

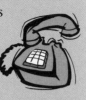

Pain that starts in the back, in the general vicinity of your kidneys, and moves to the groin could be kidney stones. The pain generally follows the path of your ureter and can last as long as three days. It's agonizing, but the pain will go away once you pass the stone. However, some stones are simply too big to pass through the body and may need medical attention.

According to the National Institute of Diabetes and Digestive and Kidney Diseases, call your doctor if you experience any of these symptoms:

- Extreme pain in your back or side that does not go away
- Blood in your urine
- Fever and chills
- Vomiting
- Urine that smells bad or looks cloudy
- A burning feeling when you urinate

Whole-wheat bread. A couple slices of whole-wheat bread contain a good amount of magnesium, a mineral known for averting stones. One study found that people who got an adequate amount of magnesium stopped getting kidney stones altogether.

LIFESTYLE REMEDIES

What you *don't* eat is just as important as what you do eat when it comes to preventing kidney stones. These tips will help you give your stones the old heave-ho.

Minimize the meat. Animal protein tends to increase levels of stone-forming minerals. Try to keep your intake less than 7 ounces per day.

Skimp on the sodium. Decreasing salt intake decreases calcium buildup in your urine and the chances of developing a stone. Experts recommend consuming only 2,300 mg per day.

Observe those oxalates. Certain foods are rich in oxalates, and too much of them can make you more at risk for a stone. See "Roll Those Stones Away," page 287, for a list of foods to avoid.

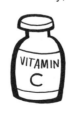

Watch the "C." Skip the daily vitamin C supplements if you take 500 mgs or more. Vitamin C increases oxalate in your urine, and too much oxalate combines with calcium and can create a stone. Getting enough C in your diet should be fine.

Forgo fad diets. High-protein diets can increase the amount of calcium in your urine, making you more likely to get a stone.

Watch what you drink. Some beverages, such as grapefruit juice and soda pop, may contribute to kidney stone formation.

Lactose Intolerance
MANAGING MILK

Lactose, the milk sugar in dairy products, can be pretty rough to digest on a good day. But our bodies manage to do it with the help of an enzyme called lactase that breaks down those tough milk sugars and converts them into glucose, or blood sugar. When lactase kicks in, milk digestion comes off without a hitch.

When there is an insufficient amount of lactase, your condition is called lactose intolerance, and it can cause some pretty miserable symptoms. Instead of being broken down, lactose instead stays intact in the intestines, absorbing fluids. When this happens, gas, cramping, heartburn, and diarrhea can result one by one or all together.

To add insult to injury, certain bacteria that call the colon home ferment the undigested lactose, causing more gas, cramping, and diarrhea.

A Common Problem

Lactose intolerance is so common that about two-thirds of the world's population suffers from it in some form. This includes:

- Between 30 and 50 million American adults

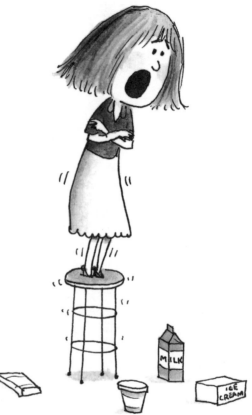

- About 50 to 80 percent of Hispanic Americans
- 60 to 80 percent of African Americans and Ashkenazi Jews
- 80 to 100 percent of Native Americans
- 95 percent of Asian Americans

Globally, Native Americans, Africans, and people of Mediterranean, Asian, and Middle Eastern descent have the highest incidence of lactose

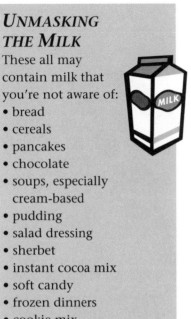
intolerance. Only about 2 percent of Americans of Northern European descent are lactose intolerant.

Most adults who are lactose intolerant usually tolerated small amounts of lactose when they were children. With aging, however, the ability to digest lactose diminishes, even for those who aren't lactose intolerant. To some degree, lactose intolerance develops in virtually everyone as they age. In other words, the body's production of lactase slows down, too.

Many people don't realize they're lactose intolerant, especially if they don't consume many milk products. Since the degree of intolerance varies with each individual, some may experience symptoms only after consuming a large amount of dairy. Others will have symptoms from a very small amount.

One way to get an idea of whether you're lactose intolerant is simply to avoid all dairy products for several weeks and see if your symptoms resolve. This isn't a conclusive method, as there may be other reasons that your symptoms don't entirely disappear. But if your symptoms do decrease, you will benefit by decreasing dairy in your diet, using a dietary aid that replaces lactase (available in most pharmacies), or using a lactose-free milk product.

For a more conclusive diagnosis, visit your doctor, who may want to order a lactose intolerance test. Before you get too discouraged, though, here are some easy remedies you can try to get some relief.

DIETARY REMEDIES

Buttermilk and goat's milk. Although they both contain lactose, some people find them easier to digest than cow's milk.

Cocoa powder. Studies indicate that cocoa powder and sugar, or chocolate powders, may help the body digest lactose by slowing the rate at which the stomach empties. The slower the emptying process, the less lactose that enters your system at once. That means fewer symptoms.

Food. People with any degree of lactose intolerance should never drink milk by itself. Always have a snack or a meal with your milk.

Hard cheese. The harder the cheese, the lower its lactose content, so cheddar and colby are good. Skip the soft cheese, including cream cheese, cottage cheese, and any product that's processed or spreadable.

Sardines. They're high in calcium, which might be lacking in your diet if you're not drinking milk or consuming calcium-rich milk products. Other high-calcium foods include canned salmon (or any other canned oily fish with bones), tofu, dark green leafy vegetables, nuts, cooked dried beans, dried apricots, and sesame seed products.

Soy milk. It's a shock after you're used to cow's milk, but it won't cause lactose intolerance. If you can't get used to the taste, try using it in recipes and products, such as pudding, where adding milk is required.

 Yogurt. Research shows that yogurt with active cultures may be a good source of calcium for many people with lactose intolerance, even though it is fairly high in lactose. According to the National Digestive Diseases Information Clearinghouse, evidence shows that the bacterial cultures used in making yogurt produce some of the lactase enzyme required for proper digestion.

JUST PLAIN YOGURT

Originally produced as a way to preserve milk, yogurt is one of the most digestive-tract-friendly foods you can eat, and its intestinal benefits have been recorded since the 16th century. The following yogurt facts pertain to regular yogurt with live cultures, not to yogurt products such as frozen treats.

- It fights the harmful bacteria responsible for diarrhea. Studies indicate that those who eat only yogurt during a severe bout may recover twice as quickly as those who are treated medically or by other means.
- It has a similar effect on the colon as fiber and can be used to maintain bowel regularity or relieve constipation.
- It is a good source of calcium and can sometimes be used in place of milk by those who are lactose intolerant because the bacteria in yogurt produce lactase.
- It helps relieve the symptoms of irritable bowel syndrome.
- A 6-ounce serving has about the same amount of calcium as 1 cup of milk.

WHEN TO CALL THE DOCTOR

- If unexplained weight loss occurs
- If the techniques you've been using to control it don't work
- If symptoms cause problems in the way you live your life
- If symptoms persist for more than a few days
- If you experience unusual pain or severity of symptoms
- If blood is present in diarrhea

FASCINATING FACT

Many women are unaware that they have lactose intolerance until they hit menopause and start consuming more milk to obtain the additional calcium they need.

DIETARY SUPPLEMENT REMEDIES

Calcium. This bone-building mineral is essential for good health. Eat calcium-rich, nondairy foods and/or take calcium supplements. Check with your doctor before you take a calcium supplement.

Probiotics. These are living organisms that reside in our intestines and keep the digestive system healthy. Increasing their numbers by taking probiotic supplements or eating foods that contain active probiotic cultures, such as some yogurts, may help you to digest lactose.

LIFESTYLE REMEDIES

Divide and conquer. Most people who suffer lactose intolerance do produce some amount of lactase. So, if that 8-ounce glass of milk you drink in the morning backfires, divide it up. Measure out ⅓ cup three times a day and see if you can handle the smaller amount.

Keep a food diary. First, cut out all milk products for 3 to 4 weeks. Then, add back small amounts of milk at a meal, ¼ to ½ cup at a time, and see what you can tolerate. Gradually increase or decrease the amount according to your symptoms.

MORE DO'S & DON'TS

- Check with your pharmacist about the medications you take. Twenty percent of prescription and six percent of nonprescription medications contain lactose as a filler.

Laryngitis
HANDLING HOARSENESS

Have you been abusing your voice? Too much vocal enthusiasm at a sports event can set you up for swollen vocal cords and no voice the next day. But that's not the only cause of laryngitis—the result of inflammation of the voice box and voice folds. More often, laryngitis is caused by an upper respiratory infection, usually viral, such as the common cold. Surprisingly, some cases of laryngitis are caused by heartburn, especially in the elderly. During the night, the acid-rich contents of the stomach come back up the throat and cause irritation.

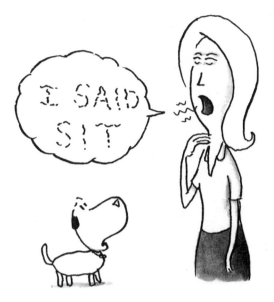

Sounds and Symptoms

When we speak, two membranes, known as the vocal chords, vibrate to produce sounds. Hoarseness, the main sign of laryngitis, is an indicator that something with the vocal chords is wrong, swollen, irritated, or infected. Besides hoarseness, symptoms of acute, or short-term, laryngitis also include a painful or scratchy feeling in the throat, a loss of range in the voice, and fatigue. You may also have the annoying feeling that you must constantly clear your throat. In heartburn-induced laryngitis, symptoms include waking up with a bad taste in the mouth, feeling like something is sticking in the throat, constant throat clearing, and hoarseness that gradually improves during the day.

DIETARY REMEDIES

Noncaffeinated tea with lemon. Any kind of tea will do, just make sure it's not too hot or too cold. The lemon will help stimulate the flow of saliva and keep your throat lubricated.
Water. Keep the throat moistened and stay hydrated by drinking your daily amount of water (eight 8-ounce glasses per

WITCH HAZEL TO THE RESCUE

The bark, leaves, and twigs of witch hazel are high in tannins, giving this plant astringent properties. Astringents are substances that can dry, tighten, and harden tissues... perfect for shrinking swollen throat tissues. A throat gargle of store-bought witch hazel and tinctures of myrrh and cloves helps reduce the pain of sore throats associated with laryngitis. Place 1 dropper full of tincture of each herb in a sip of water and rinse. If myrrh and cloves tinctures aren't available, dilute witch hazel with 3 parts water and rinse. Do not swallow the mixture.

day). Fruit juices also fit the bill, as do hot, non-caffeinated drinks, which may feel extra soothing on sore throat tissues.

HERBAL REMEDIES

Garlic. Should you have a strong stomach and no social events to attend, try the Amish treatment for sore throats and viral infections: Suck on a slice of garlic. Garlic, when sliced or crushed, releases the antimicrobial substance allicin. Allicin kills bacteria, including strep and some viruses. Slice a garlic clove down the middle and place half a clove on each side of the mouth. Pretend the cloves are lozenges and suck on them. Use as often as necessary, or as often as you can handle garlic breath.

Ginger. Fresh ginger can help soothe inflamed mucous membranes of the larynx. Try sucking on candied ginger if available or 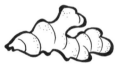 drink a cup of ginger tea. To prepare the tea, cut a fresh 1- to 2-inch gingerroot into thin slices and place in 1 quart boiling water. Cover the pot and simmer on the lowest heat for 30 minutes. Let cool for 30 more minutes, strain, and drink ½ to 1 cup three to five times a day. Sweeten with honey if needed.

TOPICAL REMEDIES

Lemon. Some folk remedies recommend sucking on a lemon to cure a sore throat. Spare yourself the face-contorting agony and try a lemon juice and salt gargle instead. Lemon is naturally acidic and helps stimulate saliva flow. The salt increases the lemon's acidity, which in turn helps kill many microorganisms prone to weak acids. To make this gargle, juice a whole lemon into a bowl and add a pinch of sea salt (or regular salt). Mix well. Add 1 teaspoon of the concentrated lemon-salt mixture to 1 cup warm water. Gargle three to four times a day as needed.

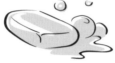

Salt. A saltwater gargle helps heal infected and inflamed vocal chords and sore throats. Add ½ teaspoon salt to 1 cup warm water and gargle several times a day as needed. Be careful to use the correct amount of salt. Gargling with an overly salty solution will only increase the irritation.

Soap and water. Laryngitis can be caused by a viral infection and is easily spread by hand-to-hand contact or by touching contaminated surfaces. Avoiding such germs is one of the best ways to prevent laryngitis. If you or someone around you has a cold, be extra vigilant about washing your hands with warm water and soap. Clean common surfaces, such as the telephone and door handles, with vinegar and a clean cloth.

Steam. Dry indoor air combined with an irritated throat can make you extra miserable. Start the day off steamy. Bring half a pot of water to boil, remove from stove, and place on a protected surface. Drape a towel over your head, lean forward over the pot, and breathe gently for 10 to 15 minutes. Be careful not to stick your face too close. Repeat in the evening before bedtime.

Vinegar. Viruses and bacteria dread an acidic environment, so make your mouth one big, albeit weak, acid bath. Gargling with vinegar can help wipe out many infectious organisms since it is a weak acid. Pour equal amounts of vinegar and

---

LOOK LIKE AN ELEPHANT, TALK LIKE A HOARSE

Here's a way to transform yourself into an elephant man or woman: Drink lots of alcohol. Excessive drinking over a long period of time causes chronic laryngitis and some unsightly elephantine features. No, you won't sprout Dumbo ears, but the folds of your vocal cords will resemble elephant skin. That explains the medical name for the condition: pachydermia—from pachyderm, the scientific term for elephant—which means thick skinned. Wrinkled and tough vocal cords result in a voice that is gravelly, hoarse, and often unintelligible.

WHEN TO CALL THE DOCTOR

- If pain accompanies hoarseness
- If the hoarseness continues for more than 72 hours
- If you have an upper-respiratory infection with fever that lasts more than a couple of days
- If you have trouble breathing
- If you notice a permanent change in the pitch of your voice, especially if you are a smoker
- If you cough up blood

water into a cup, mix, and gargle two to four times a day. You can also gargle with straight vinegar, but some people find it too strong, especially at first.

LIFESTYLE REMEDIES

Avoid alcohol. It dehydrates the body and can cause long-term vocal problems if abused (see "Look Like an Elephant, Talk Like a Hoarse," on page 295).

Cut back on caffeine. Caffeine sucks out moisture from the body. And it relaxes the muscles and valves that control the stomach's entrance (the lower esophageal sphincter), so avoid it if you have heartburn-induced laryngitis.

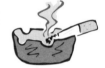

Don't smoke. Smoking and breathing secondhand smoke irritate the larynx and cause coughing, which only increases pain. Smoking is one of the most common causes of chronic laryngitis.

Run a humidifier at night in your room. Remember to clean it frequently.

When flying, stay extra hydrated. Drink more than the normal amount of water, and snack on waterlogged fruits or vegetables, such as grapes or celery sticks, when you're on an airplane.

MORE DO'S AND DON'TS

- Don't constantly clear your throat. This only irritates the vocal chords. If your throat feels like it needs clearing, try gargling with warm water or salt water instead.
- Don't whisper. It can further irritate the throat. Soothe your vocal chords by speaking in a soft, modulated voice. Better yet, don't even try to talk. Communicate in writing.

Low Immunity
MARSHALING YOUR DEFENSES

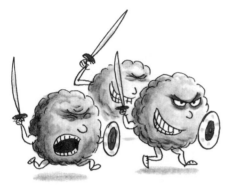
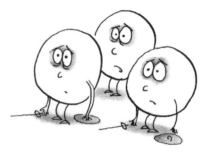

In medical terms, having immunity means that you have resistance to infection or a specified disease. So if you have low immunity, it means your immune system isn't up to par and that you have a greater chance of getting the germ-du-jour. There are many factors that affect your body's response to a foreign invader, including how you're feeling at the moment you're introduced to a suspect germ. If you consistently end up with the latest flu bug or stomach virus, your immune system may be running on empty.

The Battle for Your Body
Imagine your immune system as the front line in your body's war against foreign invaders. The vast network of glands, tissues, and cells are all soldiers working together to get rid of bacteria,

viruses, parasites, and anything that invades their turf. The major troops in this war are the lymphatic system, made of the lymph nodes, thymus, spleen, and tonsils; white blood cells; and other specialized cells such as macrophages and mast cells. Each of these troops has a specialized job in enhancing the body's ability to fight off infection.

Lymph nodes are responsible for filtering out waste products from tissues throughout the body. Under the lymph nodes' command are cells that overtake bacteria and other potentially harmful foreign bodies and crush them like ants. That's why your lymph nodes swell up like golf balls when you are actively fighting off an infection.

IS IMMUNITY INHERITED OR ACQUIRED?

The answer is...both. There are two basic types of immunity. Natural immunity is the type you inherit from your parents. If your mom and dad rarely miss a day's work and are the picture of health, chances are that you will be, too. But no matter how good your genes are, if you don't exercise or eat right and are chronically stressed, you could increase your chances of getting sick.

The second type of immunity is active immunity. Active immunity means you become immune to a disease because you had it already, like the chicken pox, or because you got a vaccination against the disease, such as your annual flu shot.

The thymus is your immune system's stealth warfare command center. You may not have heard of the thymus, but without it you would be one sick puppy. The thymus is an organ that produces many of those disease-fighting foot soldiers—the white blood cells that come to your defense against many types of infections. And the thymus produces hormones that enhance your immune function overall. So if your thymus isn't working as it should, your body may have trouble fighting off infection.

The spleen is vital to your immune defense. It produces white blood cells, kills bacteria, and enhances the immune system overall. White blood cells are your body's main defense in the battle against infection. White blood cells with names such as neutrophils, eosinophils, basophils, T cells, B cells, and natural killer cells, are all part of the vast army of disease assaulters.

When the Enemy Strikes

When something enters your body that is viewed by the immune system as harmful, your body goes into a state of heightened alert. When your immune system is healthy and all systems are go, these foreign invaders, or antigens, are typically met by a barrage of antibodies, which are produced by white blood cells. These antibodies latch on to antigens and set into action all the events that lead to the invader's eventual demise.

If things in your immune system are not working properly, you are less able to fight off foreign invaders. Eventually they set up shop in your body and you get sick. An impaired immune system can make you more susceptible to colds and other merely frustrating illnesses, and it can also make you more at risk for developing cancer.

Science is proving that getting enough of the right nutrients can help you build your immune system. Scientific studies are discovering that avoiding something as simple as a cold or something as life threatening as cancer may be affected by what you stock in your kitchen.

DIETARY REMEDIES

Almonds. Eat a handful of almonds for your daily dose of 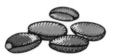 vitamin E, an immune-strengthening antioxidant. Studies have found that vitamin E deficiency causes major problems in the integrity of the immune system.

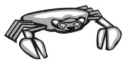 **Black tea.** Researchers at Brigham and Women's Hospital found that women who drank 20 ounces of black tea per day for two weeks had stronger resistance to infections than did a similar group of coffee drinkers. The output of interferon gamma, an infection-fighting substance, was two to three times higher.

Carrots. Carotenes, like the beta-carotene found in carrots and other red, yellow, orange, and dark-green leafy vegetables, are the protectors of the immune 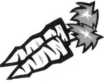 system, specifically the thymus gland. Carotenes strengthen white blood cell production, and numerous studies have shown that eating foods rich in beta-carotene helps the body fight off infection more easily.

Crab. A zinc deficiency can zap your immune system. Zinc acts as a catalyst in the immune system's killer response to

LET THEM DRING WINE

LET THEM DRINK WINE

During a cholera epidemic in Paris in the late 19th century, a French doctor discovered that people who drank wine were more immune to the dreaded disease. He asked people to mix wine into their water to protect themselves against the deadly plague.

foreign bodies, and it protects the body from damage from invading cells. It also is a necessary ingredient for white blood cell function. Nosh on 3 ounces fresh or canned crab and you've got 43 percent of your recommended daily value of this immune-enhancing nutrient.

Green Tea. The incidence of rheumatoid arthritis and other immune system disorders is significantly lower in China and Japan, which are the two leading consumers of green tea. One research study found that cells treated with green tea extract released less of the enzyme associated with arthritis, joint inflammation, and cartilage deterioration than cells not treated with the extract.

Guava. Go a little tropical with this tasty fruit and get more than twice your daily vitamin C needs. Vitamin C acts as an immune enhancer by helping white blood cells perform at their peak and quickening the response time of the immune system.

Kale. A cup of kale gives you twice the daily value of vitamin A, an antioxidant that helps your body fight cancer cells and is essential in the formation of white blood cells. Vitamin A also increases the ability of antibodies to respond to invaders.

Navy beans. Folic acid is the most common nutrient deficiency in the United States. And a folic acid deficiency can actually shrink vital immune system fighters like the thymus and lymph nodes. One cup navy beans gets you 41 percent of your recommended daily value of folic acid.

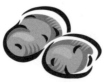

Potato. Not getting enough vitamin B6 can keep your immune system from functioning at its best. Eating a medium baked potato, skin and flesh, will provide you with one-third of most adults' daily requirements for this immune-helping vitamin.

Shiitake mushrooms. Scientists have discovered that specific components of shiitake mushrooms boost the immune system and act as antiviral agents.

Tuna. Selenium is a trace mineral that is vital to the development and movement of white blood cells in the body. A 3-ounce serving of light tuna provides 95 percent of your daily value of selenium.

Wine. A glass of red wine may help your body beat a few potentially harmful foreign bodies. Certain components in wine seem to be helpful in killing infectious bacteria, such as salmonella. But be careful: Drinking too much alcohol can cause your immune system to become depressed, leaving you more open to infection. One glass per day should do the trick.

Yogurt. Yogurt strengthens white blood cells and helps the immune system produce antibodies. One study found that people who ate 6 ounces of yogurt per day avoided colds, hay fever, and diarrhea. Another study found that yogurt could be an ally in the body's war against cancer.

CAN MULTIVITAMINS MAKE YOU STRONGER?

Getting enough of essential nutrients is a good start on the road to a healthy immune system. Generally, eating a well-balanced diet will get you on that road, but you may be thinking about taking a multivitamin to help fill in the gaps. Is it worthwhile? What should you look for?

Most nutrition experts would tell you to get the majority of your nutrients from food—mostly because there are other good-for-you components in food that a supplement may not offer. Taking a multivitamin is a good backup plan, though. If you decide to take a multivitamin, follow these tips:

- Look for a vitamin/mineral combination. You need vitamins and minerals to enhance your immune system, so be sure the product you choose has all you need.
- Don't use products that have more than 100 percent of the recommended daily allowance (RDA) or daily value (DV) of a nutrient. You're going to get most of your vitamins and minerals from your diet, so don't go overboard.
- Make sure your multivitamin meets your needs. If you need to boost your immune system, look for a multivitamin that has the vitamins and minerals discussed in the "remedies" section.
- Check the expiration date. Multivitamins may not start smelling up the place after they expire, but they can lose their potency.
- Only take what is recommended. A single dose per day is exactly what you should take. Don't take extra doses.

WHEN TO CALL THE DOCTOR

- If you have more than 4 or 5 colds per year
- If you have a chronic or ongoing infection
- If you have swollen lymph glands, even when you don't feel ill
- If you now have, or have ever had, cancer. Ask your doctor to check for signs of an impaired immune system.

HERBAL REMEDIES

Echinacea. Research has shown echinacea to boost the body's immune response. It is particularly effective at fighting viral infections, such as the cold and flu, helping your body heal faster. Take 1 or 2 capsules or tablets up to three times a day. You can also buy dried echinacea and brew it into a tea. Simmer 1 to 2 teaspoons in 1 cup boiling water for 10 to 15 minutes; drink as many as 3 cups per day.

Garlic. Garlic is well-known for its antibacterial and antiviral properties. It's even been thought to help prevent cancer. Researchers think these benefits stem from garlic's amazing effect on the immune system. One study found that people who ate more garlic had more of the natural killer white blood cells than those who didn't eat garlic.

LIFESTYLE REMEDIES

Skip the sugar. Sugar may decrease the effectiveness of white blood cells. Keep the sweet stuff to a minimum if your immune system isn't up to par.

Lose a few pounds. Being overweight has an adverse effect on your immune system. One study found that the white blood cells in overweight people were less able to fight off infection compared with their healthy-weight peers.

Try to relax. Stress can impair your immune system. Chronic stress can even shrink your thymus gland, decreasing your ability to fight off infection.

Add some activity. Exercise is a proven immune system booster. Don't overdo it, though. Too much can wear you down.

Memory Problems
SHARPENING YOUR SKILLS

Some events, and some names and faces, definitely should be forgotten. Embarrassing moments, things you wish you hadn't said or done, are memories you can relegate to the memory trash bin. Purposely forgetting is one thing, and we all try to do it on occasion. But on those occasions when memory simply fails you—when you truly don't remember a name, a job assignment slips your mind, you forget a doctor's appointment—your forgetfulness can have unpleasant consequences.

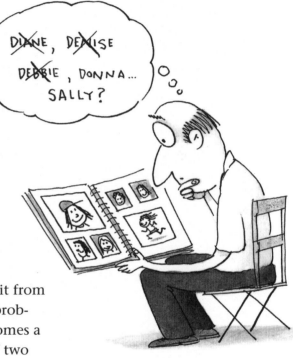

Forgetting is normal. We all experience it from time to time. And when it's an occasional problem, that's OK. But when forgetfulness becomes a chronic problem, that indicates that one of two things is happening:

1. You're not locking in the information as it's received. New information is lost in seven seconds if you don't lock it in right away.

2. You have a physical or mental condition that's preventing you from remembering. For example: Alzheimer's disease, senile dementia, hypoglycemia, severe anemia, depression, anxiety, alcohol or drug abuse, head injury, or severe viral or bacterial illness. Some prescribed medications and cancer treatment protocols make remembering a little difficult, too.

Memory is divided into two parts: short-term and long-term. The short-term memory bank holds the memory for only a few seconds, then transfers it to the long-term memory bank. If the transfer doesn't take place, the memory is lost.

If you're affected by the Seven-Second Syndrome, which is failing to lock in information once it's presented to you, there are memory-strengthening techniques that can improve that forgetfulness.

- Mnemonics. This is the skill of consciously gathering new memory (information) and connecting it to prior memory (knowledge) for easy recall. For example, if you meet someone named Webster, it might trigger you to think of Webster's dictionary. You've now connected something new, the person's name, with something you already know. The connection itself is the mnemonic.

- Acronyms. This is a word formed from a group of letters, each representing the first letter of a word that makes up a phrase. We're such an acronymic society that acronyms are assigned to just about everything, so why not join the crowd and assign your own acronyms to things you want to remember. An easy acronym that comes to mind is ASAP—as soon as possible. Maybe in your cooking ASAP can mean add salt and pepper.

- Rhymes. Rhyme and rhythm have always been terrific memory aids.

- Lists, mental images, visual prompts. These all can help you forget your forgetfulness.

Sometimes memory problems stem from nutritional deficiencies, stress, and other problems that can be controlled once you know how.

Here are some HMBs—home memory boosters—
that might just help you remember.

DIETARY REMEDIES

Blueberries. These luscious little
fruits are the richest source of antioxidants, and recent studies have
shown that blueberries may help
improve short-term memory.

Carrots. They contain carotene, which is a
memory booster. Eat them raw, cooked,
or in casseroles, or make a juice with
carrots and apricots. The apricots are
used to add a little compatible juice to
the dry carrots.

Eggs. These have lecithin, which
keeps the memory nerve cells
healthy. Lecithin is also found in
sunflower and soybean oils and can
be purchased in capsule form, too.
Studies indicate that taking up to 70 grams per
day may improve memory.

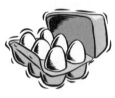

Okra. If not a memorable food, this is at least a
memory-enhancing one. So are sweet potatoes,
tapioca, and spinach. Fresh fruits, especially
oranges, and vegetables, almonds, and milk are
also good for stimulating the memory.

Pistachio nuts. If your memory loss is the result
of a thiamine (vitamin B1) deficiency, pistachio
nuts can help. One of the richest sources of
thiamine, ½ cup supplies 0.54 mg of thiamine.
The RDA for thiamine is 1.2 mg for men and 1.1
for women.

Wheat germ. Wheat germ is a good source of
vitamin E, which may help with age-related
memory loss.

THE ANATOMY OF A MEMORY

- The brain consists of more than 100 billion nerve cells called neurons.
- Each neuron has numerous fibers with tiny bulbs on the end.
- These bulbs send out chemicals called neurotransmitters that hit the walls of other brain cells.
- These other brain cells are charged by the neurotransmitters that hit them, and they send out their own neurotransmitters.
- Neurons fire off neurotransmitters millions of times each and every minute of our lives.
- Memory is controlled by these neurotransmitters.

DIETARY SUPPLEMENT REMEDIES

Vitamin B₆. A deficiency in this vitamin, also called pyridoxine, can cause memory loss. Supplementation may improve memory in older adults.

Vitamin E. Recent studies have reported improved short-term memory in older adults who took supplemental vitamin E.

HERBAL REMEDIES

Frankincense. It's not your everyday herb, but frankincense resin mixed with two common herbs—whole cloves and fresh cardamom— may remedy mild memory loss. Combine 1 teaspoon each and steep in boiling water, then inhale the steam. Do not drink! Do this for 15 minutes, two to three times per day.

Ginkgo. It's the most well-known memory herb of all. It dilates the blood vessels in the brain and increases circulation. Studies have shown better than a 50 percent increase in blood flow with the use of ginkgo, and there are indications that this herb may have properties that will lessen memory problems. However, several large studies of people age 60 and older have not found gingko to be effective in enhancing memory or warding off Alzheimer's disease or dementia.

Warning! Gingko is available in capsules in most pharmacies, but before you try any product containing gingko, consult your physician! It comes with powerful side effects, such as headache, nausea, and allergic reactions. It can cause increased bleeding, especially when taken by people using anticoagulant drugs. If you are going to have surgery, be sure to tell your doctor about your use of gingko or any other herb or supplement.

Herbal teas. Traditionally, any of these are believed to help a weak memory: sage, rosemary, marjoram, basil. Use ¼ teaspoon in a cup of boiling water. Steep for five minutes. These herbs, in an essential oil, can be added to olive oil and massaged over the neck and forehead. Add these oils to bath water, too: 5 drops to a tubful.

LIFESTYLE REMEDIES

Write it down. Post notes. Keep lists. Mark it on the calendar.

Do a daily crossword. Do the crossword puzzle in your daily paper, online, or in a puzzle book. This is a great way to exercise your brain and jog your memory.

Exercise. This stimulates circulation, which is good for the brain.

Meditate. The more you worry about memory loss, the more you are apt to suffer from it. Relax and think about other, more pleasant things.

MORE DO'S & DON'TS

- Keep a food diary. Some foods enhance mental powers, some do not. And some even make mental powers sluggish. To discover your best food choices and combinations, track your choices and reactions.
- Remember recipes. Memory is jogged by familiarity, so sit down at the table, relax, and try to recreate some favorite recipes from memory in writing. Do the same tomorrow and the following days, with the same recipes, and compare your results.

WHEN TO CALL THE DOCTOR
- If memory problems develop suddenly
- If memory problems frequently cause difficulty in everyday situations
- If memory problems begin after starting a new medication

Menopause
MAKING THE CHANGE

Well, "Aunt Flo" won't be making her monthly visit any more. The baby factory is closed. You won't be indisposed or down with the "flu" or under the weather for those few days every month. Most women look forward to the cessation of menstruation and all its associated annoyances. It happens to every woman sometime between the ages of 40 and 58—on average at age 51. But menopause isn't just closing the door on Aunt Flo. It's a process of bodily changes and a reduction in female hormones, and it occurs over several years.

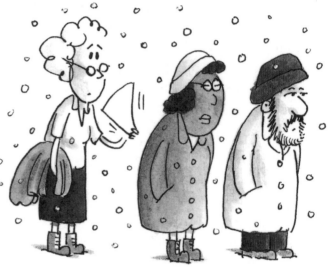

These are some of the changes prior to menopause:

- Estrogen levels begin to drop off around age 30.
- Egg production and release slow down, usually during the 40s.
- Menstrual cycles change. They become longer or shorter, lighter or heavier. Months—or only a week or two—may elapse between periods.
- Whatever happens this time will change next time.

Overall, it takes as long as six years to get through these changes and cross that menopause threshold, but once menstruation has been absent for a full year, you are pronounced "postmenopausal."

In the meantime, as menopause is galloping to the finishing line, it's dragging along a lot of symptoms: hot flashes, vaginal dryness, bladder infection, incontinence, heart palpitations, achy joints, dry or itchy skin, headache, insomnia, weight gain, thinning hair, increased facial hair, mood swings, memory problems, and change in sexual drive.

Obviously, this transition requires some medical guidance, since the consequences can be much more serious than the profuse sweating of a hot flash. There are also ways to curb some of the menopausal symptoms right in your home. And since menopause is nothing to cure, but rather to endure, curbing those problems so simply can be a big relief.

DIETARY REMEDIES

Alfalfa sprouts. Their plant estrogen may help prevent thinning of the vaginal walls. Sprinkle on a salad or use in a stir-fry. Make sure your sprouts are clean before you eat them, though. Raw sprouts can be contaminated with the *E. coli* bacteria. Flaxseed is rich in natural estrogen, too, as is soy. If you have been diagnosed with an estrogen-sensitive cancer, talk with your oncologist about whether to include estrogenic foods in your diet.

Oranges. The vitamin C in oranges is a natural immune booster. It also guards your skin against damage. Other C-rich foods include grapefruits, berries, papayas, green leafy veggies, peppers, and sweet potatoes.

Sardines. Canned sardines, with bones and oil, are rich in bone-building calcium. Because loss of bone density is a common companion to menopause and can lead to osteoporosis, calcium-rich foods are important. Low-fat dairy foods, sesame seeds, nuts, and legumes also should be added to your diet.

Soy. It comes in many forms, and they're all great at relieving symptoms such as hot flashes and vaginal dryness, preventing loss of bone density,

THE CANCER CONNECTION

Female hormones such as estrogen and progestogen have been linked to many cancers that develop in women. Those at highest risk are premenopausal, when more hormones are being produced; risk drops after menopause, when hormone levels drop off.

FASCINATING FACT
Regular alcohol consumption may be linked to an increased risk of breast cancer. It also can exacerbate the weight gain and mood swings that can accompany menopause.

and lowering cholesterol. Try adding tofu, soy milk, and tempeh to your diet.

HERBAL REMEDIES

Chamomile. Combine this with valerian to make a tea that can soothe you to sleep when you're experiencing menopausal insomnia. Drink it one hour before bed.

Evening primrose oil. It's known to be helpful in eliminating PMS symptoms, and it may also relieve menopause symptoms. Take up to 1,000 mg per day, in divided doses.

Herbal Teas. There are several that are said to reduce symptoms of menopause: red raspberry leaf, dandelion, dong quai, damiana, sarsaparilla, licorice, valerian, and black cohosh.

Parsley. Joint aches and pains are a common complaint of menopause, and parsley tea may bring relief. Steep a spoonful in a cup of boiling water for ten minutes, sweeten to taste, and drink two to three times per day. If you can stand the strong taste, add more parsley.

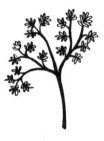

Sage. This has estrogenlike properties and can help reduce sweating and hot flashes. Steep 1 to 2 fresh leaves or a spoonful of dried sage in 1 cup boiling water for ten minutes. Sweeten with honey, add lemon if desired. Drink a cup or two every day. Or, use sage as a spice on vegetables or to season meats.

TOPICAL REMEDIES

Frozen veggies. Place the bag, wrapped in a thin towel, on the back of your neck during a hot flash.

Ice pop. Eat one to cool down during a hot flash. Or go for the ice. Use it any way that cools you off.

Olive oil. Because your face may suffer the effects of dry skin as you go through menopause, mix 1 teaspoon salt and 1 teaspoon olive oil in a small bowl, then use the mixture to gently massage your face and throat to get rid of dead skin cells and replenish lost moisture. Follow by washing with your usual face soap, then rinse.

Salt. Here's what to do to slough off the dry skin that comes with menopause. After you take a shower or bath and while your skin is still wet, sprinkle salt onto your hands and rub it all over your skin. This salt massage will remove dry skin and make your skin smoother to the touch. It will also invigorate your skin and get your circulation moving. Try it first thing in the morning to help you wake up or after a period of physical exertion. And for itchy skin, soaking in a tub of salt water can provide great relief. Just add 1 cup table salt or sea salt to bath water. This solution will also soften skin and help you relax.

Vinegar. To relieve itchy skin and/or aching muscles, add 8 ounces apple cider vinegar to a bathtub of warm water. Soak for at least 15 minutes. To cleanse and tone your face, use a mixture of half vinegar and half water. Then rinse with vinegar diluted with water, and let face air dry to seal in moisture. Make a basic skin toner using a 50–50 mixture of apple cider vinegar or white vinegar and water. Keep toner in a small spray bottle and use after your usual wash.

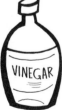

WHEN TO CALL THE DOCTOR

- If you begin to bleed after your periods have completely stopped
- If your bleeding patterns change abruptly
- If periods become extremely long or heavy
- If you experience abdominal pain
- If symptoms interfere with regular activities

LIFESTYLE REMEDIES

Avoid alcohol and caffeine. If your hot flashes seem to be triggered by alcohol or caffeine, simply stay away from them. Try substituting decaffeinated or herbal beverages. Excess caffeine also causes the kidneys to excrete more calcium, a factor in bone-thinning in postmenopausal women.

Exercise. Overall health is important in fending off the symptoms of menopause.

Relax. Stress can trigger hot flashes. Meditation, deep breathing, yoga, and other relaxation techniques can make you feel better in body and soul.

Spare the heat. Highly spiced and hot (in temperature) foods can set off hot flashes in some women.

Talk to your doctor about vitamin or mineral supplements. Don't take anything until you have your doctor's recommendation.

HOT FLASH COOL DOWNS!

Since hot flashes are the most common menopausal complaint, here are ten easy ways to cool off.

1. Layer your clothes, then remove layers as needed when the heat surges.
2. Switch your lightbulbs. Fluorescents put out less heat.
3. Wear cotton. It's a cool fabric that breathes.
4. Avoid outdoor activities during the heat of the day.
5. Have sex. Two to four times per week can stimulate hormones and reduce hot flashes.
6. Carry a fan. A small battery-operated one is convenient and portable.
7. Carry cold water. Freeze 3 to 4 inches of water in a take-along bottle, then fill it with cold water when you leave. This way you'll have cold water for hours.
8. Carry a washcloth. You never know when you'll need to pour that cold water on it and wipe your face.
9. Sleep in the buff. Hot flashes often happen while you're sleeping. They're called night sweats.
10. Skip the silk sheets. They don't breathe well. Sleep on plain white cotton. And sleep under it, too, without a blanket.

Menstrual Problems
MASTERING THE MONTHLIES

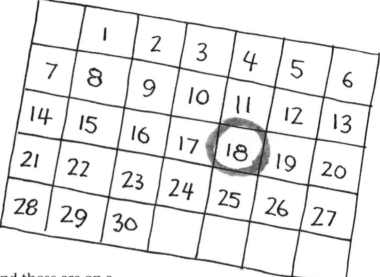

Ah, that time of the month again. It seems as if it rolls around about every other day, doesn't it? When you were young, anticipating your very first period, you were excited by that passage into womanhood. You didn't anticipate the inconvenience, pain, and associated problems: bloat, backache, leg aches, headaches, zits, cramps, and mood swings. And those are on a good menstrual day. On a bad day, bleeding is so heavy you can't move without gushing or you're too tired to breathe. When you figure out that it's more of an inconvenience than something to look forward to, you've joined the menses sisterhood.

Menstruation is the simple process of shedding the old uterine lining to make way for a new one. In other words, it's the body's way of sweeping out the cobwebs at the end of the month in preparation for the arrival of a new egg and a new cycle; all a part of the natural baby-making process with one goal in mind: conception.

Who experiences menstrual problems? At one time or another, every woman who menstruates. However, some factors make problems more likely. These include

WHAT IS A MENSTRUAL CRAMP?

It's uterine contractions caused by the release of prostaglandins, which are hormonelike chemicals. Prostaglandins also produce contractions during labor and childbirth.

MENSES FACTS

- The normal menstrual cycle varies from 21 to 35 days; the "traditional" 28-day cycle is the happy medium.
- Flow lasts from 2 to 9 days.
- 1 to 2 ounces of blood is lost throughout one normal period.
- 75 percent of all women experience some pain with menstruation; 5 to 6 percent experience incapacitating pain

- Family history of problems
- Being overweight, which is particularly associated with amenorrhea or ogliomenorrhea (see "Know Your Terminology," next page)
- Being severely underweight, also linked with amenorrhea, as is being an athlete
- Taking certain drugs
- Chemotherapy or radiation
- Medical conditions and diseases, such as polycystic ovarian syndrome (PCOS), pelvic inflammatory disease (PID), endometriosis, pelvic infection, or gynecological cancers

Most women will experience in the neighborhood of 400 menstrual cycles in their childbearing lifetime. That's a lot of cycles that can cause problems. Serious menstrual problems require medical treatment, since many can lead to infertility, infection, and in some cases, death. But some of the milder problems can be relieved with simple home remedies.

DIETARY REMEDIES

Citrus fruits. Eat or drink with your meals to enhance iron absorption into the body, since iron is easily depleted during menstruation.

Dried apricots. These are high in iron, which is important during menstruation because iron supplies can be depleted with heavy bleeding. Other iron-rich foods include liver, legumes, shellfish, and fortified breads and cereals.

Red meat. It's loaded with iron as well as zinc, which can be depleted during menses, too. Zinc is necessary for healthy bones, and a zinc deficiency may result in amenorrhea. Other iron- and zinc-rich foods: poultry, fish, green leafy vegetables.

Water. Drink plenty of it. Dehydration can cause the body to produce a hormone called vasopressin that contributes to cramps.

DIETARY SUPPLEMENT REMEDIES

Vitamin K. Women who have heavy periods may find relief by taking vitamin K supplements. This is the case even if the blood levels of the vitamin are within the normal range. If you take blood-thinning medication such as Coumadin, talk with your doctor before increasing or decreasing your vitamin K intake.

HERBAL REMEDIES

Basil. This can relieve some of the normal pain associated with menstruation because it contains caffeic acid, which has an analgesic effect. Thyme is also high in caffeic acid. Use it as a spice in cooking meat and vegetables or Italian dishes. Or steep the herb into tea, adding 2 tablespoons thyme or basil leaves to 1 pint boiling water. Cover tightly and let cool to room temperature. Drink ½ to 1 cup an hour for painful menstruation.

Chamomile. This is a reliable cramp reliever. Place ½ ounce in a 1-pint jar and cover with boiling water. Steep for one hour, strain, and drink a cup every hour or two. Use honey to sweeten to taste. This is a particularly relaxing tea just before bed.

Cinnamon. This has anti-inflammatory and antispasmodic properties that relieve cramps. Use as a tea, or sprinkle on toast or sweet rolls. If you have a heavy period, drinking cinnamon tea the day before or during your period may help.

Fennel. Another cramp cure, this spice promotes better circulation to the ovaries. Crush 1 teaspoon fennel seeds into a powder. Add to 1 cup boiling water, steep five minutes, strain, and drink hot.

KNOW YOUR TERMINOLOGY

There are lots of things that can go wrong with the menstrual cycle, and it's good to be familiar with the terms your doctor may use for the various problems. Review the following list.

- Amenorrhea: absence of menstrual periods
- Dysmenorrhea: painful menstruation with cramping
- Hypomenorrhea: scanty menstrual flow of less than 1 ounce
- Menorrhagia: excessive or prolonged menstrual bleeding
- Oligomenorrhea: episodes of menstrual bleeding occurring at more than 35-day intervals
- Polymenorrhea: episodes of menstrual bleeding occurring at less than 21-day intervals

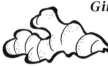

Ginger. This is a cramp reliever, and it sometimes can make irregular periods regular. Use in baked goods or to spice up vegetables and stir-fries. Tea may be the most effective form, however. Put ½ teaspoon in 1 cup boiling water, and drink three times per day.

Juniper berries. These can bring on delayed menstruation. Crush 1 teaspoon juniper berries in a coffee grinder or food processor. Place 1 teaspoon of the powder into a cup and fill with boiling water. Steep ten minutes, then take ¼-cup doses every three to four hours. Do not use for more than three weeks or if you have kidney disease.

Warning! Juniper berries can trigger preterm birth, so avoid them if you may be pregnant.

Lemon balm. This is another cramp reliever, also used for menstruation delayed by stress and tension. Lemon balm also has a mild sedative effect. Make the tea by placing 1 ounce of the herb in 1 quart boiling water, then letting it cool to room temperature. Strain and drink ½ cup per hour until the cramps are gone.

Mint. Either peppermint or wintergreen can relieve cramps. Steep into a tea and drink a cup or two per day. Try sucking on mint candy, too.

Motherwort. This herb is a folk remedy for menstrual cramps and delayed menstruation, and it has sedative properties that can relieve stress or nervousness. Place ½ ounce of the dried flowering tops in a 1-pint jar and cover with boiling water. Let stand for 20 minutes, then strain and rebottle. Take 1 to 2 ounces of the tea every two to three hours for as long as three days. Do not use if you are taking medication for a thyroid or heart condition, or if menstrual bleeding is heavy.

Mustard. A tablespoon or two of powdered mustard in a basin of nice warm water can relieve cramps, but don't drink it. Soak your feet in it to reap the relaxing effects.

Raspberry leaf. This is an old Native American cure for cramps, used by the Chippewa, Cherokee, Iroquois, Kwakiutl, and Quinalt nations. Place 1 ounce raspberry leaf in 1 pint water, then bring to a slow boil. Cover and simmer on the lowest heat 30 to 40 minutes. Cool, stir, strain, bottle. Sweeten to taste. One raspberry leaf contains 408 mg calcium, 446 mg potassium, 106 mg magnesium, 4 mg manganese, and 3.3 mg iron.

Yarrow. A tea made with this herb can stop excessive or prolonged bleeding. It can be taken during the period for bleeding relief or at the beginning to make the entire period easier.

TOPICAL REMEDIES

Hot water. Put it in a hot water bottle and place on the abdomen to relieve cramps. Or soak a kitchen towel, then wring out excess water, heat in microwave for a minute, and place on abdomen. Be careful not to burn yourself.

LIFESTYLE REMEDIES

Do the pelvic tilt to relieve cramps. Lie on your back with your knees bent and your feet flat. Tighten your abdominal muscles and your buttocks and raise your pelvis, angling it toward your head. Press your lower back to the floor, and hold the position for a few seconds. Gently lower your buttocks to the floor. Repeat several times.

Exercise regularly. This increases circulation to the pelvic region and helps clear out prostaglandins. Regular exercise can make that time of the month go easier.

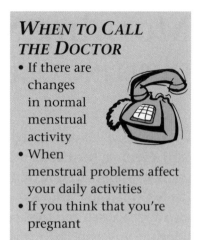

WHEN TO CALL THE DOCTOR
- If there are changes in normal menstrual activity
- When menstrual problems affect your daily activities
- If you think that you're pregnant

Morning Sickness
QUELLING QUEASINESS

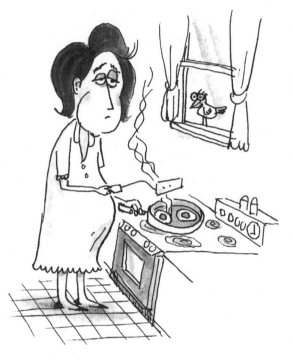

Be it the crack of dawn, high noon, or early evening, the nauseated "I am going to vomit" feeling of the mis-named "morning sickness" can strike anytime. Nausea and the accompanying vomiting associated with early pregnancy have been around since the dawn of motherhood. The ancient Egyptians wrote about the condition in 2,000 B.C. but didn't come up with a cure. The same holds true today.

Approximately 70 to 85 percent of American women will suffer from nausea, dry heaves, vomiting, or all three, usually during the first three months of pregnancy. The severity and frequency varies from woman to woman and pregnancy to pregnancy. Some lucky mothers-to-be feel wonderful from conception on. Other women vomit in the morning but feel fine the remainder of the day. But some expectant mothers suffer nonstop.

A Hormone High

Morning sickness is usually attributed to hormonal changes during pregnancy. These hormonal changes do much to maintain the health of mother and baby, but they unfortunately come with side effects, notably stomach upset. The hormone that supports your pregnancy, human chorionic gonadotropin, or HCG, is the prime suspect, as it runs at an all-time high during the first few months. Other hormones may also play a nauseating role as well, including rising estrogen and progesterone levels.

Luckily, relief is usually just a few months away since symptoms typically subside after the first trimester. In the meantime, you don't need to sit and suffer. There is no cure for nausea, but there are ways to take the edge off that unpleasant feeling. Experiment with a few cures below and find out what works best for you.

DIETARY REMEDIES

Citrus fruit. A small slice of lemon, lime, or orange added to your water or herbal tea can help ease nausea.

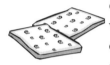

Crackers. Crackers are a pregnant woman's friend. They are portable, easy-to-digest, inexpensive, and can nip nausea in the bud. White or whole-wheat crackers, pretzels, plain popcorn, or low-salt soda crackers are your best bets. Nibble on them throughout the day and before going to bed. If nausea hits first thing in the A.M., eat crackers as your feet touch the cold floor. Better yet, stay in bed and nibble for several minutes. Sudden transitions from horizontal to vertical often trigger nausea, so go easy in the morning.

Fruits and vegetables. Water consumption is very important during pregnancy, but not all your water has to come from the tap. Foods high in water content help prevent dehydration and its partner constipation, both of which aggravate nausea. Snack on melons, carrots, celery, grapes, apples, and pears.

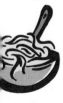

Pasta. The foods you think of as starches, such as pasta, bread, and potatoes, are easier to digest and are soothing.

Potato chips. Perhaps pregnancy is the only time in a woman's life when potato chips offer a cure … and can be consumed without guilt. For many women, munching on a

---

MORNING SICKNESS MYTHS

Myth #1: Bad bouts of morning sickness mean you'll have a girl.

Ha! Tell that to the millions of women who had morning sickness … and a boy. Morning sickness is totally unrelated to a baby's sex. What may prove true, however, is that women experiencing double the amount of morning sickness may be carrying double the amount of baby (twins!).

Myth #2: Climbing over your partner as you exit bed in the morning transfers the sickness to him and makes you feel better.

Yes, when you throw up on him, he'll feel sick too, and you might feel better for a moment, but it isn't a cure.

A SUMMERTIME DELIGHT

Raspberries. Summer months don't hold much refreshment for expectant mothers, who find the heat and humidity unbearable. But there is one cool spot in this inferno: raspberries. Red raspberry leaves have long been used to calm morning sickness, plus they make a tasty, cooling iced tea! If you're lucky enough to have raspberry bushes, gather the leaves and make them into a tea. (It's best to harvest the leaves before the berries start to appear. Make sure no pesticides/chemicals have been used on the plants.) Place 1 ounce raspberry leaves in 1 quart boiling water. Simmer for 30 minutes. Strain, cool, add ice cubes, and drink throughout the hot day.

few chips (note the word "few") at the first sign of nausea helps dissipate it. Stick to regular potato chips and stay away from the fat-free varieties that contain Olestra, the fat substitute. Olestra robs yours body of important nutrients, and it is known to cause diarrhea.

Sometimes pregnancy brings about an over-production of saliva, which can make the mother-to-be sick to her stomach. Nibbling on a handful of salt-and-vinegar chips helps dry up the saliva. Nibble only when needed. Some women may find this remedy distasteful since fat is hard to digest and can cause increased stomach upset.

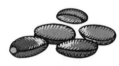

Protein-rich snacks. Nuts, peanut butter, dairy products, and other high-protein foods may help relieve nausea.

Water. Dehydration can cause nausea. Expectant mothers must drink 8 glasses of water per day.

DIETARY SUPPLEMENT REMEDIES

Vitamin B6. Many physicians recommend taking a B6 supplement to reduce morning sickness nausea. The typical dose is 10 to 25 milligrams three times per day. However, be sure to talk to your doctor before taking a supplement, and don't exceed 75 milligrams per day.

HERBAL REMEDIES

Fennel. Fennel seed is a nausea remedy from Chinese folk medicine. As with mint (see next page), fennel seed contains anesthetic constituents that may reduce queasiness. Crush 1 tablespoon fennel seeds in a coffee grinder. Place the crushed seeds in a cup and fill with boiling water. Cover and let steep for ten minutes. Drink the tea in sips to treat nausea.

Ginger. Ginger has a well-established track record as a morn- 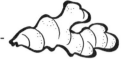 ing sickness remedy, especially in the folk medicine of New England and the Pacific Northwest. The root contains chemicals called gingerols and shogaols that relax the intestinal tract, relieving nausea and vomiting. The easiest way to get your ginger is through real ginger ale (non-caffeinated) or ginger tea. For the tea, place ½ teaspoon powdered ginger spice into a cup and fill with boiling water. Cover and let stand ten minutes. Strain and sip. Don't take more than three times daily. If needed, sweeten with just a little honey. You can also try ginger candy.

Warning! Some experts frown on using ginger during pregnancy, but others say it is OK. Limit intake to 1 gram per day for no more than four days. If you have concerns, talk to your doctor.

Lavender and thyme. Smells become more pronounced during pregnancy. Odors that didn't bother you before, like dirty laundry, can now have you reaching for a bucket. Battle smells of any sort by arming yourself with a small satchel stuffed with dried herbs. Lavender and thyme are particularly appealing since both have soothing reputations. A handkerchief scented with fresh-squeezed lemon also makes a handy remedy. Keep the satchel or hanky near the nose and breathe in deeply when odors turn your stomach sour.

Mint. The anesthetic constituents in mint work to minimize nausea by reducing the stomach's gag reflex. Make a cup of mint tea anytime you feel a wave of nausea about to crash ashore. Place 1 tablespoon mint leaves in a 1-pint jar of boiling water. Let stand 20 to 30 minutes, shaking occasionally. Strain and sip as needed.

WHEN TO CALL THE DOCTOR

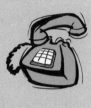

- If you are losing weight
- If the vomiting does not let up
- If you are becoming dehydrated (signs are infrequent urination and dark urine)
- If you haven't been able to keep food or drink down for 24 hours
- If you are feeling increasingly tired
- If you feel dizzy or can't focus mentally
- If morning sickness persists past the third month
- If morning sickness is accompanied by worrisome symptoms, such as headache or bleeding

Motion Sickness
TAMING TURBULENCE

It can happen almost anywhere—in the backseat of your family van, on the Tilt-a-Whirl at the county fair, on the bumpy airplane ride to grandma's, or on your Alaskan cruise. Anything that moves has the potential to give you a green hue and leave you wishing the world would put on the brakes—or at least that the plane, train, automobile, amusement park ride, or boat that's making you so ill would stop so you could die in peace. Anyone who has experienced motion sickness would agree that it is a horrible feeling—one they wouldn't want to make a repeat appearance. Thankfully, most people only deal with motion sickness on occasion. Following some simple tips can help avert those rare bouts.

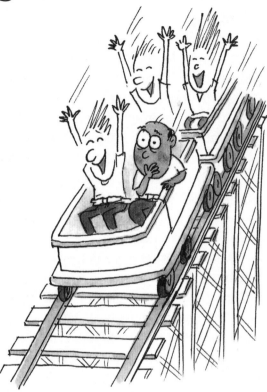

Tummy Turbulence

So why does your tummy do cartwheels every time you sail, fly, or ride? Motion sickness is purely a matter of miscommunication. When you're cruising down the road focused on a book or a person, your eyes tell your brain that you're not moving, but your inner ear tells the brain a different story. For instance, you and your girlfriends are going for a long-awaited women-only weekend. All six of you pile in your friend's minivan. You pop in the passenger seat and as soon as you get on the road, you're turned around chatting with your buddies. You see only your stationary friends sitting in the back of the van, so your eyes tell your brain that you're sitting in a room catching up with old pals. But the fluid in your inner ear is sloshing around with every bump and turn. Your brain is getting mixed signals. And in the confusion, your brain triggers your tummy and you start feeling sick. Next thing you know, you and the girls are forced to make a pit stop.

Symptoms of a Spinning Head

No one can completely avoid motion sickness. Even astronauts have bouts of nausea every now and then. For most people, motion sickness comes on fairly quickly and usually involves one of these symptoms: sweating, hyperventilation, dizziness, paleness, sensation of spinning (even after you're off the Tilt-a-Whirl), loss of appetite, and of course, nausea.

DIETARY REMEDIES

Apple juice. Drink a glass of apple juice with your pre-travel low-fat meal. Giving your body a bit of sugar with fluids before you start your journey should help you down the road. And if you start feeling ill, sipping (not gulping) some juice may help you feel better. Almost any noncitrus juice will do. Citrus juice irritates an already unstable stomach.

Crackers. Take these easily digest-ible snacks along and nibble on them every couple of hours to help prevent nausea and vomit-

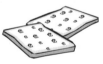

ing. An empty stomach makes it more likely that you will get sick.

Ice. Sucking on some ice chips may help calm your stomach and help divert your attention from your unsettled tummy.

Low-fat foods. If you eat a low-fat meal before you head out on your trip, you may avoid getting sick. Eating something before you leave makes your stomach more capable of

MOTION PROBLEMS? LOOK OVER THE COUNTER

There are many over-the-counter motion sickness drugs that offer relief from debilitating symptoms, but most of them are antihista-mines, which means they'll make you sleepy. If you're headed on a long flight overseas, taking a drug that makes you sleep might not be a bad thing. If you're headed to an elegant cruise ship dinner, however, you probably don't want to fall asleep before the entrée. So be wary. If you choose an over-the-counter reliever, take it 30 to 60 minutes before you're set to leave to give it ample time to work.

Other nonprescription choices for motion sick-ness are ReliefBands or BioBands. ReliefBands are FDA approved for helping motion sickness. The bands strap onto your wrist like a watch and deliver a mild electrical stimulation to your nerves, which blocks the brain signal that makes you nauseous. BioBands are based on acupressure, and they exert pressure on particular acupoints in your wrist that control nausea and vomiting.

BEST BETS FOR SICKNESS-FREE TRAVEL

Follow these travel tips and you'll be more likely to get where you're going without motion sickness misery.

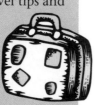

- Airplane. Sit near the front edge of a wing. And be sure to get a window seat so you can let your eyes and ears get in sync.
- Train. Sit near a window and face forward.
- Boat. A recent study discovered that where you sleep on a cruise ship isn't all that important. It's where you are when you're awake that can cause problems. Stay on deck when you can so you can spy the horizon at all times, and stay near the middle of the ship if you're sensing some rocking. There's less rocking and swaying there.
- Car. Sit in the front passenger seat so you can get a good peek at the horizon. Don't turn around if you can help it. If you struggle with sickness every time you ride, try driving.

handling the ups and downs of the road. Experts say not eating destabilizes the stomach's electrical signals, making you susceptible to nausea and vomiting.

Peppermint candies or lozenges. If you start feeling sick, get out the peppermints. Not only will you end up with fresh minty breath when you arrive at your destination, you'll also calm your queasiness. And if you're traveling with little ones, try placing 1 drop peppermint oil on their tongues before the trip. It may quash the queasies.

Tea. Sip on some warm tea if you start feeling sick. Warm beverages tend to be easier on a nauseated tummy than a tall glass of cold water. Go for the decaf brew; caffeinated drinks aren't a good idea for unstable stomachs.

HERBAL REMEDIES

Ginger. Ginger has long been an herbal remedy for queasiness, but modern science has proved this spice has merit, especially for motion sickness. One study discovered that ginger was actually better than over-the-counter motion sickness drugs. Make a ginger tea to take along with you when you're traveling by cutting 10 to 12 slices of fresh ginger and placing them in a pot with 1 quart water. Boil for ten minutes. Strain out the ginger, and add ½ cup honey or maple syrup for sweetening if you like. But ginger tea isn't the only way to get the protective and calming benefits of this herb. Studies have found that 250 to 500 mg of dried ginger taken every six hours staves off motion sickness. Your best bet is to take your dose of ginger before you travel. You could also try candied ginger: A one-inch piece should do the trick. And there's also enough ginger in gingersnaps and ginger ale to ease milder bouts of nausea.

LIFESTYLE REMEDIES

Focus on the horizon. Stay focused on the sunset, a billboard, a tree, a red light—anything outside the vehicle that isn't moving. Having a stable object to focus on helps your eyes and inner ear send the same message to your brain.

Skip the fast food. That hamburger and fries might be quick and convenient, but they won't sit well in your tummy if you have a bout of motion sickness.

Ax the alcohol. Drinking while traveling will only make you feel worse. Alcohol tends to go through the bloodstream straight to the inner ear, which throws off your equilibrium.

Put away the book (or laptop or magazine). Looking at a computer screen or a book while trees are whipping past your head will only make you sicker.

Keep busy. Listen to a book on tape or your favorite CD, or make out your grocery list in your head. Keeping your mind occupied will help you fend off nausea.

Don't worry. Motion sickness feels awful, but it's only temporary. Fretting about how bad you feel can only make things worse.

SKIP MOTION SICKNESS WITH SCOPOLAMINE?

Scopolamine is a prescription antinausea medication given to people who have trouble with motion sickness. It's available in a convenient patch form. The dime-size skin patch goes behind the ear a few hours before you leave on your trip and protects you for about 72 hours.

Scopolamine also was recently tested in nasal spray form and got rave reviews. The advantage of the nasal spray is that it works quickly. Thirty minutes after a squirt in the nose, you're ready to roll. If you're planning a trip and have a history of intense motion sickness, you may want to ask your doctor about scopolamine. Scopolamine cannot be taken by people with certain conditions, such as asthma and glaucoma.

WHEN TO CALL THE DOCTOR

If motion sickness becomes a regular occurrence or if it becomes debilitating

Muscle Soreness/Cramping
EASING THE ACHE

You've made your New Year's resolution: You are going to get in shape. Never mind that the last time you exercised was at a charity walk a few years ago and that the very expensive treadmill you bought is now buried underneath a pile of laundry. Twenty pounds and three kids ago you were an aerobics queen, so you know what it's like to feel, and look, better. So you venture into your local health club and decide to try the low/high aerobics class for people who have been out of circulation for a while. You think you can keep up with the twenty-something girls, so you grapevine and kick and half-jack with the beat for 50 minutes. By the time you get home, though, your muscles have gone on strike. The next day you can barely muster enough strength to make it out of bed, and you spend the day walking like you've been riding the range a bit too long. You'll take it slower next time. But what can you do right now to ease the pain?

Muscle Mayhem

The vast array of muscles in your body is what allows you to do something as simple as picking up a fork or as complicated as a kickboxing routine. Muscles are a complex weave of fibers that work with your brain and skeletal system to give you the agility to return that volley across the tennis court. When you're taking care to

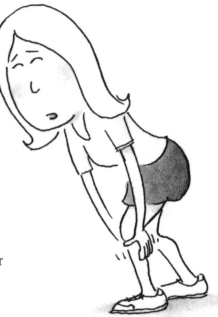

> ### THIS'LL PUMP YOU UP
> One muscle fiber is thinner than a human hair but can support as much as 1,000 times its own weight.

stretch and strengthen your muscles, they are your greatest ally. But when they don't work like they should or they get injured, you have a very painful problem on your hands.

Strains are one of the most common reasons for aching muscles. When you strain a muscle, it means you've worked it too hard, causing the muscle fibers to pull and tear. If you haven't worked out for a while and then head back full throttle without preparing your muscles for the trauma they're about to experience, or if you're an experienced exerciser and you don't warm up properly, you risk getting a strained muscle. At best, a strained muscle will leave you sore for a few days; at worst, you could end up with a more serious muscle injury.

Another common muscle malady is cramps, or spasms. Muscle cramps happen when the muscle isn't getting enough blood, and in response to the restricted blood flow the muscle shortens and tightens. The slowdown in blood flow can be caused by a variety of problems:

- A deficiency in essential nutrients for maximum muscle power, such as sodium, calcium, and potassium
- Dehydration
- Depletion of the muscles' energy supply of glycogen
- Overworked muscles
- Holding the same position for too long

Whatever the reason, when blood doesn't reach your muscles the way it should, your muscles can turn into balls of pain.

Your first priority is to give your muscles some rest and try a few home remedies that will help you feel better, fast.

NOCTURNAL NUDGES

There's nothing like a nighttime leg cramp to get you howling at the moon. Pinched nerves are the usual culprit, making your calf muscle knot up and waking you—and the rest of the house—from a peaceful slumber. Or you may simply have rolled and stretched a tendon, which caused some mixed signals to go through your spinal cord and resulted in a cramped calf muscle.

Thirty-three percent of people older than 60 have sleep-related muscle cramps at least once every two months. If you find yourself with a cramp, massage the muscle with long strokes, moving toward the heart. You may be able to avoid muscle cramps by stretching before bed (especially concentrating on the offending muscle), sleeping under lightweight covers, and being sure you get enough calcium—which is often lacking in people who get those nocturnal nudges.

HERBS THAT EASE MUSCLE ACHES

In folk medicine, some herbs have been labeled "counterirritants." These herbs stimulate blood flow to the skin and the muscles underneath. Practically speaking, counterirritants encourage healing and provide pain relief for those aching muscles. Two commonly used counterirritants in folk healing are cayenne pepper and mustard seeds.

Try this mustard plaster recipe when you have muscles aches.

1. Crush the seeds of white or brown mustard.
2. Moisten with vinegar and sprinkle with flour.
3. Spread mixture on a cloth, and cover with a second cloth.
4. Lay the moist side on the painful area, and leave on for 20 minutes. (Remove the plaster if it becomes painful.)

DIETARY REMEDIES

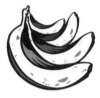

Bananas. Eat a banana or two a day and you may cut down your cramping. That's because a potassium deficiency may be to blame for muscle cramps. The adequate intake (AI) of potassium is 4.7 grams (4,700 mg) per day. One banana has 450 mg of the muscle-protecting nutrient.

Bouillon. Sipping some warm soup before heading out for a long bike ride may not sound appealing, but it may help you avoid muscle cramps. Drink 1 cup beef or chicken bouillon before you ride. It helps you replace the sodium you lose when you sweat.

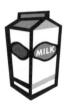

Milk. Getting adequate amounts of calcium in your diet may help curtail your cramps. Women especially seem to need plenty of calcium for muscle health. Three glasses of milk per day will meet the calcium needs of most adults.

Water. Yes, it's the elixir of life as well as your best bet for avoiding a painful muscle cramp while you exercise. When you exercise, you sweat. That sweat depletes your body of needed fluids that can cause your muscles to mutiny. Drink plenty of water before, during, and after you do your activity of choice.

HERBAL REMEDIES

Rosemary. A few leaves of rosemary can help reduce swelling in strained muscles. Use either fresh or dried leaves; fresh has more of the volatile oils. The herb has four anti-inflammatory properties, which can help calm inflamed muscle tissue and speed healing. Because rosemary is easily absorbed through the skin, placing a cloth soaked with a rosemary wash will help ease the pain. Here's how to make a rosemary wash: Put 1 ounce rosemary leaves in a 1-pint jar and fill the jar with boiling water. Cover and let stand for 30 minutes. Apply the wash to the area two or three times per day.

TOPICAL REMEDIES

Epsom salts. Jump in a hot bath with Epsom salts to ease the pain of your strain (but wait at least 24 hours before you hit the heat). Epsom salts contain loads of magnesium that is absorbed through the skin. Magnesium helps promote the healing of torn muscles. Add 2 cups Epsom salts to a tub of hot water. It also relieves any swelling.

Ice. Immediately after straining a muscle, your first order of business is to allay the swelling. The best way to keep your torn muscle from swelling is to constrict the blood vessels that run to it. The best way to do that: Ice 'em. Some athletes actually take a hop in an ice bath to soothe strained muscles, but if you're not that brave, try an ice pack on the area for 15 to 20 minutes three times per day.

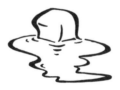

LIFESTYLE REMEDIES

Don't do too much, too fast. Start slowly and add to your workout. Some experts recommend the 10 percent rule. Add ten percent more intensity to your workout every week.

Stop. If you feel muscle pain or a cramp creeping up on you, stop what you're doing. Don't try to exercise through the pain; you'll only make things worse.

WINTERGREEN WASH

Wintergreen is a botanical precursor to aspirin, and it's helpful in relieving muscle pain. Straight wintergreen oil can be toxic to the skin, however. So create a wash using the dried herb to alleviate soreness.

1. Put 1 ounce dried wintergreen leaves in a cup.
2. Cover with 1 pint boiling water.
3. Let it stand until it cools to room temperature.
4. Apply as a wash over the sore area.

MUSCLE MANIA

There is a 3:1 ratio of muscle to bone in the human body. You have 650 muscles throughout your body and only 206 bones.

WHEN TO CALL THE DOCTOR

- If you get serious leg cramps often. It could be a signal that there's a problem with the blood flow to your muscle, or it may mean you have a nerve injury.
- If you think you may have a severe strain
- If muscle pain is accompanied by trouble breathing, dizziness, high fever, or stiff neck, or occurs after starting a new medication

Not sure if you have a severe muscle strain? Ask yourself these questions:

1. Did you feel a sharp pain at the moment you injured your muscle?
2. Does moving the muscle cause intense pain?
3. Is there localized swelling and tenderness in the area of the muscle?
4. Are you unable to use the muscle?
5. Do you have bruising or discoloration in the injured area?

If you answered "yes" to any of these questions, you may have a serious strain.

Cancel the creams. Topical sports creams, except those containing capsaicin, won't help your sore muscles because they don't do anything to the tissues underneath. And if you use a cream and place a heating pad over it, you could end up with a serious burn.

Go over the counter. Use an anti-inflammatory drug to ease the pain and stop the swelling.

Halt the heat. Don't put heat on a strained muscle in the first 24 hours after you exercise. Heat causes blood vessels to dilate and increases swelling and fluid buildup, which means your soreness will last longer than it should.

Keep moving. One of the worst things you can do for sore muscles is to stay still until the pain goes away. Walking around or doing some slow stretches returns blood flow to the muscle, making it much easier for the body to repair itself.

Keep muscles warm. In cold weather, this may help you avoid cramps.

Stretch and squeeze. When you get a cramp, stretch the offending muscle slowly. As you stretch, use one hand to gently squeeze your ball of painful muscle.

Skip the sports drinks. Unless you're running more than an hour every day, you really don't need a sports drink. Water is your best bet for replacing fluids.

Nail Problems
DOCTORING DIGITS

Most people find themselves dealing with nail problems from time to time. Nail disorders make up 10 percent of all skin conditions. So whether you've got something as frustrating as brittle nails or something more serious, such as a fungal infection, taking good care of your nails will help you put your best foot, or hand, forward.

Nail Knowledge

Though they may be a source of frustration from time to time, your nails are there for a good reason. They make it much easier to pick up a paper clip or grip a pencil. They also help support tissues in the fingers and toes and help protect your body from infection-causing bacteria. Nails are made of keratin—the same protein in your skin and your hair. Made of many layers, nails have a unique design that makes them tough and resilient. Here are their parts:

- *Nail plate.* This is the part you cut and paint and file—the tough part that is visible on fingers and toes.
- *Nail Bed.* This is the skin right below the nail. It's best if you

only see that through the translucent nail—if you've ever ripped your nail off into the nail bed, you understand. (It's quite painful!)

- *Matrix.* This is a place, invisible to the eye, underneath the cuticle that is essentially the nerve center of nail growth.
- *Lunula.* Look at the bottom of your nail. The whitish, half-moon shape where your nail disappears into the skin is actually a visible part of the matrix.
- *Cuticle.* This is the skin that wraps around the sides and base of the nail.
- *Nail folds.* The skin that frames the nail.

TRYING TO NIX THE NAIL BITING?

Biting your nails is a bad habit. It deforms the nail and can hurt the skin around the nail, opening the door to infection. If you have a nail biter in your house, you can try icky-tasting nail polish, but it probably won't do the trick. Time is the only method that seems to work for nail biters. If your child is a nail biter, don't fret; he'll probably grow out of it.

HOW DO YOUR NAILS GROW?

Fingernails grow about 1½ inches per year. Toenails grow about ½ to ¾ of an inch in a year. Your fingernails will grow faster when the weather's warm, when you're pregnant, and when they're growing back after injury.

Notorious Nail Offenders

Not paying much attention to your nails can cause you problems in the long run. And dealing with nail problems can be a painful, and yucky, business. Here is a rundown of the most common nail problems.

- *Brittle nails.* Brittle nails are less painful than many nail problems, but they're no less annoying. If you're battling brittle nails, you likely have one of two conditions—hard, brittle nails or soft, brittle nails. Both make you more likely to have nails that split and break easily. Hard nails can be caused by using nail polish removers too often (don't use more than twice a month and avoid those with acetone), being in a too-dry environment (like indoor heat), or not wearing gloves while dealing with harsh chemicals or detergents. If you have hard, dry nails, you need to moisturize them, just as you would dry skin. Soft, brittle nails, on the other hand, are caused by exposing the nails to too much moisture—either using too much hand lotion or keeping your hands in water too long. Soft nails need to be kept dry. As you get older your skin gets drier and you encounter more problems with brittle nails.

- *Fungus.* Fungal infections make up 50 percent of all nail disorders. Toenails are more susceptible than fingernails because toenails live in a warm, moist, fungus-loving environment. Fungal infections may cause the nail plate to separate from the nail bed (ouch!) and cause very unpleasant-looking debris, usually white, green, yellow, or black, to build under the nail plate.

- *Ingrown nails.* Ingrown nails are another common nail offender. Not properly trimming your nails can make you more likely to get an ingrown nail, but wearing too-snug shoes can also be a contributing factor. A nail becomes ingrown when the corner of the nail curves downward into the skin, causing a very painful condition. Ingrown nails are more common on toenails, but fingernails are not immune to the problem.
- *Nail trauma.* You slam the car door on your finger, or you bash your thumbnail with a hammer. As blood rushes to the surface of your nail, it forms a bruise. This type of injury can open the door to other infections and needs to be watched carefully.

It'd be nice if drinking a glass of milk made your nails grow more quickly, but the reality is there's nothing you can eat or drink that will make your nails grow longer or stronger. Neither eating gelatin nor taking vitamin and mineral supplements will make your nails any stronger or grow any faster. But there are some home staples that will help you keep your nails at their healthiest and alleviate frustrating nail problems.

TOPICAL REMEDIES

Baking soda. Clean your nails and soften cuticles by scrubbing them with a nailbrush dipped in baking soda.

TIPS FOR NATTIER NAILS

Taking good care of your nails is your best bet to avert nail problems. Try these tips for healthier nails.

- Take time to trim. Short and square nails are the least likely to chip or rip. Cut nails straight across with manicure scissors or nail clippers.
- Don't be a file fanatic. Use an emery board instead of a metal file; it's gentler on the nails. Don't file down deep into the nail folds or you could set yourself up for more fragile nails. And don't file too much, as you can do more harm than good.
- Leave your cuticles alone. Don't push back the cuticle with orange sticks, pumice pencils, or any other cuticle cutters or pushers.
- Don't share. When you share nail-grooming equipment, you may also share germs.
- Remember the power of polish. Nail polish makes your nails look nice and can protect them from damage. But avoid polish that contains formaldehyde, and give your nails a polish vacation now and then. Stick with a once-a-week schedule, or less, for applying and removing polish. Acetone in nail polish removers can cause dry, brittle nails.
- Don't mess with hangnails. If you get a hangnail, don't rip it or bite it off. Clip the dry part and then apply an over-the-counter antibiotic ointment.

WHEN TO CALL THE DOCTOR

- If a fungal infection does not respond to over-the-counter antifungal medications
- If your ingrown toenail is very painful and pus develops or you see redness that seems to be spreading
- If you have diabetes and any toenail problems
- If the bruise under your hammer-hit nail puts too much pressure on the nail; the doctor may need to drain it

These may signal a more serious problem:

- Pale or bluish nails can mean anemia.
- Yellowish nails may mean diabetes.
- White nails can indicate liver disease.
- Half-pink, half-white nails can mean kidney disease.
- Thick yellow nails that are growing slower than usual can indicate lung disease.
- Nails shaped like the back of a spoon may signal cardiopulmonary disease or asthma.
- Nails that dip inward may signal anemia.
- A dark spot may be a sign of skin cancer.

Bath oil. Soak brittle nails in oil for 15 minutes before trimming to prevent splitting and breaking.

Salt. Soaking painful ingrown nails in a warm saltwater solution will help ease the pain and relieve swelling. Add 1 tablespoon salt per quart of water and soak for 30 minutes. A saltwater soak can also make tough nails easier to trim. Try soaking nails in the same solution for five to ten minutes before trimming.

Vinyl gloves. Wetting your hands too often or exposing them to harsh detergents or chemicals can cause brittle nails. Wearing vinyl gloves—especially if you sprinkle a bit of baby powder in them—keeps your hands dry and safe from abrasive materials.

Water. Hard brittle nails need some moisture. Soak your nails in lukewarm water and then slather on a moisturizer with phospholipids, urea, or lactic acid.

LIFESTYLE REMEDIES

To avoid fungal infections:

- Change your socks often.
- Don't go barefoot in a public shower.
- Keep your nails clean and dry.
- Use an antifungal spray on your feet and in your shoes.

To avoid or treat ingrown toenails:

- Apply an antibiotic ointment to the infected area.
- Don't wear shoes and socks that are too snug.
- Put small pieces of cotton under the edge of the ingrown nail. That will help the nail grow above the skin.
- Trim toenails straight across.

Nausea and Vomiting
HALTING THE HEAVES

It happens to everybody. No one gets a free pass. But that doesn't make the misery of nausea and vomiting any easier on your system.

Nausea is a warning signal; it means stop eating, let your stomach rest. Vomiting is a warning signal, too; it means something doesn't belong in your stomach and it's time to get rid of it. In other words, nausea and vomiting are two ways that your tummy protects itself.

Who Dunnit?
Usually nausea and vomiting are self-limiting. Once the cause is removed, the symptoms go away. So what causes these unsettling symptoms? There are many possibilities, including

- something you ate or drank
- a medication you took
- food poisoning
- early pregnancy
- a stomach disorder
- a viral or bacterial infection
- migraine headache
- head injury
- inner ear infection
- stress
- recreational drug use

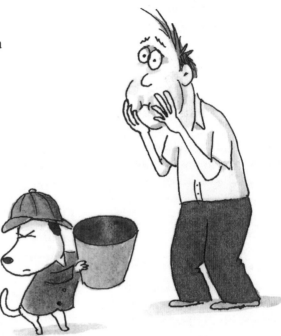

- binge-purge eating disorders
- visual disturbances
- fear

The bottom line is that nausea and vomiting are not caused by any single factor. And they're not illnesses in themselves—they're symptoms of something else going on with your body.

When to Halt the Heaves
Although your first inclination after vomiting is to find some way to stop it from happening again, this emetic

BACK IN THE SWING OF EATING

When vomiting starts, eating stops. You don't feel like eating, and there's no reason to eat since your stomach is rejecting your attempts to fill it. Eventually you do have to start again, though, and unless you're a glutton for more gut-wrenching punishment, starting out easy is best. Here's how to resume eating after a bout of vomiting.

- Try clear liquids first. You can take them during your bout of vomiting, although they may come back up. When you can keep them down, consume only clear liquids such as water, broth, flavored gelatin water, and noncitrus fruit juices for 12 hours.
- After 12 hours, switch to bland foods: rice, cooked cereal, clear soups with rice or noodles, cottage cheese, baked potatoes, flavored gelatin. Eat these for 24 hours.
- After a day of bland foods, add mild foods back into your diet, such as baked or broiled lean meats and steamed vegetables. Skip greasy and spicy foods for a few more days just to make sure your stomach is ready to handle them.

rush is really your friend because it often does get rid of whatever is ailing you. On occasion, however, nausea and vomiting drag on. You may be able to cope with ongoing nausea, but there are risks to repeated vomiting. If you vomit a lot or for many days, you can become dehydrated. And if vomiting accompanies morning sickness, the nutritional flow to the developing fetus may be disrupted.

Because nausea and vomiting are usually just sideshows and not the main event, under most circumstances they can be remedied right in your home without too much fuss or muss. Here are several ways to put them in their place.

DIETARY REMEDIES

Cranberry juice. Avoiding solid food for a day is sometimes recommended when you're nauseated and vomiting, but don't give up the fluids. Drink cranberry juice during your fast. It's generally easy on your digestive tract.

Lemon juice. Mix together 1 teaspoon honey and 1 teaspoon lemon juice. And this cure comes with a folkish instruction: Dip your finger into the mix and lick it off so that you take it in slowly.

Lime juice. For an immediate nausea/vomiting stopper, mix 1 cup water, 10 drops lime juice, and ½ teaspoon sugar. Then add ¼ teaspoon baking soda and drink.

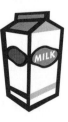 *Milk.* Don't drink it straight. Instead, try this vintage milk-toast recipe for a bland food that's easy to eat when combating nausea and vomiting. Heat 1 cup milk until hot but not boiling.

Put it in a bowl. Then take 1 piece of toast, slightly buttered, and crumble it into the milk. Eat slowly.

Onion. Juice an onion to make 1 tea- spoon. Mix with 1 teaspoon grated ginger and take for nausea.

Peppermint candy. Peppermint anesthetizes the stomach, which reduces the gag reflex and stops vomiting. Suck on a piece or two to rid yourself of the symptoms.

 Popcorn. Air pop a cup or two and place in a bowl. Do not add butter or salt. Instead, pour enough boiling water over the popcorn to cover it, then let it stand for 15 minutes. Popcorn is a carbohydrate that's especially necessary if you've been vomiting or skipping meals, and the added water is good for dehydration.

Soda crackers. Chewing on a few of these can help quell nausea.

Vinegar. To stop the nausea of morning sickness, stir 1 teaspoon apple cider vinegar into 1 glass of water and drink.

HERBAL REMEDIES

Aniseed. This helps cure nausea and vomiting. Brew aniseed into a tea by putting ¼ teaspoon in ½ cup boiling water. Steep for five minutes. Strain and drink once per day. Or sprinkle some aniseed on mild vegetables such as carrots or pumpkin. If your stomach will tolerate fruits during or just after a bout of nausea or vomiting, try aniseed on baked apples or pears.

Cinnamon. Steep ½ teaspoon cinnamon powder in 1 cup boiling water, strain, and sip for nausea. Do not try this remedy if you're pregnant.

NAUSEA-FRIENDLY FOODS

Even though you're queasy, you have to eat something. Isn't that what your mother always told you? Well, she was right. Nausea and vomiting can lead to dehydration and a depletion in vital nutrients, so unless you're fully engaged in a bout of vomiting, here are some foods that might go down easily: rice, cooked cereal, crackers, puddings, low-fat milkshakes, fruit salad, and cottage cheese. Also, try mixing a little white rice with cottage cheese. It has little visual appeal and it tastes pretty bland, but it digests easily.

FASCINATING FACT

Smell can exacerbate nausea and bring on vomiting. If you're feeling a little queasy, stay away from cooking smells, especially fried and spicy foods. Also skip the foods about which you have negative thoughts. Just the thought of those foods really can make you sick.

APPLY A LITTLE PRESSURE

Try these acupressure techniques:

For Nausea: On the inside of your wrist, from the point at which it bends, measure toward your elbow three finger widths. Press this area firmly with your thumb for one minute, then repeat but this time move only two finger widths. Repeat on opposite wrist.

For Vomiting: Start at the inside of your wrist and measure toward your elbow two thumb widths. Massage this area with your thumb, using deep circular motions, for one minute. Breathe deeply as you massage. Repeat on the opposite wrist.

Clove. Brew a cup using 1 teaspoon clove powder in a teacup full of boiling water. Strain out any clove that might be remaining, and drink.

Cumin. Steep a tea with 1 teaspoon cumin seeds and a pinch of nutmeg to soothe tummy troubles.

Fennel. Crush 1 tablespoon seeds and steep for ten minutes in 1 cup boiling water. Sweeten to taste with honey. Sip as necessary for nausea.

Ginger. This is the best stomach woe cure of all. Taken in any form, it will relieve nausea. Try ginger tea, gingerbread, or gingersnaps, just be sure they are made with real ginger, not artificial ginger flavoring. For travel, take along ginger sticks or crystallized ginger instead of travel sickness pills or patches. Studies show ginger to be more effective than the potion you purchase at the pharmacy. Skip the ginger ales, though, unless they have real ginger content. Much of today's ginger ale is missing its curative ginger.

Mint. Mint tea relieves nausea. Simply steep about 1 tablespoon dry leaves in 1 pint hot water for 30 minutes; strain and drink. Don't toss out the leaves when you drink the tea. Eat them! Eating boiled mint leaves can cure nausea too.

TOPICAL REMEDIES

Try a cold compress. A cold compress on your head can be comforting when you've been vomiting.

LIFESTYLE REMEDIES

Hit the bed. Rest is the best cure for whatever's causing your nausea or vomiting.

Buy bismuth. If you must take an over-the-counter remedy, try one that contains bismuth, such as Pepto-Bismol. It will coat the stomach and relieve discomfort. Skip the fizzy seltzer stuff, though. It contains aspirin, which may be an irritant.

Stick to clear liquids. When your stomach is upset, it doesn't need the additional burden of digesting food. Liquids that are room temperature are easier to digest, and they will help prevent dehydration.

Just rinse, don't gargle. This will freshen your breath too.

OTHER HERB HEALERS

These may not be readily available at home, but once you try them, your kitchen may never again be without them.

- **Catnip.** If kitty takes a little nip of the weed regularly, maybe that's why she's never nauseated. To cure your nausea, add 2 tablespoons catnip leaves to a pint jar of boiling water and steep for 30 minutes. Strain and drink. Catnip should not be used if you're pregnant or nursing, or if you've been diagnosed with gynecological conditions because it can lead to excessive menstrual bleeding.

- **Chamomile.** In a tea, this can soothe nausea. Place 2 tablespoons in a pint jar and fill with boiling water. Steep for 30 minutes, strain, and sip. For a nice flavor, eliminate 1 tablespoon chamomile and replace with 1 tablespoon fresh mint.

- **Yarrow.** For a tea to fight nausea, place 1 tablespoon dried yarrow leaves in a pint jar full of boiling water and let steep for 20 to 30 minutes. Strain and drink. Don't use yarrow if you're pregnant.

- **Horehound.** A cup of horehound tea is said to be effective at fighting nausea that's brought on by stress. Take 2 teaspoons of the dried herb and add to 1 cup boiling water. Steep for ten minutes and drink three times a day. Avoid using during pregnancy.

WHEN TO CALL THE DOCTOR

Call 9-1-1 immediately:

- If you're experiencing abdominal pain, blurred vision, muscle weakness, difficulty speaking or swallowing, or muscle paralysis. This could be botulism.

- If with nausea and vomiting you are sweating, are dizzy, have especially teary eyes or excessive saliva, or experience mental confusion or abdominal pain 30 minutes after eating. This can signal pesticide poisoning or other deadly contamination.

- If you vomit blood or your vomit contains material that resembles coffee grounds

Call your doctor for:

- Bloody or tarry stools
- Symptoms of dehydration
- Swelling or pain in the abdomen or rectum
- Symptoms that recur
- Symptoms that last more than two to three days
- Symptoms accompanied by a fever of 101.5 degrees Fahrenheit or higher

Nosebleeds
STOPPING THE FLOW

Nosebleeds can run the gamut from a tiny trickle to a big gush. It may be disturbing to see blood drip from your otherwise placid nose, but there is usually no need to worry. Nosebleeds are typically harmless annoyances. It may look like you're losing lots of blood, but the amount is usually insignificant.

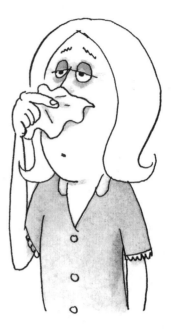

The inner nose is one of the more sensitive parts of the body. Lined with hundreds of blood vessels that reside close to the surface, the nostrils don't take kindly to being harassed and will bleed with little provocation, which can come from a number of sources. These are the main reasons your nose might bleed:

- Trauma, such as a fall or a sports-related injury
- Dry air
- High altitudes
- Nose picking
- Sneezing
- Nose blowing
- Rubbing the nose
- Allergies
- Upper respiratory infection
- Age (With age, nasal tissues tend to dry out and shrink, making them more fragile and prone to bleeding.)

Nosebleeds can also be caused by tumors, but this is a rare occurrence.

The main way to stop a nosebleed is to firmly but gently pinch your nostrils closed, holding them tightly together for five to ten minutes. Lean forward to prevent blood from running down the throat. In addition to this first line of treatment, there are other means to help stop a nosebleed as well as to prevent one.

DIETARY REMEDIES
Dark green leafy vegetables. These are high in vitamin K, which is essential for proper blood clotting.

Oranges and orange juice. Keeping those blood vessels in top form is one way to prevent them from breaking so easily. Vitamin C is necessary to the formation of collagen, which helps create a moist lining in your nose. So drink and eat foods rich in vitamin C to help stave off nosebleeds.

Water. Dry winter air and thin, dry, mountain air can dry out the nose in no time. Being well hydrated helps. Always drink 8 glasses of water per day, but have a few more during the driest times and in the driest places.

Shellfish. Zinc is a nutrient known to help maintain the body's blood vessels. Eat oysters, crab, and lobster, which are all high in zinc. Fortified breakfast cereals and cashews are also good sources.

TOPICAL REMEDIES

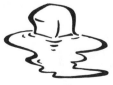

Baking soda. Used for nasal irrigation. See "Salt" on page 342.

Cotton. Some folk remedies require you to place various objects on different parts of your head to cure a nosebleed. (See "Myths," page 343.) One such folk cure that seems to work involves a simple piece of cotton. Place it inside your upper lip against the gum during a nosebleed. What's the secret behind this cure? Location, location, location. A major blood vessel that supplies the interior of the nose runs right through the upper lip. The slight pressure of the cotton wad can help stop bleeding.

Ice. Ice is nice for stopping bleeding by constricting the blood vessels, and for reducing

TAKING A NOSE DIVE

New scuba divers often are alarmed when they experience a nosebleed. Although many blame the salt water, the real problem usually stems from inadequate equalization of the sinuses and middle ear. Without proper equalization during descent, the delicate blood vessels in the lining of the nose can burst. Divers with sinus troubles, allergies, past nose injuries, or a deviated septum may find equalization a problem and experience nosebleeds more frequently. A slow, gentle descent into the deep blue with frequent equalization can help prevent the flow of red.

HIGH ALTITUDE NOSEBLEEDS

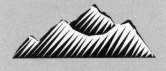

For some people, a trip into the mountains turns into a bloodbath of sorts. Bloody noses are a common complaint among skiers, hikers, and other outdoor enthusiasts who venture high into the hills. Mountain air isn't one of nature's more gentle substances. It's dry, thin, and typically cold. When such abrasive air touches the tissue lining the inside of the nasal cavities—a paper-thin membrane loaded with blood vessels—you may be seeing red soon.

An easy cure: Before hitting the slopes (or trail), dab a protective coating of petroleum jelly (Vaseline) inside your nostrils. If that doesn't do the trick, head back to the lodge, order a hot beverage, and carefully inhale the steam.

inflammation (if the nose is injured). Place crushed iced into a plastic zipper-type bag and cover with a towel. (A bag of frozen vegetables works fine, too.) Place the compress on the bridge of the nose and hold until well after the bleeding stops, but no longer than 15 to 20 minutes.

Salt. Nasal irrigation, commonly used by allergy sufferers to rid the nasal passages of mucus, dust, and other gunk, also helps soothe and moisturize irritated nasal membranes. You'll need 1 to 1½ cups lukewarm water (do not use softened water), a bulb (ear) syringe (typically found with baby products in the pharmacy), ¼ to ½ teaspoon salt, and ¼ to ½ teaspoon baking soda. Mix the salt and baking soda into the water, and test the temperature. To administer, suck in the water using the bulb, and squirt the saline solution into one nostril while holding the other closed. Lower your head over the sink and gently blow out the water. Repeat this, alternating nostrils until the water is gone. You can also buy a neti pot, a device used for nasal irrigation, at drugstores.

Steam. Take every opportunity to breathe steam, be it from your morning tea or from a mini steam bath. To do the latter, boil ½ pot water and put it on a sturdy surface. Place a towel over your head, lean forward, and breathe gently through your nose. Don't lean in too far or you'll burn your sniffer! Try a mini steam bath twice a day.

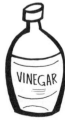

Vinegar. Take a cloth or cotton ball and wet it with white vinegar. Plug it in the nostril that's bleeding. Vinegar helps seal up the blood vessel wall.

DIETARY SUPPLEMENT REMEDIES

Vitamin E. Keep your nasal membranes moisturized by applying vitamin E several times per day. Open a capsule, coat your pinky finger or a cotton swab, and gently wipe it just inside your nostrils. This is especially good to do before going to sleep.

LIFESTYLE REMEDIES

Be nice to your nose. Resist the urge to blow it or touch it after a nosebleed.

Pick flowers, not your nose. Fingers only irritate the nose. Use a soft tissue or nasal irrigation if you need to remove debris.

Blow gently, one nostril at a time, and only when necessary.

Don't smoke. Smoking irritates and dries out nasal passages. Stay out of smoky environments, too.

Treat your allergies. Constant sneezing and blowing the nose due to hay fever is tough on those delicate nasal membranes. Stop sniffling and see a physician for allergy treatment remedies.

WHEN TO CALL THE DOCTOR

- If your nose gushes blood and can't be stopped after five minutes
- If you have high blood pressure, diabetes, or blood-clotting problems
- If your nosebleeds become frequent, since this may indicate a blood clotting disorder or hypertension
- If blood runs down your throat instead of out your nose
- If the nosebleed is the result of a nose, face, or head injury

MYTHS: THE NOSE DOESN'T ALWAYS KNOW

There are as many oddball nosebleed cures as there are noses. We DON'T recommend trying any of these at home.

- **Just a reminder!** Tie a string around your left pinky to stop bleeding.
- **You'll look pretty.** Wear a necklace of red beads to prevent nosebleeds.
- **What a workout.** Raise and hold both hands above your head.
- **Cool off!** Place a cold wet rag or paper towel on the back of your neck.
- **Look out below!** Drop a nail down your back.
- **The luck of the weekend.** You'll have good fortune if your nose bleeds on Friday.
- **A balancing act.** Keep a silver piece under the upper lip to ease a nosebleed.
- **A certain poison.** Leave rusty nails in cider vinegar until the rust is removed. Drink this liquid to cure a nosebleed.
- **Smack away.** Chew gum to stop a nosebleed.
- **A spicy solution.** Wear two nutmegs on a red string to prevent nosebleeds.
- **Simple arithmetic.** Count to 20, and the bleeding will stop.

Oily Hair
STRIPPING YOUR STRANDS

You just washed your hair this morning, and now you look like you went four quarters on the court with Shaquille O'Neal. But you weren't playing basketball; you were just going about your daily business. That means the sebaceous (oil) glands in your scalp are working overtime and you've got greasy, stringy, and sometimes smelly hair.

Don't get mad at those glands for doing their job. Oil protects your hair shafts from breaking, keeps your scalp in good condition, and gives your hair that nice, healthy-looking sheen. Unfortunately, sometimes it's overzealous.

So why does the dipstick measure too much oil? Several factors can be responsible, including:

- Heredity: If one of your parents had oily hair, chances are you will too.
- Hormonal fluctuations: In adult women, it may come with the menstrual cycle or using birth control pills. In teens it's just part of the ever-embarrassing teenaged experience—oily hair, zits, the works. When the hormones simmer down, the problem usually evens out.
- Bulking up: Excessive oil is a side effect of using androgenic hormones to increase body mass.
- Hair texture: Fine hair is often oilier than coarse hair because it takes up less room on the scalp. This means people with fine hair

FASCINATING FACT
Oily hair exacerbates facial acne.

are usually crowned with lots more of it than people with coarse hair. And the more hair there is, the more oil because each follicle is supplied with two to three oil glands.

Diet's Not to Blame

Take notice that diet is not one of the oil-producing culprits listed. That's because diet doesn't play much of a role in the development of oily hair, contrary to what many people believe. Eating french fries won't send the grease directly to your scalp—unless you rub your french fries through your hair.

The good news about oily hair is that it's rarely a serious medical problem. And one of the best treatments for the condition is a daily shampoo and a thorough rinse. It may be best to save the shampoo for morning, since sweating while you sleep and the pressure of your head on the mattress or pillow can put your oil glands in overdrive. You'll find lots of shampoo and rinse varieties to experiment with in the home remedies that follow.

TOPICAL REMEDIES

Alcohol. Any kind of alcoholic beverage has a nice drying effect. The higher the alcohol content the better. Mix a shot glass full with a couple cups of water and rinse through your hair. Yes, you have to rinse it out. And don't drink the rinse water!

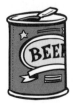

Beer. Beer can have a drying effect, and it cleans right down to your scalp. It also leaves your hair with a healthy shine.

A FUNGUS AMONG US

Recent medical research has pinpointed the cause of some very stubborn dandruff. It lives in the hair follicles, making the scalp very oily, and the scaly dandruff that results is a real greaser. Traditional remedies for oily hair won't treat this stuff, however, because it's a hair fungus called *pityrosporum ovale,* and it will probably take a prescription shampoo or pill to clear it up. But here are some things you can do to get yourself ready to fight this slick bother.

- Strengthen your immune system. Fungi do some of their best work when the body's immunity is low, so arm yourself with these immune-boosting foods: broccoli, sweet potatoes, red meats, whole-grain breads, oranges, sunflower seeds, onions, scallions, and rice.
- Go for the garlic. It's a strong antifungal.
- Be cautious about your hair-grooming habits. Don't contaminate anybody else with your towel, comb, or brush. And don't recontaminate yourself, either. Wash hair accessories thoroughly after use with hot water and soap.

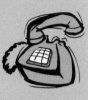
Cider vinegar. Soak your hair in a small basin of water with ¼ cup cider vinegar—or put the concoction in a spray bottle and rinse through your hair, then wash out with warm water. This helps control nasty shampoo buildup. However, don't do this if you dye your hair, because it may dull the color.

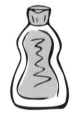

Lemon juice. Mix the equivalent of the juice from 1 lemon with 1 cup water and rinse through your hair, then rinse with warm water. Lemon juice can help control shampoo buildup, too. If you color your hair, don't do this.

Tea. Rinse your hair in diluted tea. Tea contains tannic acid, an astringent, which can cut the oil.

LIFESTYLE REMEDIES

Don't use conditioners after you shampoo. They just coat the hair, which won't help control the oil. If your ends are split and you must condition them, add conditioner only to the ends of your hair, not your whole head. Use a conditioner especially designed for oily hair.

Don't brush your hair 100 strokes. Every time you drag that brush through your hair, you're pulling oil out of the scalp and distributing it throughout your hair.

Shampoo daily. Use a shampoo that is designed for oily hair.

Rinse thoroughly. Soap residue causes dirt and oil to build up more quickly.

Oily Skin
TONING DOWN THE SHINE

The blame-game is easy when it comes to oily skin. Glistening, glowing, shiny skin happens because of two factors: hormones or heredity, neither of which you have much control over.

Oily skin is often a genetically inherited trait. If Mom or Dad or Grandma had a shiny face, chances are you will, too. On the other side of the coin, hormones also play a big role in oil production. As a fair-faced child, your facial glands (sebaceous glands) were quite small and didn't produce much oil. Then puberty hit. Just around the time you wanted to be "in," out popped the hormones encouraging those small glands to grow and produce copious amounts of oil. But teenagers aren't the only ones agonizing over their faces. Oily skin can continue throughout life, especially if hormones and heredity are both to blame.

The Male Factor

There's one more player in the blame game. Blame oily skin on men, or more specifically, the male hormone androgen that controls oil production in the skin. It sounds odd, but even women's bodies (the ovaries and the adrenal glands) produce male hor-

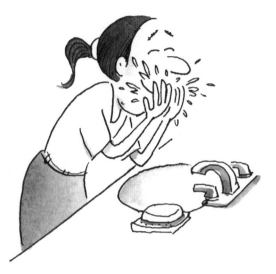

mones. Many women notice that their skin feels oilier around their menstrual cycle and during menopause. This is due to fluctuating levels of androgen.

Although you can't change your genes, there are plenty of ways to combat oily skin.

TOPICAL REMEDIES

Almonds and honey. The luscious combination of succulent almonds and sweet honey works well as a gentle facial scrub for removing oils and dead skin cells. Mix a small amount of ground almonds with

WHEN OILY WAS IN
To be greasy was once fashionable, at least in ancient Egypt circa 1400 B.C. Upper-class women placed a large cone of perfumed grease atop their heads. As the desert sun beat down, the grease dripped down onto their skin. By the end of the hot day, their skin glistened, glowed, and smelled fragrant.

DON'T BLAME OILY SKIN
Although people often blame oily skin for their acne, it's not oily skin's fault! Acne is caused when oil gets trapped below the skin's pores and becomes contaminated with bacteria. Many people with oily skin don't have blocked pores; instead the oil spouts right to the surface and shines.

honey to make a paste. Gently massage the paste into your skin with a comfortably hot washcloth. Rinse with cool water.

Apples. This homemade oil-ridding facial requires some creative cooking. Mix ½ cup mashed apple, ½ cup cooked oatmeal, 1 slightly beaten egg white, and 1 tablespoon lemon juice into a smooth paste. Apply to your face for 15 minutes, then rinse with cool water.

Baking soda. Liquid soap users can add ½ teaspoon baking soda into the mixture. Rub gently onto oily areas such as the nose and chin. This gentle abrasive works well in getting rid of blackheads as well as oil. Rinse with cool water.

Cornstarch. Cornstarch dries up oily patches. Mix 1 to 3 tablespoons cornstarch with enough warm water to make a paste. Rub on your face, let dry, and then shower or rinse off with lukewarm water in the sink. Try this once per day for best results.

Lemons. Mix equal parts lemon juice and water, pat on face, and let dry. Rinse first with warm water followed by cool water for a refreshing treat.

Limes and cucumbers. Citrus fruits and some veggies refresh the skin and help reduce oils. Mix ½ teaspoon lime juice with an equal amount of cucumber juice. Apply a few minutes before showering.

Milk of Magnesia. This makes a nice facial mask for oily skin. Use the flavorless variety, and apply a thin layer to your face. Leave on during the day. If that seems too noticeable, apply at night.

Salt. This is nature's best desiccant. Place lukewarm water into a small spray bottle and add

1 teaspoon salt. Close your eyes, then squirt some of this salt spray on your face once during the day. Blot dry.

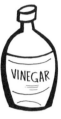 ***Vinegar.*** A good way to exfoliate the skin is with white or apple cider vinegar. Apply using a cotton ball before bedtime. Leave it on for five to ten minutes and then rinse with cool water.

Use this remedy for three weeks to see improvements. If your skin is super sensitive, dilute the vinegar with four parts water. For a summertime treat, chill the vinegar or freeze it into ice cubes and apply as a cooling facial.

HERBAL REMEDIES

Aloe vera. Slice open a leaf and smear the gel onto the face up to three times per day. Let dry. (Keep a small amount in the refrigerator for a refreshing face-lift!)

Witch Hazel. Moisten a cotton ball with witch hazel and dab on your face twice per day to remove residue and tighten pores.

LIFESTYLE REMEDIES

Go au naturale. The less makeup you wear, the better for your complexion. If you do wear makeup, use water-based, hypoallergenic products.

Keep your hands off your face during the day. Hands deliver excess oil and dirt.

Pull hair back from the face. Often oily hair and oily skin go together.

Use tissues or special oil-absorbing papers. These remove excess oil between cleanings.

More isn't better. Wash your face with plenty of soap and comfortably hot water just twice per day. The body responds to obsessive washing by producing more oils.

WHEN TO CALL THE DOCTOR

- If you have severe acne
- If you notice a sudden change in your skin

PIMPLE BE GONE!

A lone pimple always seems to pop out right before your big speech, the big party, or any other "big" social event. Leave it to the oil glands to clog up at the most stressful of times. If you feel a big pimple coming on, ice it immediately. Hold an ice cube covered in a towel on the spot for a few minutes. Repeat during the day. The ice eliminates the redness and inflammation that are so embarrassing.

Osteoporosis
BOLSTERING YOUR BONES

More than 34 million Americans are at risk for osteoporosis because of low bone mass, and more than 10 million have already been diagnosed with this bone-degenerating disease. Women make up an astounding 80 percent of those who are affected by osteoporosis. Though most people associate osteoporosis with older people, the disease strikes young and old alike. Osteoporosis does become much more common as you age—affecting 55 percent of women older than 50.

Bone Up on Osteoporosis

As you grow, your bones get stronger and longer. By the time you reach the age of 20, you've got 85 to 90 percent of your adult bone mass. By the time you reach your 30th birthday, your bones are at their strongest. If you were able to take a look inside your bones during those peak years, you'd see a hard outer shell and something that looks like a honeycomb on the inside. About 80 percent of your bone mass is that tough, hard outer bone, which is called cortical bone. The rest of your bone make-up is the honeycomblike material called trabecular bone. After you hit age 30, your bone mass begins to decline. Trabecular bone is typically the first to lose critical density, and as you get older, cortical bone mass also declines, but at a somewhat slower pace.

DON'T FORGET THE GUYS

Men have 25 percent more bone mass than women, but they begin to lose bone mass as they age, just like women. However, the process is much slower in men. Any man older than 65 could be at risk for osteoporosis.

Osteoporosis literally means "porous bones." That means someone diagnosed with the disease has lost so much density that there's not much there to hold their bones together, putting them at greater risk for bone breaks and fractures. The National Osteoporosis Foundation calls osteoporosis the "silent disease" because there are virtually no symptoms of bone loss. Unless you're aware of the risk factors and take action, you may not know you have the disease until some benign bump on the garage door turns into a fracture.

Who Gets Osteoporosis?

When you think of osteoporosis, you probably picture a petite, silver-haired Caucasian woman. In reality, that woman *could* be the poster child for the disease—being Caucasian or Asian, female, small-framed, and underweight are major risk factors for thinning bones. So is being post-menopausal. That's because estrogen is vital to bone strength, keeping bones strong by stimulating bone-building substances called osteoblasts and suppressing bone-destroying substances called osteoclasts. Estrogen also helps the body absorb and use calcium more efficiently. As women approach menopause, estrogen production steadily declines, and the protection it provides against osteoporosis is lost. But one of the greatest risk factors for osteoporosis is something you can't see and you can't control—heredity. Other risk factors include not getting enough calcium, having an eating disorder, using certain medications such as corticosteriods, not exercising, smoking, and having certain health problems, such as gastrointestinal disease, cancer, alcoholism, diabetes, lupus, and rheumatoid arthritis.

THE CALCIUM CONNECTION

You've heard it over and over: "Drink milk for strong bones." But what's the big deal? Why is calcium so vital for your bones? For one, your body contains more calcium than any other mineral, and 99 percent of that calcium is in your bones. When you eat or drink calcium, it goes into your bones and then gets taken out for other bodily functions.

Making sure you get enough calcium means you have enough to feed your bones and some reserve for times when your nervous system needs a little of the mineral to help pass messages from your brain to your big toe. You also need a reserve for times when you simply don't get enough in your diet. Most milk is fortified with vitamin D, which helps the body absorb calcium.

Thankfully, there are many ways you can combat and even reverse the damaging effects of this bone-thinning disease, and the earlier you start the better. Why not try some of the following bone boosters in your home?

DIETARY REMEDIES

Apples. Boron is a trace mineral that helps your body hold on to calcium—the building block of bones. It even acts as a mild estrogen replacement, and losing estrogen is instrumental in speeding bone loss. Boron is found in apples and other fruits such as pears, grapes, dates, raisins, and peaches. It's also in nuts such as almonds, peanuts, and hazelnuts.

Bananas. Eat a banana a day to build your bones. Studies have found that women who have diets high in potassium also have stronger bones in their spines and hips. Researchers think this is related to potassium's ability to keep blood healthy and balanced so the body doesn't have to leech calcium from the skeleton to keep blood up to par.

Broccoli. Eat ½ cup broccoli to get your daily dose of vitamin K. Studies are finding that postmenopausal women with low levels of this vital vitamin are more likely to have osteoporosis.

Margarine. Slather a teaspoon of low trans fat margarine on your toast for a dose of vitamin D. Vitamin D helps the body absorb calcium, a necessary ingredient to bone health.

Milk. When it comes to strong bones, getting enough calcium is a must. One cup of milk can provide 300 mg of the 1,000 to 1,200 mg of calcium

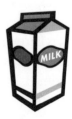

the government recommends you get every day. But milk is not the only calcium-rich food on the market. Other foods high in calcium include salmon, blackstrap molasses, tofu, turnip greens, and dried figs.

Orange juice. Grab a glass of OJ to get your vitamin C. Necessary for the body processes that rebuild bones, getting enough vitamin C is vital to preventing osteoporosis. Grab some calcium-fortified orange juice and get a healthy dose of bone-building nutrients.

Peanut butter. A recent review of studies on nutrition and osteoporosis found that magnesium was a vital component in strengthening, preserving, and rebuilding bones. You can get 50 mg of magnesium by eating 2 tablespoons of peanut butter.

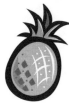 *Pineapple juice.* Drink a cup of pineapple juice and give your body some manganese. Studies are finding that manganese deficiency is a predictor of osteoporosis. Other manganese sources are oatmeal, nuts, beans, cereals, spinach, and tea.

Tofu. Soy is showing promise as a potential bone strengthener. Soy contains proteins that act like a weak estrogen in the body. These "phytoestrogens," or plant-based estrogens, may help women regain bone strength.

DIETARY SUPPLEMENT REMEDIES

Calcium. If you don't get enough calcium in your diet, be sure to use a supplement to help prevent osteoporosis. See "Calcium Boosters," page 355, for information about selecting a supplement.

EXERCISE AND STRONG BONES

Eating a bone-building diet and exercising are the two most powerful tools you have in your fight against osteoporosis. Doing any kind of exercise is helpful in building your bones, but there are specific types that will help you boost your bone strength.

- Weight-bearing exercise. Walking briskly or running can put a force two to three times your body weight on your bones. Women who walk regularly have stronger bones than women who don't exercise. Try adding in some walking or other weight-bearing activity, such as tennis.

- Strength training. You can build bone strength and substantially cut your risk of fracture from osteoporosis by lifting weights a couple of times per week. Aim for exercises that focus on the hips, spine, and arms, three vulnerable areas for osteoporosis sufferers. A study in which women age 50 to 70 lifted weights twice a week for a year found they developed the bone density and muscle strength of women 20 years younger.

WHEN TO CALL
THE DOCTOR

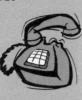

- If you are at risk for osteoporosis. There are tests that can determine your bone density, and your doctor can advise you about prevention and treatment of the disease.
- If you have sudden pain in your back, which may indicate a fracture in a bone in the spine

SODA DOESN'T STEAL

A prevailing myth about osteoporosis is that the phosphorus in carbonated drinks can cause your bones to deteriorate. That's simply not true. Too much phosphorus can hinder your body's absorption of calcium, but soda doesn't have enough phosphorus to cause any problems. Soda may steal your appetite for more nutritious drink or food, but it won't rob your bones.

LIFESTYLE REMEDIES

Abstain from alcohol. Alcohol interferes with the way your body absorbs calcium.

Cut the caffeine. Caffeine is a diuretic, and some experts believe drinking too much can cause your body to excrete too much calcium. Don't drink more than 2 cups of coffee or 4 cups of tea per day.

Don't smoke. Nicotine works like alcohol in railroading your body's need to absorb calcium.

Get some sun. To up your supply of vitamin D, be sure to catch a few rays. Spending 5 to 10 minutes a day in the sun without wearing sunscreen will give you an adequate supply without causing your skin to suffer.

Keep your weight on track. Here's one time when having a few extra pounds works to your advantage. Women who are underweight for their height are at a higher risk of getting osteoporosis.

Restrict your salt. Salt may actually steal calcium away from your bones.

Strengthen your muscles. Strengthening your muscles helps support your bones. Take a can of beans—or any one-pound can—and do a few bicep curls. These cans are a perfect weight for beginners and will help you begin to build a little muscle.

CALCIUM BOOSTERS

For people who need some calcium insurance, there are plenty of calcium supplements on the market. Look for supplements containing calcium citrate or calcium carbonate.

- Calcium citrate. This type of calcium is better absorbed by the body and doesn't require you to eat when you take it. Look for a brand that contains vitamin D.
- Calcium carbonate. When you're browsing through calcium supplements, this is probably the type of supplement you'll come across most. You can get it in capsules, tablets, and even chocolate chews. You do need to eat something when you take these supplements to allow your body maximum absorption. This form is common in many over-the-counter antacids, such as TUMS.

To maximize the benefit of taking calcium supplements

- Spread them out. Your body can't absorb more than 500 mg of calcium at a time, so don't take a supplement that contains more than that. And if you need to supplement with more than 500 mg, take them at different times of the day.
- Calcium at night. If you only take one supplement per day and it's made of calcium carbonate, take it with dinner or before bed. Your digestion is slower when you're asleep, so taking it then will ensure your body absorbs the calcium and vitamin D. If you have heartburn, though, you might want to take your supplement at another time of day.
- Try this test if your supplement doesn't have a code saying it meets United States Pharmacoepia (USP) standards: Place one supplement tablet in a cup of vinegar. Stir the tablet every five minutes. If it doesn't disintegrate within 30 minutes, don't take it. It probably won't dissolve in your tummy either.

Overweight
GETTING FIT

Diet. Mention that little four-letter word to any woman anywhere in the world and you'll get the same reaction—disgust. If you really want to know the intensity of feeling behind the word, order a slice of cheesecake and eat it in front of a woman who has been on a diet for a few weeks. Shouldn't be too hard to find one—approximately 40 percent of women are dieting at any given moment. You are likely to end up with heel marks on your forehead and a plate of half-eaten cheesecake in your lap.

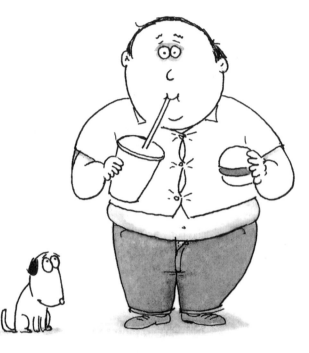

Battle of the Bulge

According to recent statistics, more than 66 percent of the population is overweight. Of those, about half—some 72 million people—are obese.

Because of the alarming number of adults and kids packing on the pounds, Americans are discovering that traditional diets don't work. In fact, the four-letter word that caused so much angst for women over the years is getting the boot. The latest thinking on losing weight is that you don't have to deprive yourself to shed pounds. It's simply a matter of using your noodle (the one on your shoulders, not on your plate) to learn how to eat healthy.

Eating smart and exercising are your best bets to paring down to a healthy weight. For most people that means making a complete lifestyle change—not one that means no more cheesecake, ever, but one that knows how to incorporate that cheesecake into an overall healthy eating style.

Are You or Aren't You?

So how do you know if you're overweight or obese? First you need to calculate your body mass index (BMI). This is the method the government uses to determine who's at a normal weight, who's overweight, and who's obese. The National Heart, Blood, and Lung Institute Web site has a handy BMI calculator (www.nhblisupport.com/bmi/). To do the work yourself, divide your weight in pounds by 2.2 to convert your weight to kilograms. Then divide your height in inches by 39.37 to convert it to meters. Multiply your height in meters by itself and then divide your weight in kilograms by that number. Say you weigh 150 pounds and you're 5'7" (67 inches). Your BMI figures would look like this:

> 150 divided by 2.2 = 68.2
> 67 inches divided by 39.37 = 1.70
> 1.70×1.70 = 2.89
> 68.2 divided by 2.89 = 23.59

A normal BMI is between 19 and 24.9. A BMI between 25 and 29.9 is considered overweight. And a BMI over 30 is considered obese.

Weighing the Risks

Being overweight or obese zaps your energy level and can make everyday tasks an ordeal. Carrying around excess pounds also is a risk factor for some serious conditions. The National Institutes of Health say being overweight or obese can increase your risk for diabetes, heart disease, high cholesterol, stroke, high blood pressure, gallbladder disease, osteoarthritis, sleep apnea, and some forms of cancer.

You may think that the best way to cure being overweight is to stay out of the kitchen, but that's simply not true. In fact, the best thing you can do for yourself in your quest to lose weight is to create a healthy kitchen. Stocking your kitchen

CAN YOU BE FIT AND FAT?

Sounds like an oxymoron, but you can be considered overweight by BMI standards and be in perfectly healthy condition. For example, a muscular six-foot-tall football player can weigh in at 250 pounds—well over his "ideal" weight. He's obviously in good shape. He just has loads of muscle, and muscle weighs more than fat. So don't look at the scale as your only indicator of good shape. You have to consider your overall lifestyle.

FILL UP ON FIBER

Fiber is a complex carbohydrate that your body can't digest. It's found mostly in fruits, vegetables, whole grains, beans, nuts, and seeds. Because fiber is hard to digest, it sticks around in your system, making you feel full longer. Fiber has many other benefits—it helps your digestive system run smoothly, helps reduce cancer risk, helps control blood sugar in people with diabetes, and lowers cholesterol. In your quest to create a healthy diet, try to include fiber-rich choices with every meal.

GET WITH THE LABEL LINGO

There are loads of products on your grocery store shelf that claim they are "fat free" or "reduced fat." But what exactly does that mean? Here's the lowdown.

- Fat free. There's so little fat in the product that it's not worth noting on the package.
- Low fat. There's fewer than three grams of fat per serving.
- Reduced fat. The product has at least 25 percent less fat per serving than the full-fat version of the product.
- Light. Those light potato chips have one-third fewer calories or 50 percent less fat than the regular kind.
- Lean or extra lean. This label is reserved for packaged seafood, game, cooked meat, or cooked poultry. Lean ground beef contains less than 10 grams of total fat per 3-ounce serving. Extra lean ground beef has less than 5 grams of total fat per 3-ounce serving.

with healthy foods and fat-reducing utensils can help you shed the pounds.

DIETARY REMEDIES

Applesauce. When you're baking muffins or cakes, substitute applesauce for half of the oil, margarine, or butter. If your recipe calls for ½ cup vegetable oil, use ¼ cup applesauce and ¼ cup oil.

Evaporated skim milk. This is a great cream substitute. You can use it in everything from recipes that call for cream to your coffee.

Extra lean ground beef. You can shave off some fat by choosing leaner varieties of ground beef. Look for beef that says 90 percent lean or higher on the package.

Frozen yogurt. Want some ice cream but don't want the fat? Try some frozen yogurt. Most kinds of frozen yogurt are lower in fat than ice cream—just watch your serving size and check the nutrient label to be sure. A calorie is a calorie, regardless of its source.

Fruit. Fruit gives you a natural sweet fix and is loaded with good-for-you vitamins and minerals. Some good choices for your fruit basket include apricots, cantaloupe, 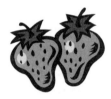 grapefruit, oranges, peaches, and strawberries.

Low-fat salad dressing. There are many flavorful, low-fat salad dressings available. And a low-fat version can save you fat and calories.

Low-fat frozen dinners. There are loads of healthy frozen dinners on the market these days. Stock your freezer with some in-a-hurry healthy choices, and you won't be as tempted to zip through the drive-through.

Nonstick cooking spray. Spraying your pans with nonstick cooking spray instead of coating them with vegetable oil can save you 27 grams of fat and 230 calories.

Olive oil. Getting more monounsaturated fats into your diet can help keep your cholesterol under control and may help you shed pounds. Because it's mostly monounsaturated fat, olive oil is a much healthier choice than, say, butter.

Sharp cheddar cheese. Using a little of flavorful cheeses such as sharp cheddar in your recipes will help you lose fat without losing taste.

Skim milk. Whole milk has 8 grams of fat per cup, skim milk has none. And you get just as much calcium and vitamin D. If you've been drinking the heavier stuff, it may take a while to get used to the different texture (skim milk

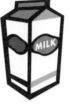

WHEN TO CALL THE DOCTOR

- If you are overweight or obese and are ready to lose weight safely. Most doctors take a team approach to medical intervention in weight loss. You'll typically have a doctor, a registered dietitian, and an exercise physiologist on your team. When it comes to giving advice, be sure that each person sticks to their specialty.
- Sudden, rapid weight gain or loss. (See "Uncontrolled Weight Gain," page 361).

THE HEALTHY PLATE

The Food Guide Pyramid is still the gold standard when it comes to healthy eating. The American Dietetic Association recommends getting 2 to 3 servings of meats, poultry, or fish; 2 to 3 servings of milk, yogurt, and cheese; 2 to 4 servings of fruit; 3 to 5 servings of vegetables; and 6 to 11 servings of breads, cereals, rice, and pasta (at least half should be whole grain). But what's a serving? And how does that work in the real world? It's actually easier than it sounds.

- Bread, cereal, rice, and pasta. One serving size equals: 1 slice of bread, 1 small roll or biscuit, ½ hamburger bun, 6 small crackers, ½ cup rice or pasta, or 1 ounce dry cereal.
- Fruit. One serving size equals: 1 whole medium fruit such as an apple, banana, or orange; ½ grapefruit; ½ cup berries; or ¼ cup dried fruit.
- Vegetables. One serving equals: ½ cup cooked veggies, ½ cup chopped raw veggies, or 1 cup leafy raw veggies such as spinach.
- Milk, yogurt, and cheese. One serving equals: 1 cup milk, 8 ounces yogurt, 1½ ounces natural cheese, or 2 ounces processed cheese.
- Meat, poultry, fish, dry beans, eggs, and nuts. A serving size equals: 3 ounces cooked lean meat, poultry, or fish (without skin); 1 egg; ½ cup cooked beans, peas, or other legumes; or two tablespoons peanut butter.

CAN A PILL REALLY CURE OBESITY?

The answer is a resounding, "Nope!" Prescription weight-loss medications, which have come into vogue in recent years, are not magic beans. But for people who are considered obese (have a BMI of 30 or more), they might offer some help.

Prescription weight-loss pills tend to work on two theories. One type, such as the drug Orlistat, keeps the body from holding onto fat in the small intestines. Other drugs, such as Meridia, trick the brain into thinking the stomach is full. The problem with these drugs is that they become less effective over time, and some people who take them may end up regaining the weight. They also can create problems with blood pressure and heart rate. And they may produce unpleasant side effects such as flatulence, oily stools, urgent bowl movements, and even incontinence.

Unless your doctor really thinks these are a good idea for your specific case, it's best to avoid them.

is more watery). Try going from whole milk to two percent and slowly making your way to skim.

Vegetables. These are near-miracle foods for losing weight and staying healthy. The American Dietetic Association recommends getting at least five servings of vegetables per day. 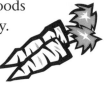 Some smart choices: broccoli, carrots, potatoes, spinach, sweet potatoes, tomatoes.

LIFESTYLE REMEDIES

Don't count calories. You'll drive yourself crazy if you keep tabs on every morsel that enters your mouth. Just learn how to make healthy choices and watch your portion sizes.

Eat every meal. Skipping a meal will not help you lose weight. In fact, it may slow down your metabolism and set you up for scarfing down a plate of brownies in a moment of weakness.

 Give up the alcohol. The average American gets 10 percent of their calories from alcohol. Think of the savings if you don't have a cocktail.

Keep an eye out for fat. Eating less fat is crucial for a healthier diet. It helps keep your weight down and keeps your body healthier—reducing your risk of heart disease and some cancers. Why is fat such a problem for people trying to lose weight? Fat packs in nine calories per gram, while carbohydrates and protein have only four calories per gram. That means the more fat you eat, the more calories you pile on, and the greater chance you have for putting on a few pounds. The American Dietetic Association recommends getting around 30 percent of your calories from fat.

Resist magic cures. There is only one proven way to lose weight—eating a healthy, low-fat diet and exercising. If anyone promises that you'll lose a pound a day, that a "miracle" food will help you lose pounds, says you need an artificial food or pill to lose weight, offers diets or gadgets that can get rid of fat from one part of the body, or says you have to eat their organization's food to lose weight, don't buy into it.

Seek out support. A group of friends or an organized outfit such as Weight Watchers can be vital ingredients in meeting your weight-loss goals. They can provide accountability and support, and they can help you learn how to make healthier choices.

PSYCHOLOGICAL REMEDIES

Don't try to be Cindy Crawford. Only a very small portion of the population is meant to look like a supermodel. Be sure that you are realistic when you think about weight loss. Aim for a weight that is healthy for you.

Be patient. Though you wish with all your might that those ten pounds would slough off overnight, it just won't happen. A healthy weight-loss goal for a week is about ½ pound. And give yourself time to adjust your habits. It takes time to make a change.

Be kind. Don't belittle yourself if you indulge in a dessert once in a while. Treat yourself every now and then, and those "forbidden" foods won't be so tempting.

UNCONTROLLED WEIGHT GAIN

You gain 10 pounds in a month. Unless you've been sleepwalking to the refrigerator for a midnight snack, you can't think of any changes in your eating or exercise habits that would cause you to pile on that weight so quickly. Some conditions, such as hypothyroidism, and some drugs, such as insulin, steroids, and hormone replacement therapies, can cause you to gain weight without even trying.

If you suddenly gain weight and have any of the following symptoms, you might want to call your doctor and ask about hypothyroidism.

- Feeling tired all the time
- Increased sensitivity to cold
- Joint and muscle aches
- Decreased appetite
- Constipation
- Heavy menstruation
- Dry, rough skin
- Coarse hair or unusual hair loss
- Trouble concentrating and remembering

Poisonous Plant Rashes
LIMITING THE SPREAD

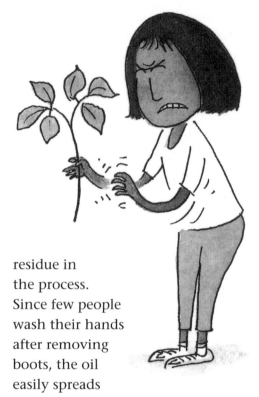

Contact with poison ivy, poison oak, or poison sumac often goes hand in hand with camping and other outdoor activities. Outdoor enthusiasts by the tentful have had to cut trips short after an unfortunate encounter with one of this threesome. The problem stems from the plant's colorless oil, called urushiol. Whenever one of these plants is cut, crushed, stepped on, sat on, grabbed, rolled on, kicked, or disturbed, the oil is released. Once on the victim, the toxic oil penetrates the skin and a rash appears within 12 to 48 hours after exposure. This is a true allergic reaction to compounds in the urushiol. The rash starts as small bumps and progresses into enlarged, itchy blisters. No body part is immune to the oil, although areas most often irritated are the face, arms, hands, legs, and genitals.

Don't Touch!

Touching the oil after initial contact is what spreads the rash—something easily done. For example, you unknowingly walk over poison ivy and the oily residue sticks like glue to your hiking boots. Later, you remove the boots, unwittingly touching the residue in the process. Since few people wash their hands after removing boots, the oil easily spreads from the hands, to the face, and even to the genital area should you make the unfortunate decision to use the bathroom. The damage is done by the time the rash breaks out. Touching the rash once it appears does not spread the oil—or the rash.

Warning! Since poison plant oils don't just disappear, it's crucial to wash anything that has had contact with the victim or the oil, including clothing, boots, pets, other people, sleeping bags, fishing poles, walking sticks, etc. Use gloves when cleaning pets, people, and objects that may have had contact with the oil.

Outdoor expeditions need not be ruined if people learn to recognize the terrible threesome. Here are some pointers:

- **Poison ivy.** Poison ivy plants have serrated, pointed leaves that appear in groups of three leaflets. The leaves are green in summer but are reddish in spring and fall. Their appearance can vary, and poison ivy plants are found everywhere in the United States. In the East, Midwest, and South, it grows as a climbing vine. In the West and northern states, poison ivy resembles a shrub. Poison ivy rarely appears above 5,000 feet.
- **Poison oak.** Like poison ivy, poison oak has leaves of three, and the shrub's size differs depending on location. In the Southeast, it appears as a small shrub, while in the West, poison oak appears as a large shrub. It has greenish-white berries and oaklike leaves.
- **Poison sumac.** The leafy one of this threesome is poison sumac, a small shrub with two rows of 7 to 13 leaflets. Sumac prefers the swampy bogs of northern states and swamps in southern states. Its leaves are smooth-edged and remain red; the plant has cream-colored berries. Unlike poison ivy and oak, poison sumac does not produce leaves in groups of three.

Even experts can be fooled by the poisonous three, so here's some relief from home.

HERBAL REMEDIES

Aloe vera. According to folk medicine, aloe vera sap helps treat poison ivy

ON-THE-GO REMEDIES

Before heading off into the wild, grab a few items from home for a poisonous plant first-aid kit. Include a small bag of baking soda, a container of vinegar or rubbing alcohol, a bar of plain soap, an old but clean towel, and a water bottle.

OVER-THE-COUNTER ITCH RELIEVER

Calamine lotion has long been used to take the itch out of poisonous plant irritation. Calamine contains zinc oxide and acts as a drying astringent to reduce the swelling of the rash. It's also a mild disinfectant, which helps prevent infection.

rash through its anti-inflammatory constituents. Break off a leaf and apply the sap to the affected area. Allow to dry and gently wash off. Reapply every two hours.

TOPICAL REMEDIES

Baking soda. Concoct a paste of baking soda and water, and spread it on the affected area. Freshen the application every two hours for a total of three applications each day. Before going to bed, pour a cup of baking soda into a lukewarm bath and take a soak.

Coffee. If you have any leftover (cold) coffee in your cup, pouring it on a poison ivy rash may be a good way to get rid of the coffee and the rash. Appalachian folk medicine followers believe in washing the affected area with a cup of cold black coffee. Coffee beans contain chlorogenic acid, an anti-inflammatory. This coffee cure hasn't been proven, as there haven't been any studies done on it.

Soap and water. Waste no time in getting the poisonous plant victim in contact with soap and water. Quickly, but gently, wash the affected area with lukewarm water and mild, plain soap. Air-dry the skin. Any towels used for cleaning should be washed immediately in hot water and detergent since the oil can linger.

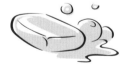

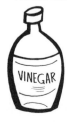

Vinegar. Be it from plant, insect, or allergic reaction, itches of all sorts are tamed by a simple vinegar rinse. First wash the affected area with soap and lukewarm water, then rinse. Apply vinegar with a cotton ball, rub gently, and rinse. Or, add a cup of vinegar to your bathwater and soak away the itch.

LIFESTYLE REMEDIES

Cover up. When working and playing outdoors in prime poisonous plant territory, wear long pants, long-sleeved shirts, protective footwear, and if gardening, gloves.

Remember the pet connection. Often a mysterious case of rash can be traced to the furry family member who diligently patrols the outdoors: Fido or Fluffy. The oil gets on the animal's fur and is transferred to you via petting.

Consider using IvyBlock. This product protects you by absorbing urushiol before it irritates the skin. It can be applied before heading out into potential poison plant territory.

TRUE OR FALSE?

Burning poison ivy will get rid of it.
False. Never burn poison ivy, especially in an enclosed environment such as a fireplace or firepit. The oil, urushiol, is carried in the smoke and can seriously irritate your eyes, skin, and lungs.

Dead plants don't give you a rash.
False. Yes, they do. Even after a plant is dead, the oil lives on for years and can give you a rash.

You can catch a poison ivy rash like you can a cold.
False. Once you develop a rash, it can't be passed from person to person.

Scratch a rash and it spreads.
False. What may happen, however, is that you develop a nasty infection from irritating the skin.

The "leaves of three" motto always holds true.
False. Never assume poison ivy and poison oak come with three leaves. Leaflets may come in groups of five, seven, or even nine.

Immunizations exist for poison ivy.
True. Immunizations exist, but the procedure takes time, effort, and commitment on the part of patient and doctor. Plus, there are side effects. Immunizations aren't recommended for the general public. Bush firefighters and others working in daily close contact with poison ivy should consult an expert and get the facts.

Poison ivy and oak are related to the cashew.
True. Sounds nutty, but it's true.

Bleach helps cure a poison ivy rash.
False! If there is one remedy you should never try, it's pouring bleach onto your skin. Expect a nasty burn and then some.

Eat a poisonous leaf to desensitize yourself.
False. Eating a poisonous leaf will not desensitize you, but it will make you very ill.

Spring and summer are poison ivy/oak/sumac season.
False. Urushiol, the oil that causes the reaction, doesn't take winters off. Even in colder months when the plants are bare, the twigs can still cause a powerful reaction.

Poor Appetite
AROUSING HUNGER

"What do you mean you're not hungry?" You've probably heard this response when you declare no desire to eat. Humans have a physical need for food and nourishment, so when an appetite is lacking, something is usually amiss... and that alarms people who care about you.

A poor appetite can stem from many factors. Perhaps the most common causes are emotional upset, nervousness, tension, anxiety, or depression. Stressful events, such as losing a job or a death in the family, can also make the appetite plummet. Diseases such as influenza and acute infections play a role in appetite reduction, as do anorexia nervosa and fatigue. Illegal and legal drugs, including amphetamines, antibiotics, cough and cold medications, codeine, morphine, Demerol, and some cancer-treatment drugs can also take a toll on the appetite. Sometimes poor eating habits, such as continuous snacking, can lead to a reduced appetite at mealtimes. A poor appetite can also be one symptom of a serious disease.

Fortunately, for minor cases of poor appetite, the kitchen is the best place to get the appetite back into gear.

THE RIGHT SPOT

If you visit an acupuncturist, they might press on a point on your head to control your appetite. This point is located in the hollow just in front of the external opening of the outer ear.

DIETARY REMEDIES

Bitter greens. Mama always told you to eat your greens. If she knew you weren't eating properly, she might add, eat your "bitter" greens. Bitter greens consist of arugula, radicchio, collards, kale, endives, escarole, mizuna, sorrel, dandelions, watercress, and red/green mustard greens...in other words, all those leaves you find in fancy restaurant salads. Stimulating digestion is the name of the game with bitter greens. They prompt the body to make more digestive juices and digestive enzymes. Bitter foods also stimulate the gallbladder to contract and release bile, which helps break fatty foods into small enough particles that enzymes can easily finish breaking them apart for absorption. This is important because fats carry essential fatty acids, such as heart-healthy omega-3s, along with fat-soluble vitamins A, D, E, and K and carotenoids such as beta-carotene.

Water. The wonders of water never cease. Water helps control the appetite, especially when you drink the recommended daily amount: 8 glasses! Don't skimp, even if you don't feel like drinking.

HERBAL REMEDIES

Caraway. The early Greeks knew caraway could calm an upset stomach and used it to season foods that were hard to digest. Today, unsuspecting cooks who simply love the flavor of caraway continue the tradition by adding caraway to rye bread; cabbage dishes, such as sauerkraut and coleslaw; pork; cheese sauces; cream soups; goose; and duck. The Germans make a caraway liqueur called Kümmel and serve it after heavy meals. One

THE FRENCH CONNECTION

The culinary-minded French have a highly seasoned stew of meat or fish called ragout. The name is derived from the French verb meaning, "to stimulate the appetite of."

Dandelions help stimulate digestion, thanks to a bitter substance called taraxacin that promotes the flow of bile from the liver and hydrochloric acid secretions from the stomach. Dandelion also helps the body to absorb nutrients and eliminate wastes more efficiently. Don't use dandelions from any lawns that may have been sprayed with chemicals or fertilizers. Dandelions are also available in some groceries and fruit and vegetable markets. Here is a recipe to get you started:

Sautéed Dandelions
Add young dandelion leaves to a stir-fry, or sauté them with mushrooms, onions, and shredded kale and cabbage in some sesame oil. The greens cook quickly, even on low heat, so don't overcook them. (They'll be mushy and distasteful.) Remove from heat, add a dash of sesame oil and balsamic vinegar, and garnish with sesame seeds. Serve as a side dish or over rice.

Warning! Avoid dandelions if you have too much stomach acid, ulcers, diarrhea, irritable bowel syndrome, or ulcerative colitis.

of the easiest ways to enjoy caraway is with a good helping of sauerkraut. Sauté ½ medium onion in 1 to 2 tablespoons butter. When onions turn deep golden brown, add 1 can sauerkraut and its liquid along with 1 or 2 tablespoons brown sugar and 1 teaspoon caraway seeds. Let the mixture simmer (covered) for 1 hour. Serve as a side dish with meat, poultry, or sausage.

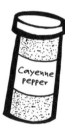

Cayenne pepper. Nothing revs up the old digestive engine like cayenne. Cayenne pepper has the power to make any dish fiery hot, but it also has a subtle flavor-enhancing quality. There is some evidence that eating hot pepper increases metabolism and the appetite. Add a few shakes of cayenne pepper to potato salad, deviled eggs, chili, and other hot dishes such as stews and soups.

Fennel. Fennel, like its cousin caraway (both belong to the *Umbelliferae* family of herbs), is a familiar digestive aid, both for relieving stomach upset and for boosting the appetite. For a delicious, nutritious salad topped with an orange-fennel dressing, see the Recipe Box on opposite page.

Ginger. Ginger helps stimulate a tired appetite, both through its medicinal properties and its refreshing taste. Try nibbling on gingersnaps or sipping ginger ale made with real ginger. Ginger tea is also a way to start the day off on an appetizing note. To make, place ½ teaspoon powdered ginger into a cup and fill with boiling water. Cover and let stand 10 minutes. Strain and sip. Don't take more than three times daily. If needed, sweeten with just a little honey.

Warning! Pregnant women should consult a doctor before taking ginger.

Mint. Peppermint refreshes the palate and revives the appetite. Make a cup of mint tea and enjoy anytime you don't feel like eating. Place 1 tablespoon mint leaves in a 1-pint jar of boiling water. Let stand 20 to 30 minutes, shaking occasionally. Strain and sip as needed. If you're tired of teas, make a glass of mint lemonade by adding a few sprigs to the lemonade mixture and letting it sit for 10 minutes before sipping.

LIFESTYLE REMEDIES

Head home to comfort foods. A poor appetite can be perked up by foods you adored as a child.

Watch that stress level! Keeping stress inside destroys your appetite. Relieve stress by talking to someone, getting a massage, soaking in a warm bath, or taking a mini-vacation.

Exercise. Take a vigorous walk each day, and your appetite will soon kick in.

WHEN TO CALL THE DOCTOR

- If your appetite doesn't improve in several days
- If emotional problems are causing you not to eat
- If you are experiencing unexplained weight loss or gain

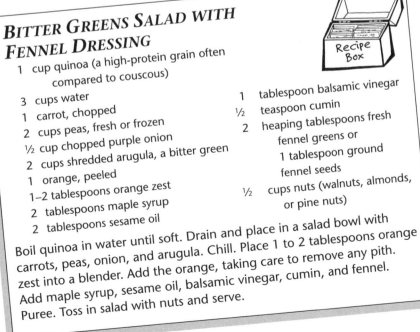

BITTER GREENS SALAD WITH FENNEL DRESSING

Recipe Box

1 cup quinoa (a high-protein grain often compared to couscous)
3 cups water
1 carrot, chopped
2 cups peas, fresh or frozen
½ cup chopped purple onion
2 cups shredded arugula, a bitter green
1 orange, peeled
1–2 tablespoons orange zest
2 tablespoons maple syrup
2 tablespoons sesame oil

1 tablespoon balsamic vinegar
½ teaspoon cumin
2 heaping tablespoons fresh fennel greens or 1 tablespoon ground fennel seeds
½ cups nuts (walnuts, almonds, or pine nuts)

Boil quinoa in water until soft. Drain and place in a salad bowl with carrots, peas, onion, and arugula. Chill. Place 1 to 2 tablespoons orange zest into a blender. Add the orange, taking care to remove any pith. Add maple syrup, sesame oil, balsamic vinegar, cumin, and fennel. Puree. Toss in salad with nuts and serve.

Postnasal Drip
TURNING OFF THE FAUCET

You may wake up with a sore throat, a hacking cough, or simply clearing your throat every morning—or you may just feel as if something has settled in the back of your throat. Any of those experiences could mean that you've got postnasal drip.

On any given day, you've got one to two quarts of mucus running down the back of your throat. That's an awful lot of slime, but it serves a significant purpose. Mucus acts as a broom, cleaning out the nasal passages. It flushes away bacteria, viruses, and other infection-causing invaders and clears out foreign particles. Mucus also helps humidify the air that travels in your body, keeping you and your insides comfortable. Unless you think about it (like while reading this book) you probably don't even notice all that mucus making its way down your throat. But if you become acutely aware of mucus in the back of your throat, or feel as if someone has turned on a faucet in your head, you're probably dealing with postnasal drip.

What Fuels the Faucet?

Postnasal drip happens when mucus production goes awry. There may be

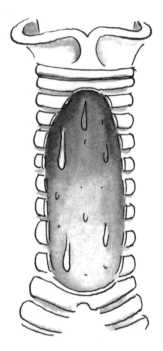

an overproduction of mucus, which gives you that typical drip, drip, drip feeling in the back of your throat. The mucus is clear, thin, and very runny. At the other extreme is thick, sticky mucus that is yellow or green. This kind of mucus occurs when mucus production slows down and thickens, hanging around in the throat.

Many factors can trigger a change in mucus production, including:

• *Allergies.* If you can tell spring is coming by the amount of tissue on your dashboard, you've probably got a hay fever allergy—one of the most common causes of postnasal drip.

- **Air pollution.** Some major pollutants in smog, such as nitrogen dioxide and sulfur dioxide, can make your mucus go haywire.
- **Cold air.** When you step outside on a cold wintry day, your nose is likely to start dripping. The same increase in mucus production happens when you're in any cold, dry environment.
- **Colds and flu.** Your nose runs during a cold or the flu to get rid of unfriendly bacterial or viral invaders. So, if you think about it, postnasal drip is actually a great defense. Try to remember that when your nose is raw from blowing it.
- **Deviated septum.** This is a technical term that means the cartilage that divides the nose into two sides has moved. It may be an innate structural problem, or it may be caused from that thwack in the nose you got while playing patty-cake with your one-year-old. Whatever the cause, a deviated septum can alter mucus flow.
- **Dusty or smoky conditions.** Dust and smoke can dry out your nose and make it tough to produce an adequate amount of mucus, so the mucus you do produce gets thicker. As a result, you end up clearing your throat every few seconds.
- **Getting older.** Another one of the joys of passing years is that your mucus production slows down and your mucus gets thicker. That's why you hear older men hacking

POSTNASAL DRIP OR POST-DINNER REFLUX?

You wake up in the morning hacking and harumphing. You have a sour taste in your mouth, and you are so hoarse at the breakfast table you can barely speak, but by dinner you don't have any problems. You might not have postnasal drip but rather a leaky stomach. Once you lie down in bed, your stomach may leak into the esophagus, causing last night's dinner to come back to your throat. If you think heartburn might be the link to your sore throat and morning hack-fest, elevate the head of your bed six to eight inches, eat at least two hours before bed, and don't stuff yourself. You might also try cutting back on alcohol and caffeine. To get some relief before bed, take an antacid to block stomach acid from making its way back to your throat.

SAY NO TO NASAL SPRAYS

Sure you feel better after squirting an over-the-counter nasal spray up your honker. These sprays restrict blood flow to your nasal passages, reducing inflammation and swelling. But if you use these sprays for more than a few days, you may make your problem worse. Avoid nasal sprays that contain phenylephrine, hydrochloride, oxymetazoline, and xylometrazoline. Saline nasal sprays are the only exception; they are safe to use and won't exacerbate your problem.

when they wake up. Thicker mucus takes some time to get moving through the throat. Swallowing muscles get weaker as you get older, too, so you may not be able to get rid of mucus as well as you once could.

- *Nasal or sinus polyps.* Okay, so polyps is not a word you really like to hear, especially when they're growing in your nose. But polyps are typically noncancerous growths that simply obstruct or change mucus flow.

- *Pregnancy.* A change in hormones seems to cause postnasal drip problems in some pregnant women.

- *Sinus infections.* Your doctor calls it "sinusitis." Infection in the four cavities surrounding your nose can make you miserable. Sinuses can become swollen or blocked, and bacteria set up shop, causing a mean infection. Thick green or yellow mucus is a good indication that you have a sinus infection. Don't let this one go without seeing a doctor. Antibiotics are the only way to completely clear it up.

- *Some medicines.* Antihistamines, diuretics, and some tranquilizers can dry up mucus production. When those commercials say that a product gives you "dry mouth," you can bet it gives you a dry nose and throat as well.

Most problems with postnasal drip are merely irritating and eventually will go away. But you can alleviate some symptoms with home remedies.

DIETARY REMEDIES

Water. Drinking enough water is a commonsense defense against postnasal drip. It keeps your mucus thin and your body, including your nasal passages, well hydrated. Drink at least eight 8-ounce glasses of water a day.

TOPICAL REMEDIES

Baking soda. If you're willing to do anything to clear up your mucous problem, try this remedy. Mix 1 cup warm water, 1 teaspoon salt, and a pinch of baking soda. Get a nasal syringe and squirt the mixture into your nostril, closing off the back of your palate and your throat. Tilt your head back, forward, and to each side for eight to ten seconds in each position to get the solution through all four of your sinus cavities. After you swish everything around, blow your nose. Try squirting in three or four bulbs full of the solution on each side of your nose. If you don't have a bulb syringe, you can snort the mixture out of your cupped hand. Try this process up to six times per day when you're dealing with postnasal drip. If you want to avoid future problems, do it twice per day.

Salt. Gargling with salt water can help soothe your sore throat. Add ½ teaspoon salt to 1 cup water and gargle away.

WHEN TO CALL THE DOCTOR

- If your mucus is thick and yellow. You may have a sinus infection, which will require an antibiotic.
- If you have a chronic problem with postnasal drip

Premenstrual Syndrome (PMS)
SUBDUING SYMPTOMS

It's that soon-to-be time of the month, and all of a sudden you start doing the Jekyll–Hyde switch. Your mild, calm demeanor is replaced by rages, and your emotions become unstable. Sometimes you feel out of control. At this time of the month, friends and loved ones may go out of their way to avoid you.

These mood swings, along with a host of other symptoms such as water retention, breast swelling and tenderness, depression, irritability, fatigue, food cravings, and headaches, are known as premenstrual syndrome (PMS). They typically begin a few days to a week before menstruation and end when the menstrual period begins.

Researchers believe that about three out of four women of childbearing age experience PMS in some form. Symptoms and severity vary from mild and manageable to severe and disruptive. Some women only have one symptom, while others have a whole constellation of problems. PMS can be downright brutal for about 10 percent of women with a diagnosis of severe PMS, also known as premenstrual dysphoric disorder. They're the

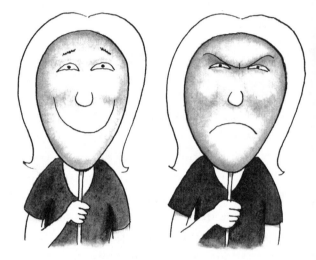

ones who experience many symptoms to a debilitating degree, causing serious problems on the job and in interpersonal relationships.

What Causes PMS?
Well, doctors don't really know what causes PMS, but they believe it is a result of hormonal changes, particularly in estrogen, that occur around the menstrual cycle. Some believe that PMS mood swings may be related to deficiencies in vitamin B6 and magnesium. One theory of PMS suggests that its symptoms are due to an ovarian hormone imbalance of either estrogen or progesterone.

Even though it's not fully understood, PMS is now recognized as a legitimate condition, not something that's all in women's heads. There are medications available that can mitigate or stop many of the harshest symptoms. Like so many other conditions, though, there are simple home treatments that can help relieve symptoms. So try them and see what happens. If you're a PMS sufferer, you know that anything that might help is worth a try.

DIETARY REMEDIES

Almonds. These tasty nuts are rich in magnesium, which is important for normal hormonal function. A lack of magnesium 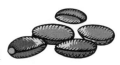 may cause muscle cramps. Other magnesium-rich foods include green vegetables, breakfast cereals (skip those sugary ones), and potatoes.

Avocados. These contain natural serotonin, which may supplement the mood-lifting brain chemical naturally produced by the body. Dates, plums, eggplants, papayas, plantains, and pineapple are also sources of serotonin.

 Bananas. Rich in potassium, they can relieve the bloating and swelling of water retention that comes with PMS. Other foods such as figs, black currants, potatoes, broccoli, onions, and tomatoes are potassium-rich, too.

Cherries. An Ayurvedic remedy to relieve PMS symptoms, including bloating and mood swings, is to eat 10 fresh cherries on an empty stom- ach each day for one week before the start of the menstrual period.

DON'T DO DIURETICS

Feeling a little bloated? Are your ankles puffed up enough to make three instead of two? Bloat and water retention are common symptoms of PMS, but avoid the common cure-all diuretics. They can wash away essential minerals, such as potassium, that are helpful in fighting PMS symptoms. (Heart palpitations can be a PMS side effect, and potassium evens out heart rhythm.) Instead, try natural diuretics such as parsley or dandelion tea or fresh, steamed asparagus. Limit salt and alcohol intake, too. And be sure to drink plenty of water.

Chicken. It's rich in Vitamin B6, which may be depleted in women who suffer from PMS. Vitamin B6 may help relieve depression by raising levels of serotonin, a mood-enhancer, in the brain. Other B6-rich foods include fish, milk, brown rice, whole grains, soybeans, beans, walnuts, and green leafy vegetables.

Oatmeal. It breaks down slowly and gradually releases sugar into the bloodstream. This slow, steady release combats the cravings that come with PMS. Whole-wheat bread, whole-wheat pasta, brown rice, and fruit produce the same effect.

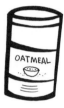

Sunflower seeds. They're rich in omega-6 fatty acid, which may be low in women who suffer from PMS. Pumpkin and sesame seeds are also loaded with omega-6 fatty acids.

Turkey. It supplies tryptophan, an amino acid that converts into serotonin, a mood-enhancer. Cottage cheese is another source of tryptophan.

SUPPLEMENTS WITH A PMS PUNCH

Studies show that symptoms of PMS may be relieved by certain vitamin and mineral supplements. Check with your doctor before you take any of these. They all can have serious side effects.

Vitamin/Mineral	Daily Dosage
Vitamin E	400 IU
Vitamin B6	50–100 milligrams
Calcium citrate	1,000 milligrams
Magnesium	300–500 milligrams

HERBAL REMEDIES

Black pepper. Add a pinch to 1 tablespoon aloe vera gel, and take three times per day with meals to relieve symptoms such as backache and abdominal pain. Aloe vera gel taken with a pinch of cumin works well too.

Chasteberry. This herb has a reputation among herbalists as one of the best PMS symptom-beaters. As an extract, put 15 drops under your tongue, twice per day. As a tea, add 1 tablespoon chasteberry and 3 tablespoons red raspberry leaves to 1 quart boiling water. Steep 20 minutes, strain, and drink 2 cups per day. Chasteberry can alter hormone levels, so don't use if you are pregnant, nursing, taking birth control pills, or being treated for hormone-sensitive cancer. It can also affect the dopamine system in the brain, so avoid chasteberry if you are taking dopamine-related medications such as levodopa.

Cinnamon. Good sleep habits are important in the treatment of PMS, and a brew of cinnamon tea is relaxing just before bed. Sweeten to taste with honey. Chamomile tea is a relaxing bedtime choice, too.

Dong quai. Also called Chinese angelica, this herb stabilizes hormone levels. Take it as a tea, starting a few days before PMS symptoms set in. How do you know when that will be? Familiarize yourself with the symptoms found on page 374, and mark your symptom onset on your calendar. In a month or two, you'll see the pattern. When you do, start taking dong quai tea several days prior to that. Stop as soon as your period starts. And don't restrict your notes to the symptom list found here. Since there are 150 known symptoms, also write down anything different that you experience

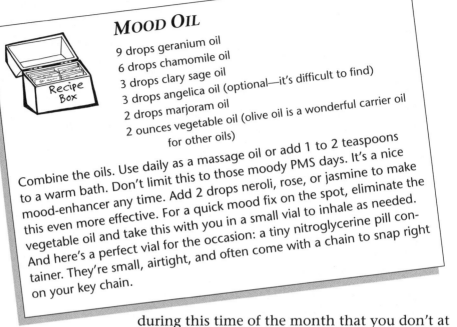

MOOD OIL

9 drops geranium oil
6 drops chamomile oil
3 drops clary sage oil
3 drops angelica oil (optional—it's difficult to find)
2 drops marjoram oil
2 ounces vegetable oil (olive oil is a wonderful carrier oil for other oils)

Combine the oils. Use daily as a massage oil or add 1 to 2 teaspoons to a warm bath. Don't limit this to those moody PMS days. It's a nice mood-enhancer any time. Add 2 drops neroli, rose, or jasmine to make this even more effective. For a quick mood fix on the spot, eliminate the vegetable oil and take this with you in a small vial to inhale as needed. And here's a perfect vial for the occasion: a tiny nitroglycerine pill container. They're small, airtight, and often come with a chain to snap right on your key chain.

during this time of the month that you don't at other times.

Warning! Dong quai has the potential to cause bleeding complications in people who take the blood-thinning drug warfarin.

Evening primrose oil. This is beginning to get recognition from traditional medical sources as a possible PMS reliever, although research is mixed on its effectiveness. Take 3,000 mg per day, in divided doses. Begin taking it ten days before your period is expected to start.

Rose petals. A simple tea of fresh or dried petals may cure irritability or agitation. Simply steep a few in 1 cup boiling water. Petals can be added to fruit and vegetable salads, too.

TOPICAL REMEDIES

Ice. If you're suffering tension or extreme anxiety, a nice cooling drink may be relaxing. Or wrap some ice in a kitchen towel to use

as a cold compress on aching muscles and PMS headaches.

Kitchen towel. Soak it in water, wring it out, then warm it up in the microwave for a minute. Moist heat is soothing, so apply this to your belly when you're having abdominal or ovarian cramps. Be careful not to burn yourself.

LIFESTYLE REMEDIES

Crunch on carbs. Fresh fruits, vegetables, and whole-grain cereals and breads can reduce the cravings that come with PMS. They also help elevate mood. Eat smaller meals, then snack on these carbohydrates every three hours: popcorn (skip the butter), pretzels, and rice cakes. Consume about 100 calories per snack.

Cut the caffeine. And that goes for coffee, cola, and chocolate. Caffeine contributes to breast pain and anxiety, two of the leading PMS complaints.

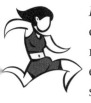

Exercise. Endorphins, which are brain chemicals responsible for improving mood, are released during aerobic exercises such as walking, running, and swimming. Increase your exercise regimen, working out once a day starting the week before your period to help relieve or prevent PMS symptoms.

Forgo fats. Fats—especially saturated fats—may make PMS symptoms worse. Limit fat to less than 20 percent of your daily calories.

Sleep tight. Interruption in regular sleep rhythms can interfere with your regular cycle and cause irritability and fatigue.

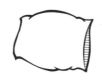

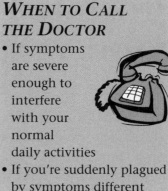

WHEN TO CALL THE DOCTOR
- If symptoms are severe enough to interfere with your normal daily activities
- If you're suddenly plagued by symptoms different from your regular PMS symptoms, especially abdominal, ovarian, or breast pain

Prostate Problems
PAMPER YOUR PROSTATE

A sad fact of growing older for the male gender is that most men older than 60 (and some in their 50s) develop symptoms of prostate problems. The three most common disorders are benign prostatic hyperplasia (BPH), a noncancerous enlargement of the prostate; prostatitis, an inflammatory infection; and prostate cancer. BPH is so common that some physicians consider it a normal consequence of aging.

The prostate's main role is to produce an essential portion of the seminal fluid that carries sperm. This walnut-shaped gland that surrounds the tube that carries urine away from the bladder and out of a man's body starts to grow larger around puberty and continues to grow and grow. This enlargement doesn't usually cause symptoms until after age 40, and it usually doesn't cause problems until age 60 or later.

An enlarged prostate presses on the urethra, creating difficulties with urination and weakening the bladder. Some of the symptoms of prostate problems include

- difficulty urinating
- frequent urination, especially at night
- difficulty starting urination
- an inability to empty the bladder
- a dribble of urine despite the urgent need to urinate
- a burning sensation when urinating
- uncontrolled dribbling after urination
- pain behind the scrotum
- painful ejaculation

Ignoring prostate problems is a bad idea. Left untreated, prostate problems can get progressively worse, become more painful, and can lead to dangerous complications, including bladder and kidney infections.

Changes in diet can help relieve some prostate discomforts and, in some cases, may reduce the chances of developing prostate cancer.

DIETARY REMEDIES

Corn silk. This has been used by Amish men for generations as a remedy for the symptoms of prostate enlargement. When fresh corn is in season, cut the silk from 6 ears of corn. (Corn silk can be dried for later use too.) Put in 1 quart water, boil, and simmer for ten minutes. Strain and drink a cup. Drink 3 cups per week.

Fish. Fish help fight prostate cancer and tumor growth. Try to get 2 servings per week of fish that are high in omega-3 oils (the good oil) such as tuna, mackerel, or salmon.

Pumpkin seeds. These are used by German doctors to treat difficult urination that accompanies an enlarged prostate that is not cancerous. The seeds contain diuretic properties and plenty of zinc, which helps repair and build the immune system. Pumpkin seeds taste best plain. Remove the shells and don't add salt. You can also try a tea. Crush a handful of fresh seeds and place in the bottom of a 1-pint jar. Fill with boiling water. Let cool to room temperature. Strain and drink a pint of pumpkin seed tea per day.

Soy. Soy-based foods contain phytoestrogens, which are thought to help reduce testosterone production, which is believed to aggravate prostate cancer growth. The phytoestrogens are believed to limit the growth of blood capillaries that form around tumors of the prostate.

WHEN TO CALL THE DOCTOR

- If you experience one or more of the symptoms listed on page 380
- Every year, for an annual prostate cancer test

Tomatoes. Studies have shown that as little as 2 servings of tomatoes (including cooked tomatoes) per week can help cut the risk of prostate cancer by half. Tomatoes are full of lycopene, an antioxidant compound that helps fight cancer.

Watermelon seeds. The Amish use watermelon tea to flush the system out and help with bladder problems and prostate problems. Collect watermelon seeds in a cup. When you have ⅛ cup fresh seeds, put them in a 1-pint jar and fill with boiling water. Let the tea cool, strain, and drink 1 pint of tea every day for 10 days.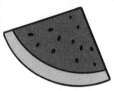

DIETARY SUPPLEMENT REMEDIES

Saw palmetto. Several small studies suggest that saw palmetto may be effective at treating BPH symptoms, although other studies have found no benefit. Palmetto extracts can be purchased at a health food store. Consult your physician for recommended dosages. Saw palmetto has some possible side effects, including breast tenderness (even in men) and reduced sexual desire.

Stinging nettle. Stinging nettle has been used in Europe for hundreds of years, and studies have shown it to reduce symptoms of prostate problems (but not to reduce the size of an enlarged prostate). Nettle helps by influencing the action of hormones in the body. Take stinging nettle in extract form (as capsules). Check with your physician for the correct dosage. Nettle may interact with drugs prescribed for high blood pressure, diabetes, heart disease, and arthritis, so make sure to consult with your doctor about potential drug interactions. Do not self-treat prostate problems using herbs or any other home remedy.

Psoriasis
SOFTENING THE SCALES

Imagine having an unwanted guest show up on your doorstep. No one knows who invited him, and no one really wants him there. He's one of the most annoying people you've ever met, and his personality is so abrasive, you're embarrassed to take him anywhere.

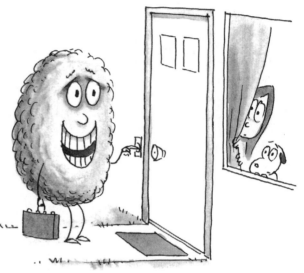

If you have psoriasis, or know anyone with this frustrating skin condition, you know that it's much like that uninvited guest. It shows up in the form of dry, inflamed, red, scaly patches of skin. Not only are psoriasis flare-ups aggravating, they make people with the condition so self-conscious about their appearance that they're reluctant to go to the grocery store without ample covering. Probably most frustrating of all is that there's no magic formula to kick this guest out of town indefinitely. You have to learn how to deal with flare-ups as they come and take good care of yourself and your skin.

The Psoriasis Puzzle

Normally, your skin cells go through a month-long life cycle. New cells are formed deep within the skin, and over a period of about 28 to 30 days they make their way to the top of the skin. By that time, your old skin cells die and are sloughed off by everyday routines such as showering and toweling off.

The skin of a person with psoriasis, however, goes into fast-forward when the immune system sends out faulty signals that speed up the skin's growth cycle. The entire skin cell process happens in three or four days, causing a buildup of dead skin cells on the surface of the skin. Thankfully, this quickening of skin cells usually happens in patches, mostly on the scalp,

THE SKIN THEY'RE IN

Psoriasis affects 7.5 million Americans. It occurs equally in men and women. Though most people may link psoriasis with the elderly, the average age of a first-time psoriasis sufferer is between 15 and 35 years. The condition can occur in every stage of life from birth to old age. In fact, 10 to 15 percent of people who get psoriasis are younger than 10 years old.

lower back, elbows, knees, and knuckles. The technical term for these dry, irritating, scaly patches is plaques.

Psoriasis is one of the most prevalent autoimmune diseases in the United States, affecting some 7.5 million people. In about 32 percent of psoriasis cases, there's a family history of the condition, which means there is a significant genetic link. Doctors do know that there are specific lifestyle factors that can trigger psoriasis or make symptoms worse. Drinking alcohol, being overweight, stress, a lingering case of strep throat, anxiety, some medicines, and sunburn all tend to make psoriasis even more unbearable.

Psoriasis isn't contagious, though it looks like it might be. Some people end up with mild cases of the condition that produce small patches of red scales. Others are plagued by psoriasis—it covers large areas of their body with thick scales. Some people even get psoriasis in their nails, which causes the nails to become pitted and malformed, and even to break away from the skin. In some 10 to 30 percent of cases, a type of arthritis called psoriatic arthritis develops.

Though there is no way to get rid of psoriasis, you can help your body recover more quickly and ease your symptoms with some simple home remedies.

TOPICAL REMEDIES

Apple cider vinegar. Add 1 cup apple cider vinegar to 1 gallon water. Soak a washcloth in the mixture and apply it to the skin to ease itching.

Baking soda. To ease the itch, mix 1½ cups baking soda into 3 gallons water. Apply to your itchy patches with a washcloth soaked in the solution.

Epsom salts. Add a handful of these healing salts to your bath. They'll keep swelling down and bring healing to your psoriasis.

Mineral oil. This is another time-proven skin soother. Add a bit to your bath and soak your aching skin.

Olive oil. An old favorite for easing psoriasis outbreaks is mixing 2 teaspoons olive oil with a large glass of milk and adding the concoction to your bathwater. Or if you are dealing with psoriasis on your scalp, massage some warm olive oil on your scaly patches. It will help soften the dead skin and make it easier to remove.

Plastic wrap. After you douse your patches in moisturizer, wrap them in plastic wrap to help hold the moisture in. Change the wrapping often.

Salicylic acid. Shampoos and creams that contain salicylic acid may help to get rid of annoying scales. Use according to package directions, because overuse can cause irritation and temporary hair loss.

Try tar. Coal tar shampoos, creams, and bath items are a long-used treatment for psoriasis. They seem to work by helping to loosen scales, which makes them easier to slough off. Try an over-the-counter brand. Follow directions carefully, because coal tar may cause irritation and can be carcinogenic in high concentrations.

Choose soap carefully. Use "superfatted" soaps that contain moisturizers, or go for soap-free cleansers. They'll both be kinder to your skin.

Medicate the itch. Over-the-counter cortisone creams or antihistamines may help ease some of the itch and inflammation.

Vegetable oil. Get in the tub and add a cupful of vegetable oil to your bath to ease your psoriasis.

HELP IS ON THE HORIZON

According to the National Psoriasis Foundation (NPF), many Americans with psoriasis have given up on finding a treatment for their disease. But the NPF, whose main goal is to raise public awareness of the disease and support ongoing research into psoriasis, offers some rays of hope. Because psoriasis is driven by the immune system, researchers are looking at immune-suppressing drugs as a treatment for psoriasis. Other treatments include UVA and UVB laser delivery systems and combination therapies that utilize older treatments in different ways.

WHEN TO CALL THE DOCTOR

• At the first sign of a psoriasis-like patch. Psoriasis can mimic more serious skin conditions and even certain types of skin cancer.

White vinegar. Vinegar helps ease the itch. Add a cup to your bathwater.

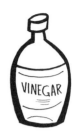

DIETARY SUPPLEMENT REMEDIES

Fish oil. Some studies have found a link between intake of omega-3 fatty acids in fish oil to improvement in psoriasis patches. Fish oil helps boost immune function, and since psoriasis is an immune-mediated disease, researchers believe it could improve symptoms. There are also commercial creams available that contain fish oils or derivatives of the oils. Be sure to discuss the options with your doctor.

HERBAL REMEDIES

Cayenne. Capsaicin, the substance that gives cayenne pepper its heat, blocks the communication system of sensory nerves. Studies have found that a cream containing capsaicin helped relieve itching and got rid of psoriasis plaques. Look for a cream containing .025 to .075 percent capsaicin—no more than that or you risk burning your skin. It takes about a week for the cream to work.

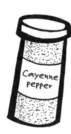

LIFESTYLE REMEDIES

Keep skin supple. Moisturize to help minimize swelling, make your skin more flexible, and make scales less apparent. Look for moisturizers that are thick and lock moisture into the skin—ingredients like lactic acid seem to work best. Or use cooking oils, lard, or petrolatum. Apply moisturizer right after a bath or shower to hold onto natural oils and water.

Make the indoors tropical. Humidify your house to make you more comfortable during a flare-up.

Seasonal Affective Disorder
LOOKING FOR LIGHT

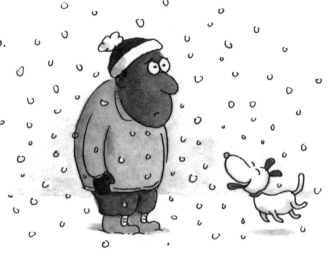

Ho hum. Another day, so much to do. But you can't seem to drag yourself out of bed. In fact, with Ma in her kerchief and Pa in his cap, the only thing you'd really like to do is snuggle in between the covers for your long winter's nap.

If that's a description of the way you feel every winter, you could be suffering from seasonal affective disorder, or SAD. It affects millions of people during the winter months when there is less sunlight. In rare cases, SAD can occur in the summer.

In addition to a depressed mood, symptoms of SAD include cravings for carbohydrates, inability to concentrate, irritability, lethargy, weight gain, and a lack of interest in sex.

Although the link between the gray, short days of winter and SAD is well-established, no one knows why some people are affected and others are not. Current thinking associates SAD with too much melatonin, the hormone that causes you to be sleepy. Normally, sunlight stops melatonin production in the body, and darkness starts it. When adequate sunlight is missing, as it usually is in the winter months, that wanna-go-to-sleep hormone kicks into overtime production because there's nothing around to tell it to turn itself off. Some medical researchers compare SAD

THE PINEAL GLAND
The pineal gland is an odd little organ, smaller than an aspirin tablet, that regulates our daily rhythms. It's our biological clock. When light is absent, the pineal gland activates two of its natural enzymes to turn the hormone serotonin into melatonin. Serotonin is what keeps us from being depressed, stops us from craving sweets and carbohydrates, and regulates normal sleep patterns. When melatonin kicks in, these normal serotonin activities are reversed, because the pineal gland gets insufficient sunlight.

SAD FACTS

No one can say for sure why some people suffer due to decreased sunlight, but these statistics tell the SAD story:

- SAD affects as much as 20 percent of the U.S. population.
- The incidence of SAD increases from the South to the North; 1 percent of the residents in Miami suffer SAD, 10 percent of the people living near the U.S.-Canadian border suffer SAD, and 28 percent of those in Fairbanks, Alaska, have it.
- SAD is extremely rare in people living within 30 degrees latitude of the equator.
- Three out of four people with SAD are female.
- People are most likely to first experience SAD symptoms between the ages of 18 and 30.
- SAD runs in families.

FASCINATING FACT

Seasonal affective disorder is typically a condition of winter, but symptoms may start as early as September and continue all the way through April.

to hibernation. During the winter, many animals store up carbohydrates, crawl into a cozy cave, resist the mating urge, and snooze until spring. Sounds pretty primal, but that's exactly the way people who suffer SAD react, only in a modified version.

Another theory is that SAD is a result of a delay in the timing of the body clock. In SAD patients, the body's lowest temperature occurs at 6 A.M., rather than at 3 A.M., as it should normally. As a result, they are awakening when physiologically it is the middle of the night. When treated with light from 6 A.M. to 8 A.M., these patients experience a shift in minimum temperature to an earlier time and an associated shift in mood.

Doctors often treat SAD with antidepressants. For some, they work. For others, the side effects are overwhelming, often worse than the condition itself. So if you've got SAD, look at home for some relief.

DIETARY REMEDIES

Apricots. This fruit gradually raises serotonin levels and helps keep them there, as do apples, pears, grapes, plums, grapefruits, and oranges.

Avocados. They are high in natural serotonin, which seems to suppress appetite. Also high in natural serotonin are dates, bananas, plums, eggplant, papayas, passion fruit, plantains, pineapples, and tomatoes.

Brown rice. The sugar in this rice is slow to release into the bloodstream, which helps blood sugar levels stay constant instead of going through highs and lows. Drastic changes in blood sugar can lead to weight gain, which is a side effect of SAD. Other foods with a similar effect on blood sugar are whole-wheat bread and whole-wheat pasta.

Cereals. Cooked cereal, unsweetened muesli, and bran flakes are slow to release sugar into the bloodstream, which helps raise serotonin levels. (See "The Pineal Gland" on page 387 for the role of serotonin.

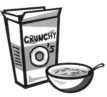

Cottage cheese. It's high in tryptophan, which is lacking in people with SAD. Other foods just as high in tryptophan are turkey, fish, and eggs.

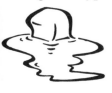

Ice. When you can't get going no matter what you do, try sucking on some ice. Its chill can give you a wake-up call. Or, splash your face and wrists with ice water.

Legumes. These help maintain an even serotonin level throughout the day and night.

Shellfish. These are high in tyrosine, which forms chemicals that act on the brain cells to improve concentration and alertness, both of which become sluggish with SAD. Other foods high in tyrosine are fish, chicken, skinless turkey, cottage cheese, plain yogurt, skim milk, eggs, tofu, and very lean ham, pork, and lamb.

Turkey. Protein foods such as turkey, low-fat cottage cheese, chicken, and low-fat dairy products can reduce the carbohydrate cravings of SAD as well as control the weight gain that occurs during SAD months.

HERBAL REMEDIES

Herbal teas. Any herbal tea is a better choice than teas with caffeine. Your reduced energy level may cause you to turn to caffeine for a boost, but it can also cause

WHEN TO CALL THE DOCTOR

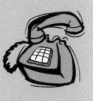

- When you have your first SAD symptom. Other ailments, including underactive thyroid gland, low blood sugar, chronic fatigue syndrome, chronic viral illness, and some strains of flu, mimic SAD and must be ruled out.
- When symptoms, including depression, prevent you from performing your normal daily activities
- If you experience thoughts of hurting or killing yourself

anxiety, muscle tension, and stomach problems, so opt for herbal. Chamomile, peppermint, and cinnamon are pleasant-tasting choices. Drink a cup instead of giving in to your carbohydrate cravings.

Peppermint oil. Or lemon oil. Steep in water and inhale. These are stimulating and may give you a little extra zip.

LIFESTYLE REMEDIES

Curtains. Open them, or remove them, especially where you have a southern exposure.

Cut trees and bushes away from your windows. Remove heavy drapes that block the light.

Dirty dishes. If your sink is near or under the window, save all your dishes from the night before and wash them the next day, during the brightest sunlight.

Exercise. Aerobic exercise has a positive effect on moods. Try walking, jogging, biking, or swimming. Even better, exercise in the sun or near a nice, sunny window.

Light Therapy. For some SAD sufferers, sitting in front of a light box or wearing a light visor for 30 minutes a day can reduce symptoms. Talk with your doctor about whether light therapy is appropriate for you.

Take a walk in the sun. Morning or early afternoon sun is the best.

Vacation in a warm, sunny climate during the winter months.

Sore Throat
RELIEVING RAWNESS

It's scratchy, tender, and swollen, and you dread the simple task of swallowing. But you must swallow, and when you do, you brace yourself for the unavoidable pain. If you've got a sore throat, you're in good company; everybody gets them, and millions of people trek to the doctor's office for treatment every year.

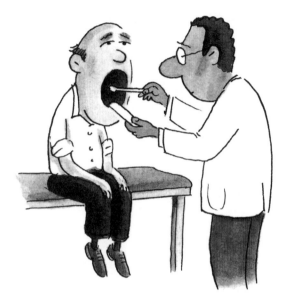

The mechanics of a sore throat are pretty simple. It's an inflammation of the pharynx, which is the tube that extends from the back of the mouth to the esophagus. The following are the leading causes of sore throat:

- Viral infection (colds, flu, etc.). Often accompanied by fever, achy muscles, and runny nose, viral infections can't be cured, but their symptoms can be treated. A sore throat from a viral source will generally disappear on its own within several days.
- Bacterial infection, especially from streptococcal bacteria (strep throat). Symptoms are much like those of a viral infection but may be more severe and long lasting. Often a bacterial infection is accompanied by headache, stomachache, and swollen glands in the neck. A strep infection is generally treated with antibiotics because permanent heart or kidney damage can result. Culturing the bacteria is the only way a doctor can determine the cause of the sore throat.

Although those are the primary reasons for a sore throat, there are others, including:

- Smoking
- Acid reflux
- Allergies
- Dry air, especially during the night, when you may sleep with your mouth open

FASCINATING FACT
Don't add boiling water to vinegar. The boiling water drives off volatile acetic acid, which, along with the added water, dilutes the vinegar too much.

- Mouth breathing
- Throat abuse: singing, shouting, coughing
- Polyps or cancer
- Infected tonsils
- Food allergy

Whatever the cause, you want a cure when your throat's on fire. In some cases, medical attention is definitely required to cure the underlying infection. But there are soothing remedies to be found at home that can stand alone or work side-by-side with traditional medicine to stifle that soreness.

DIETARY REMEDIES

Cider vinegar. This sore throat cure is found in several different remedies. Here are a few of the more popular ones:

For sipping: Mix 1 tablespoon each of honey and cider vinegar in 1 cup warm water.

For gargling: You'll need 1 teaspoon salt, ½ cup cider vinegar, and 1 cup warm water. Dissolve the salt in the vinegar, then mix in the water. Gargle every 15 minutes as necessary.

AMISH ONION & HONEY SORE THROAT SOOTHER

6 white onions, finely chopped
1 cup honey
juice of 1 fresh lemon
2 tablespoons olive oil

Sauté onions in olive oil until transparent, stirring often. Stir in honey (use brown sugar if recipe is for children under 2 years of age). Add lemon juice. Continue to cook over low heat until mixture thickens. Remove from heat, pour in glass jar. Take 1 tablespoon as often as needed.
Store in refrigerator.

For soaking: Soak cheesecloth or gauze in ⅔ cup warm water with 2 tablespoons cider vinegar. Wring out and apply to the throat, covering it with dry gauze or an elastic bandage. Wear it all night.

Horseradish. Try this Russian sore throat cure. Combine 1 tablespoon pure horseradish or horse-radish root with 1 teaspoon honey and 1 teaspoon ground cloves. Mix in a glass of warm water and drink slowly.

Juice bar. This is cold and soothing to a hot throat. Don't suck, though. Sucking may irritate the throat even more. Simply let small pieces melt in your mouth.

Lemon juice. Mix 1 tablespoon each of honey and lemon juice in 1 cup warm water. Sip this mixture.

Lime juice. Combine 1 spoonful with a spoonful of honey and take as often as needed for a sore throat.

Onions. This tear-promoting veggie contains allicin, which can kill the bacteria that causes strep. Eat them raw or sautéed. And check the Recipe Box on the opposite page for a sore throat soother.

Raspberries. These can make a great gargle (see Recipe Box page 396). If you also have a fever, the gargle can be used as a fever-reducing drink. Do not drink any liquid you have used as a gargle.

Salt. Yes, when your mother told you to gargle with salt water, she knew what she was talking about. It cuts phlegm and reduces inflammation. Dissolve ½ teaspoon salt in ½ cup warm water, and gargle every three to four hours.

LARYNGITIS? SHUSH!

If you've got laryngitis, don't whisper. Whispering is just as rough on your vocal chords as shouting. To get that voice back, talk quietly or be silent. And moisturize those vocal chords to help them heal. Drink 8 to 10 glasses of water per day, drink ginger tea, and inhale steam.

Water. Gargle with 4 parts water to 1 part three-percent hydrogen peroxide two to three times a day. Also, sip plain water throughout the day to prevent your throat from becoming dry.

HERBAL REMEDIES

Chamomile. Make a tea by adding 1 teaspoon chamomile to 1 cup boiling water. Steep for ten minutes, strain, then gargle three to four times a day. Make a poultice by mixing 1 tablespoon chamomile flowers in 2 cups boiling water. Steep five minutes, then strain. Soak a clean towel in the warm solution, wring it out, and apply to throat. Remove when cold and reapply as often as necessary.

Garlic. This Amish remedy can treat or prevent sore throats. Peel a fresh clove, slice it in half, and place 1 piece in each cheek. Suck on the garlic like a cough drop. Occasionally, crush your teeth against the garlic, not to bite it in half, but to release its allicin, a chemical that can kill the bacteria that causes strep.

Horehound. This is a great remedy for sore throats, but it's not a common herb found on most shelves. If you do happen to find it, make a tea with 1 tablespoon horehound leaves and 1 cup boiling water. Steep, strain, and gargle. You can also suck on some horehound hard candy. Avoid using during pregnancy.

Marjoram. Make a soothing tea with a spoonful of marjoram steeped in a cup of boiling water for ten minutes. Strain, then sweeten to taste with honey.

Sage. This curative herb is a great sore throat gargle. Mix 1 teaspoon in 1 cup boiling water.

Steep for ten minutes, then strain. Add 1 teaspoon each cider vinegar and honey, then gargle four times per day.

Turmeric. Try this gargle to calm a cranky throat. Mix together 1 cup hot water, ½ teaspoon turmeric, and ½ teaspoon salt. Gargle with the mixture twice per day. If you're not good with the gargle, mix ½ teaspoon turmeric in 1 cup hot milk and drink. Turmeric stains clothing, so be careful when mixing and gargling.

TOPICAL REMEDIES

Beets. Make a poultice by grating 2 to 3 tablespoons red beets and covering them with 2 cups boiling water. Soak a clean towel in the warm solution, wring it out, and apply to the throat. Remove when cold and reapply as often as necessary. Beets will stain the cloth (and your skin) so use a towel that you don't mind turning reddish purple.

Steam. With or without herbs, inhaling steam can relieve the discomfort of a sore throat. Heat a pot full of water, remove from heat, make a tent with a towel, and place your face over the steam. Then breathe. Adding 1 to 2 drops eucalyptus oil can also be soothing.

LIFESTYLE REMEDIES

Drink plenty of fluids, especially fruit juices. Nix the colas and scratchy foods, such as chips and pretzels. They'll just aggravate an already irritated throat.

Rest. This will allow your body to build up the defenses to fight off whatever's causing your sore throat.

WHEN TO CALL THE DOCTOR

- If you have a swollen throat and are having difficulty breathing, call 9-1-1 or seek immediate emergency treatment
- If your sore throat lasts more than four days
- If you suspect a serious infection such as strep
- If you have a fever of more than 103 degrees Fahrenheit or any fever lasting more than three days
- If you have a skin rash
- If swallowing is very painful
- If the sore throat is accompanied by an earache
- If you have achy joints
- If you have blisters or pus in your throat
- If you're spitting up bloody phlegm
- If the sore throat prevents you from performing normal activities
- For any sore throat in infants, young children, people with weakened immune systems, or older people

A Singer's Rules

To prevent a sore throat or ease one that you have, take this advice from professional singers, whose livelihood depends on the condition of their throats:

- Avoid crowds, especially during flu season.
- Wear a scarf around your throat on cold, damp, or windy days.
- Don't sleep in a draft.
- Suck on sugarless hard candy or chew sugarless gum for relief from a dry throat.
- Drink a little of a Singer's Friend Tea before you perform (even if you're not singing at the Metropolitan Opera tonight, this is still a good throat soother):

  2 tablespoons lemon juice
  2 teaspoons honey
  1 cup warm water
  Some singers will add 1 teaspoon minced garlic, but only if it's a solo performance!
  Mix and sip slowly, while warm.

Raspberry Gargle

2 cups ripe red raspberries
2½ cups white wine vinegar
1 cup sugar

Place berries in a bowl and cover with the vinegar. Cover, and refrigerate three days. Place the mixture in a saucepan, add sugar, and bring to a gentle boil. Simmer 15 minutes, remove from heat, and cool. Strain through a sieve, pressing down the berries to retrieve as much juice as possible. Store in a bottle, refrigerate, and use as needed.

Recipe Box

Stomach Upset
TACKLING TUMMY TROUBLES

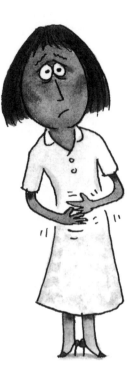

You and your wife celebrated your promotion with dinner at your favorite barbecue joint. You've been working hard for months, so you deserve to indulge. On the way home you groan and mutter that you wish you had stopped after that first barbecue platter. Your wife shrugs her shoulders. You both know the price for your revelry will be a painful night of bloating, gas, and heartburn.

Sometimes your tummy can turn on you even when you haven't been making one too many trips to the buffet table. It's important to know what's normal tummy trouble and what's something to take more seriously.

The Digestive Dance

When you eat something, the digestive process begins right away in your mouth. Your salivary glands produce digestive juices that lubricate your food and prepare fat for digestion. The food travels through your esophagus into your stomach, where digestive juices continue to break food down even further so it can travel on to the small intestine. The pancreas and liver secrete other digestive juices that flow into the small intestines. In the small intestine, vital nutrients including vitamins, minerals, water, salt, carbohydrates, and proteins are sucked out of the food and absorbed into your body. By the time your dinner makes its way to the large intestines, it's mostly bulk and water. The large intestines absorb the water and help you get rid of the excess.

STOMACH? YOU ARE HERE

You're on *Who Wants to Be a Millionaire* and Regis asks the million dollar question: Where is your stomach located? If you're like most people, you'd say in the center of your abdomen. Unfortunately, you'd be out a lot of money if you made that your final answer. The stomach is actually much higher than you think. It's located below the diaphragm, just to the left of your sternum.

Sometimes things in the digestive system go awry and cause indigestion, a catchall term that means you simply have trouble digesting your food. When you eat too much, or you eat the wrong foods, you may get one of a number of indigestion symptoms, including nausea, vomiting, heartburn, bloating, or gas.

Those unpleasant feelings may send you running to the drugstore for relief, and if they do, you've got plenty of company. The American Gastroenterological Association says that digestive problems are one of the most common reasons Americans take over-the-counter medications. Indigestion can be a symptom of something more serious, such as gastritis, an ulcer, severe heartburn, irritable bowel syndrome, or diverticulitis. However, if it's just the result of over-doing it at dinner, try some of these home cures for relief.

DIETARY REMEDIES

Apples. Adding fiber to your diet will help alleviate stomachaches and keep your digestive system healthy. One study of fiber's effect on the tummy discovered that people who ate fiber-rich foods at the first sign of a tummyache cut their chances of getting a full-blown upset stomach in half. If you haven't been eating much fiber, be sure to start slowly. Jumping in with loads of fiber-rich foods after living on burgers and fries will give you a mean case of gas. Add fiber gradually over a few months and drink plenty of water to avoid overloading your system. To get started, grab an apple and nosh away, but remember to eat the peel—that's where you get most of your roughage.

Baking soda. Make your own antacid with baking soda. Mix ½ teaspoon baking soda in ½ glass water and drink away. Remember to read the antacid instructions on the baking soda label before you take this home remedy. Avoid this remedy if your doctor has advised you to cut back on salt.

 Bananas. If you have a sensitive tummy, bland foods such as bananas seem to ease the pain. One study found that half the people who took banana powder capsules every day for two months eased their tummy pain. You can get similar results by eating a banana—or better yet a plantain banana—every day.

Crackers. You haven't eaten anything all day, and you can't understand why your stomach is churning and burning. The answer is probably overactive stomach acids. Your best bet is to eat something but to stick with something bland, such as nibbling on crackers.

Rice. If an overflow of stomach acid bothers you, try eating ½ cup cooked rice with your dinner. It's a complex 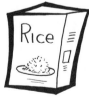 carbohydrate that keeps the stomach busy churning, diverting excess acid. Plus it's a bland food that tends to be easy on the stomach.

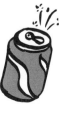 ***Soda pop.*** Sipping on a can of decaffeinated soda can help settle your stomach. This trick is especially useful if you've eaten too much. The carbonation in the soda causes you to burp, which can relieve the discomfort of an overfull belly.

LIFE AND TIMES OF YOUR LUNCH

You ate tuna fish on rye at noon, and that tuna will be with you for a while before it's digested. Take a look at how long food takes to get from entrance to exit.

- Esophagus: One bite slides down the esophagus in eight seconds.
- Stomach: Carbohydrates take two hours to digest. Proteins take four hours. Fatty foods stick around for six hours.
- Small Intestines: Foods stay in this winding road for three to five hours.
- Large Intestines: That sandwich will stay in the large intestines for 4 to 72 hours before it makes its departure.

TAKE SOMETHING BITTER AND MAKE YOUR STOMACH BETTER

Folk medicine has a grocery list of herbs that can ease stomach trouble and help your digestive system work like a dream, or at least a lot better than it has been. One of the most frequently recommended categories of digestive aids is a bitter tonic. These tonics help stimulate the digestive system by kicking in stomach acid and liver bile, which improve digestion and help the body better absorb essential nutrients. Some of the most frequently prescribed bitter tonic herbs are wormwood, chamomile, goldenseal, Oregon grape root, gentian, and boneset. Take note: Don't try a bitter tonic if you have heartburn or any other kind of pain accompanying digestion.

Water. Drinking water is your best bet for avoiding tummy trouble. It helps move things through the digestive system smoothly. Try drinking at least six to eight 8-ounce glasses of water every day.

DIETARY SUPPLEMENT REMEDIES

Antacid. Antacids can help neutralize stomach acids, which can cut that burning sensation you feel when you have an empty stomach. But be careful what kind of antacid you choose. Though they help keep those stomach acids calm, antacids can cause other trouble if you're not careful. Most have calcium or magnesium as a main ingredient. If you tend to be constipated, try an antacid with magnesium listed first on the list of ingredients. If diarrhea is more bothersome for you, pick an antacid with calcium listed first.

HERBAL REMEDIES

Caraway seeds. These seeds act similarly to fennel seeds. They help with digestion and gas. You can either make a tea from the seed or you can do what people in Middle Eastern countries have done for centuries—simply chew on the seeds after dinner. Caraway seed tea: Place 1 teaspoon caraway seeds in a cup and add boiling water. Cover the cup and let stand for ten minutes. Strain well and drink as many as 3 cups per day—be sure to drink on an empty stomach.

Catnip. This herb has long been known as an aid for tummy trouble, and it's been used to treat digestive problems, stomach cramps, and gas for hundreds of years. Like chamomile, catnip has sedative properties that help you—and your stomach—relax. Sip a cup of catnip tea when you are experiencing stomach upset: Place 1 teaspoon dried catnip in a cup and pour boiling water over the herb. Let the tea steep for ten minutes. Strain and drink as much as 3 cups per day on an empty stomach. Catnip should not be used if you're pregnant or nursing or if you've been diagnosed with gynecological conditions, because it can lead to excessive menstrual bleeding.

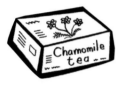

Chamomile. This herb is well-known for its soothing properties, and it indeed eases stomach cramps and gas, helping the stomach relax. To make your own chamomile tea: Put 1 tablespoon chamomile flowers in a cup. Pour boiling water over the flowers and let sit for ten minutes. Strain and drink the warm tea on an empty stomach up to three times per day.

Cinnamon. This aromatic spice stimulates the digestive system. Make a tea by stirring ¼ to ½ teaspoon cinnamon powder into 1 cup hot water. Let the tea stand as long as 5 minutes and drink.

Fennel seeds. This remedy is one of the most prescribed for gas and stomach cramps by medical herbalists. Try a fennel tea for your stomach: Place 1 teaspoon fennel seeds in a cup and add boiling water. Cover the cup and let stand for ten minutes. Strain well and drink as many as 3 cups per day—be sure to drink on an empty stomach.

Ginger. Ginger has a long-time reputation for helping stomach ailments of all types—particularly 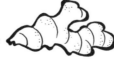 nausea and gas. Ginger helps food flow smoothly through the digestive tract, allowing the body to better absorb nutrients. Drink a cup of ginger tea to get your stomach back on track. To make your own ginger tea:

WHEN TO CALL THE DOCTOR

- If you have excessive abdominal cramping that doesn't go away after 30 minutes or gets worse with time. You may have an intestinal obstruction.
- If you have vomiting, fever, extreme nausea, or abdominal cramping. You could have food poisoning or an ulcer.
- If your stomachache lasts longer than a day
- If your indigestion is accompanied by pressure in the chest, nausea or vomiting, sweating, or breathing trouble. You could be having a heart attack and should seek emergency medical atention.

Add ½ teaspoon ground ginger to a cup of hot water, let stand for up to three minutes, strain, and drink.

Mint. A folk remedy for indigestion, mint (in the form of peppermint or spearmint) can soothe a troubled tummy. Mint helps food move through the intestines properly and eases stomach cramps. Sip a cup of mint tea for relief: Put 1 teaspoon dried mint in a cup and add boiling water. Cover the cup and let it stand for ten minutes. Strain and drink as much as 3 cups of the warm tea per day. Be sure to drink it on an empty stomach.

Thyme. Thyme stimulates the digestive tract, helps with stomach cramping, and relieves gas pressure. Try some thyme in a bottle (or cup): Place 1 teaspoon dried thyme leaves in a cup. Fill the cup with boiling water, and let stand, covered, for ten minutes. Strain and drink on an empty stomach as often as three times per day.

TOPICAL REMEDIES

Hot water. Heat some water on the stove and pour it into a hot water bottle. Put the soothing heat on your stomach after you eat to help increase circulation to the abdominal area. Improved circulation may help improve digestion.

LIFESTYLE REMEDIES

Ax the alcohol. Alcohol is a stomach irritant.

Banish the aspirin. Aspirin and nonsteroidal anti-inflammatory drugs such as ibuprofen have been known to cause ulcers. If you're prone to tummy trouble, avoid both of these drugs.

Cut the coffee. Coffee causes stomach irritation in some people.

Don't skip meals. Acid will build up in your stomach and may leave you with an aching tummy.

Stress
PUTTING PRESSURE IN ITS PLACE

Stress. We all know what that's about, don't we? The traffic in your life is jamming up. Everything is fast-paced, high-pressured, loaded with responsibility. Some people thrive on that roller-coaster rhythm, but others don't, and the stresses in their lives begin to take a toll, physically and mentally. The stresses alter body chemistry and affect immunity.

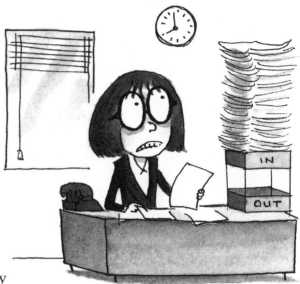

During a stressful event, the body shifts into red-alert mode, and the fight-or-flight response kicks in. Immediately, the endocrine system boosts its production of stress hormones such as epinephrine, nor-epinephrine, and adrenocorticotropic hormone (ACTH). As stress levels continue to increase, the blood pressure, heart rate, and amount of cholesterol released in the blood climb, and the hypothalamus releases endorphins, your body's own natural pain killers.

Your body can recover from occasional stresses. But when stress is chronic—when the body stays in red-alert mode for prolonged periods—health begins to suffer. Excessive amounts of stress hormones reduce the immune system's ability to fight disease. Constant surges in blood pressure and cholesterol production can damage

EXPERIENCE THE ESSENCE

Essential oils are beneficial in treating many problems. To relieve symptoms of stress, add 5 or 6 drops of lavender oil to a nice warm bath and allow yourself a 30-minute stress break. To beat that stress when you can't take a bath, put a few drops of the oil in a small glass (not plastic) bottle and carry it with you. Dab the oil on a handkerchief or tissue and inhale when you feel stressed. You can find 1-ounce glass dropper bottles at most pharmacies. Other stress-reducing oils: chamomile, sandalwood, geranium, cypress, juniper, rose, clary sage. Or add 1 to 2 drops of any of these essential oils to ½ cup warmed sesame oil to use for a wonderfully relaxing massage.

blood vessels and increase heart disease risk. The constant unleashing of powerful stress hormones can contribute to insomnia, migraines, backache, exhaustion, increased stomach acid, irritability, psoriasis outbreaks, sexual dysfunction, infertility, and stroke. What's more, highly stressed people may be at greater risk for a range of ailments, from the common cold to heart disease.

So, how's your stress level? If you answer yes to these questions, then read on. You may benefit from some of the home remedies for stress.

Stress on the job:

1. Are you overworked, underappreciated, or both?
2. Does it take everything you've got, physically, mentally, or both, just to make it from 9 to 5?

Stress at home:

1. Do you have enough time for the fun things?
2. Do people expect more from you than you want to give?
3. Are there some important relationships that should be better?
4. Are there some changes you'd really like to make in yourself?

If you find yourself muttering "yes" to half of these, you're stressed. To what degree depends on your ability to cope with stress. If you need a little relief, here it is.

DIETARY REMEDIES

Celery. The phytonutrients called phthalides found in celery have a widely recognized sedative effect, so eat your celery raw or chopped into a salad.

Cherries. They soothe the nervous system and relieve stress. Eat them fresh or any way you like them.

Lettuce. This stress-reducing veggie has a calming effect. A small amount of lactucarium, a natural sedative, is found in the white, milky juice that oozes from the lettuce when the stalk is snapped.

Oats. Besides fighting off high cholesterol, oats produce a calming effect that fights off stress. Use them in bread recipes and desserts or for thickening in soups. Or just eat a bowl of oatmeal! See Recipe Box, below, for a healthy oatcake recipe.

Pasta. When you're faced with eating a late-night meal, choose pasta. It causes a rise in the brain chemical serotonin, which has a calming effect on the body. Rice produces the same effect.

Whole-wheat bread. It's high in the B vitamins, which sustain the nervous system. Other B-rich foods include whole-wheat pita bread, whole-grain

FASCINATING FACT
If you're a pet lover, you know that quality time with Fluffy or Fido makes you feel better. Researchers believe that the pet effect has real health benefits, too, especially as a stress-buster. In fact, studies indicate that pet-lovers with heart disease have a higher survival rate than those with heart disease who don't have a pet in their lives. Why? Cuddling a pet seems to lower heart rate and blood pressure.

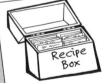

EASY OATCAKES

6 ounces regular oatmeal
½ teaspoon salt
½ ounce butter, softened
Additional oatmeal

Mix oatmeal and salt in bowl. Add butter and 5 ounces boiling water, and mix into a sticky dough. Let it stand for five minutes to allow oatmeal to expand. Then, sprinkle flat surface with a few tablespoons of oatmeal, turn dough out onto it, and knead lightly. Roll dough out as thinly as possible, sprinkling with more oatmeal to prevent sticking, then cut into circles, squares, or desired shapes. Bake at 325 degrees Fahrenheit for 15 to 20 minutes until dry and crisp but not browned. Use as you would a cracker.

MAKE 'EM LAUGH

Can you laugh stress away? Maybe not completely, but a hearty chuckle helps. In addition to making you feel better, laughing has other benefits.

- Laughing uses 15 facial muscles, and it's a great muscle toner.
- When you're laughing, your pulse and breathing speed up. This increases the amount of oxygen carried in the blood, giving your vital organs a vital boost in energy.
- After you laugh, there's a period of muscular relaxation, and for those who suffer arthritis or nerve pain, this can bring physical relief.
- For asthmatics and others who suffer lung problems, laughing increases air exchange in the lungs, increasing oxygen circulation and clearing out mucous plugs.
- Laughing exercises the heart muscle.
- Laughing boosts the immune system by increasing circulation. This helps the body fight off infection. The boost to circulation also reduces the risk of blood clots responsible for heart attack and stroke.

cereal, pasta, and brown rice. For a good stress-fighting diet, about 60 percent of your daily calories should come from these starchy foods, divided among your meals. Whenever possible, choose whole grains over refined grains.

HERBAL REMEDIES

Cardamom seeds. These are said to freshen the breath, speed the digestion, and cheer the heart, and they also bust the stress. To make a tea, cover 2 to 3 pods with boiling water and steep for ten minutes. Cardamom pods can be added to a regular pot of tea, too, in order to derive the calming effect. Also, crush the pods and add to rice or lentils before cooking, or use in a vegetable stir-fry. If you like the taste, cardamom seeds are a good addition to cakes and biscuits. Instead of pods, you can use 1 teaspoon powdered cardamom, which is available in the spice section of the grocery store.

Peppermint. Drink a cup of peppermint tea before bed to relieve tension and help you sleep. Chamomile, catnip, and vervain work well, too. Place 1 teaspoon of the dried leaf in a cup of boiling water. Sweeten with honey and sip before bed. To reap the fullest benefits, sipping this soothing tea should be the last thing you do before you tuck yourself in for the night. (Avoid catnip if you are pregnant or nursing.) During the day, if you don't have time for a cup of tea, try a peppermint. Read the label for a good variety, though. One with peppermint, sugar, and little else is best. The more extra ingredients that go into the candy, the less the relaxing benefit.

Tarragon. A tarragon tea calms the nervous system. Add ½ teaspoon dried tarragon to 1 cup boiling water. Or use it fresh, snipped into salads or vegetables. It's a good seasoning for creamy soups, too, or added to a salad dressing of balsamic vinegar with a dash of honey.

TOPICAL REMEDIES

Baking soda. A soothing bath in baking soda and ginger can relieve stress. Add ⅓ cup ginger and ⅓ cup baking soda to a tub of hot water and enjoy the soak.

Salt. Try this muscle-soothing bath to wash that stress away. Mix ½ cup salt, 1 cup Epsom salts, and 2 cups baking soda. Add ½ cup of the mix to your bathwater. Store the dry mix in a covered container, away from moisture.

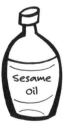

Sesame oil. For a nice relaxation technique, warm a few ounces and rub it all over your body, from head to toe. Sunflower and corn oil work well, too. After your massage, take a long, hot soak in the tub.

LIFESTYLE REMEDIES

Choose control. You can't control everything in your life, but that doesn't mean you should relinquish all control. Take control where you can. You'll find that a little control can go a long way in fighting stress. Make a list with two headings: "Things I Can Control" and "Things I Can't Control." When you see it in print, you'll be surprised how much of your life is already under your control. That, in itself, should relieve some stress.

WHEN TO CALL THE DOCTOR

- When you're experiencing symptoms. Stress symptoms mimic the symptoms of other serious illness, including thyroid disease; therefore it's vital that your doctor determine the cause of your problem.
- When stress interferes with normal daily activity, and home treatments do not work. There are medications available that can remedy symptoms.
- When stress causes any kind of chest pain, even mild pain

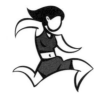

Exercise. The endorphins released in 20 minutes of aerobic exercise have a feel-good effect that reduces stress.

Find your purpose. Knowing your purpose can relieve stress, and if nothing special comes to mind, create a purpose. Volunteer at a homeless shelter, or make new friends at a nursing home. When you involve yourself in something other than your stress, it will actually decrease.

Nix the artificial stimulants. Caffeine, nicotine, alcohol—they may seem to relieve stress, but the effect is only temporary. In the long run, they can make you anxious and cause you more health problems.

Relax. Take some deep breaths. Give your stressed-out muscles a break, and soak in a nice warm tub or listen to relaxing music. Indulge in a flight of fantasy, read a book, meditate or pray, or take up a hobby. Squeeze your stress away. Make your own inexpensive stress ball by filling a small balloon with baking soda, then tying off the opening. Simply squeeze to reduce stress.

Seek support. It's easier to cope when someone is there to hold your hand.

Sunburn
SHIELDING YOUR SKIN

A sunburn is one of the most common hazards of the great outdoors. The unappealing and painful lobster look results when the amount of exposure to the sun exceeds the ability of the body's protective pigment, melanin, to protect the skin. What makes sunburn different from, say, a household iron burn? The time factor. A sunburn is not immediately apparent. By the time the skin starts to become red, the damage has been done. Pain isn't always instantly noticeable, either. You may feel like you're glowing after two hours sitting poolside without sun protection, but just wait awhile. You'll change your tune (not to mention color) when the pain sets in, typically 6 to 48 hours after sun exposure. Like household burns, sunburns are summed up by degree. Mild sunburns are deep pink, punctuated by a hot, burning sensation. Moderate sunburns are red, clothing lines are prominent, and the skin itches and stings. Severe sunburns result in bright red skin, blisters, fever, chills, and nausea.

Being burned to a crisp can lead to serious consequences later in life. In fact, one severe, blistering sunburn

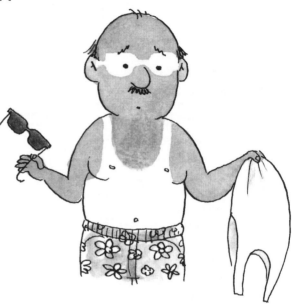

during childhood doubles your chances of developing melanoma, a potential deadly form of skin cancer. Sunburn also raises the risk of other types of skin cancer such as basal cell and squamous cell carcinomas. If cancer doesn't frighten you, then the specter of developing premature wrinkling and age spots just might.

Obviously, covering up and applying a waterproof sunscreen with a high SPF (sun protection factor) is the best way to prevent sunburn. However, if you slip up and expose your tender flesh to the fierce sun, these home remedies should help you chill out.

WAYS OF THE RAYS

Here on Earth, we're exposed to two types of ultraviolet rays: UVA and UVB. Unlike visible light, these rays are shorter in wavelength, are higher in energy, and fall outside the visible spectrum (so you can't see what's hitting you). When these high-energy rays strike your skin, they generate free radicals, which can damage DNA. UV damage can be short-term (a painful burn) or long-term (premature aging of the skin and skin cancer). What's the difference between UVA and UVB rays?

UVA: Ultraviolet A

- a longer wavelength
- penetrates the deep layers of the skin and produces damaging free radicals
- linked to premature aging of the skin
- can pass through window glass in cars, houses, and office buildings
- most common ray used in tanning beds

UVB: Ultraviolet B

- a shorter wavelength
- doesn't penetrate deeply into the skin
- can cause significant damage to DNA
- the primary cause of sunburn and skin cancer
- cannot pass through windows

DIETARY REMEDIES

Water. As the sun fried your skin, it also dehydrated it. Be sure to replenish liquids by drinking plenty of water while recovering from a sunburn. Being well hydrated will help burns heal better. You'll know you're hydrated when your urine runs almost clear.

TOPICAL REMEDIES

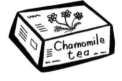

Baking soda. Adding a few heaping tablespoons of baking soda to cool bathwater makes a sunburn-soothing remedy. Just keep your soaking time down to 15 to 20 minutes. If you soak any longer, you risk drying out your already lizardlike skin. When you've emerged from the bath, resist the urge to towel off. Instead air-dry and don't wipe the baking soda off.

Chamomile tea. Brew dried chamomile in a tea and sponge onto affected areas. Make the tea by combining 1 teaspoon dried chamomile with 1 cup boiling water, or use a prepackaged chamomile tea bag. Cool and apply. Do not use chamomile if you have pollen allergies, or else you may suffer a skin reaction atop the burn.

Cornstarch. Sunburns often strike where skin meets bathing suit. Sensitive and hard-to-reach spots you've neglected to smear with suntan lotion (along bikini lines, underneath buttock cheeks, or around the breasts and armpits) often fall victim. These burn spots then have to face daily irritation from tight elastic in bras and underwear. To ease chafing, cover the burned area with a dusting of cornstarch. Don't apply petroleum jelly or oils, which can exacerbate the burn by blocking pores. If the burn is blistering, however, don't apply anything.

Milk. Cool off with a cold glass of milk. Don't drink it; put it right on your body. Soak a facecloth in equal parts cold milk and cool water, wring it out, and gently press it on the burned areas.

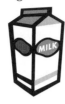

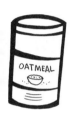

Oatmeal. Oatmeal added to cool bathwater offers wonderful relief for sunburned skin. Fill up the bathtub with cool water, not cold water since that can send the body into shock. Don't use bath salts, oils, or bubble bath. Instead, scoop ½ to 1 cup oatmeal—an ideal skin soother—and mix it in. Another option is to buy an oatmeal powder found in the pharmacy. Follow the packet's directions. As with the baking soda, air-dry your body and don't wipe the oatmeal off your skin.

Potatoes. The plain old potato makes for a wonderful pain reliever. It's a time-tested technique known throughout the world. Take two washed potatoes, cut them into small chunks, and place them in a blender or food processor. Blend or process until the potatoes are in liquid form. Add water if they look dry. Pat the burned areas with the

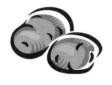

WHAT'S WITH THE WHITE NOSE?

There's no need to rush out and buy a fancy sunscreen to shield yourself from harmful rays. Sun protection is as close as your medicine cabinet. Remember that tube of zinc oxide tucked in the back? This thick white pasty substance is one of the best forms of skin protection, especially for protruding parts of the face such as the nose and ears. Zinc oxide, a natural mineral, contains particles that scatter, reflect, or absorb solar radiation, making it ideal for sunny climates. In fact, you've probably seen zinc oxide in action: Many lifeguards smear their noses with it. It's a complete cover up. If you'd rather not have your nose glowing white, there are now transparent zinc oxide ointments that may be more cosmetically appealing. Zinc oxide is also an ingredient in some sunscreens. Check the label.

PICKING THE RIGHT PLANT

There are 240 species of aloe, only four of which are recognized as being of nutritional or medicinal value to humans. When buying an aloe vera plant for sunburn relief, make sure it is the *Aloe barbadensis miller* variety. Fortunately, this is the most common variety.

The aloe vera plant grows in the dry regions of Africa, Asia, Europe, and the Americas. The cactuslike plant with

long, needle-sharp leaves filled with a clear, viscous fluid is a member of the lily family. Use only the clear liquid to treat sunburn.

WHEN TO CALL THE DOCTOR

- If there is extensive blistering with the sunburn
- If you feel nauseated or weak, run a fever, or have chills
- If a moderate or severe sunburn covers the facial area, hands, feet, or genital area

THE ALLURE OF ALOE

Aloe vera (aloe means a "shining bitter substance") has long been prized as a plant with healing qualities. The ancient Egyptians were particularly fond of the plant and referred to it as the "plant of immortality." They valued the plant so much that aloe was included among the funerary gifts buried with the pharaohs.

pulverized potatoes. Wait until the potatoes dry, then take a cool shower. A less messy method is to apply the mash to a clean gauze and place it on the burn. Change the dressing every hour. Continue applying several times per day for a few days until the pain is relieved.

Vinegar. Adding ½ cup vinegar to your cool bathwater can also take the sting out of the sunburn.

HERBAL REMEDIES

Aloe vera. The thick, gel-like juice of the aloe vera plant can take the sting and redness out of a sunburn. Aloe vera causes blood vessels to constrict. Luckily, this healing plant is available at your local nursery or even in the grocery store's floral department. (See "Picking the Right Plant," page 411.) Simply slit open one of the broad leaves and apply the gel directly to the burn. Apply five to six times per day for several days.

LIFESTYLE REMEDIES

Avoid these hours. Try not to go out in the sun between the hours of 10 A.M. and 3 P.M., because that's when the sun's rays are the strongest.

Learn the cloud cover myth. Don't think you're protected if the skies are cloudy. Damaging rays aren't inhibited by clouds, and you can still get burned. So wear sun protection or cover up even when it's cloudy.

Use a waterproof sunscreen if you'll be swimming or if you'll be sweating a lot. Reapply frequently (follow the directions on the label).

Check your meds. If you're taking any medications, be sure to check about side effects from sun exposure. Some medications, such as tetracycline, cause a rash on areas exposed to the sun.

Teething
CUTTING THROUGH PAIN

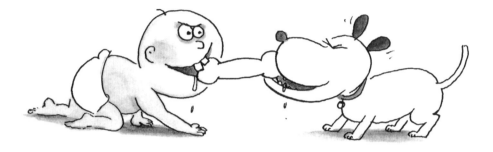

Just when you thought your bouncing bundle had started sleeping through the night, she decides to wake up the neighborhood with a 3 A.M. concert. You wander bleary-eyed into her room, wondering what in the world is the matter. You pick her up and hold her for a bit. As soon as you sit in your trusty rocker, your little miss sticks your finger in her mouth and starts gnawing. She's been doing this for a few months, but tonight you feel something firm and hard protruding out of her bottom gums. Her first tooth!

Teething Time

Your baby's first tooth is certainly a time for rejoicing. It's a real milestone in her life. And it also explains why your kid has been a drool factory, why she's been sticking anything and everything into her mouth lately, and why she's been so cranky. By the time that first tooth cuts through the gums, your baby has endured swollen, painful, inflamed gums for days or even months. They don't call it "cutting" teeth for nothing. Getting those first teeth is an ordeal for any kid.

Babies actually have tooth buds in place, resting right under the gums, before they're born. Those teeth then push their way through the gums, making their debut anywhere from four to eight months of age. The process of getting primary teeth continues until close to the third birthday. Your sweet pea will probably get her bottom front teeth first, followed by her top front teeth. Don't fret if she has huge gaps between teeth or if the teeth grow in a little crooked. Things will straighten out over time. By the time your little one is finished getting

DODGE THAT DROOL

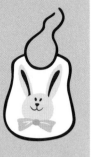

When the teething process hits high gear, baby steps up saliva production and becomes a drool machine. By the end of the day, your baby has soaked through his shirt, his pants, his sheets, your shirt, your pants, and almost every rag you have in the house. That overproduction of drool can sometimes irritate baby's face, cheeks, neck, and chest, giving him a mean rash.

To keep baby dry and drool-free, keep a cloth-covered bib on him at all times, except nap time and bedtime, and use it to wipe up any excess. Change the bib frequently. Also keep a cloth diaper or towel nearby to wipe any drool that may get on parts unreachable by the bib. If your baby's skin is sensitive to his saliva, try coating vulnerable parts with some petroleum jelly. That'll act as a drool repellent and keep your little dumpling clean and free from rashes.

that first set of teeth, she'll have 20 munching, crunching teeth. These will stay in place until she's ready for permanent teeth, sometime around her sixth birthday.

Teething is, of course, just a part of life. But there are some things you can grab at home that will ease your baby's discomfort and make her a happy camper—at least for a while.

DIETARY REMEDIES

Applesauce. Cold foods like straight-from-the-fridge applesauce taste good and are gum-friendly.

TOPICAL REMEDIES

Baby bottle. One trick for making baby happier during teething is to put water in a baby bottle and freeze the bottle upside down (so the water is frozen at the nipple). Give it to the baby when he gets fussy and let him chew on the cold, comforting nipple for a while.

Bagels. Refrigerate an ordinary bagel and it becomes your very own homemade teething ring. It's great for babies to gum on while they're getting teeth in and can help ease that teething ache.

 Bananas. Stick a banana in the freezer and then let baby put the soothing, sweet treat to her gums.

Dishcloth. Put a clean wet dishcloth or towel in the refrigerator and let it get nice and cold. Then give it to junior and let him gnaw away on the cloth. This will help ease inflamed gums and will feel good in baby's mouth.

Ice. Wrap some ice in a dishtowel and let baby suck on the towel. The cold ice will keep swelling down and ease baby's pain. But don't let

her suck on just the ice—it can be harmful to the baby's gums.

Spoon. Take a tip from the American Dental Association—stick a spoon in the fridge for a few hours and then let baby have at it. The cold metal against her gums will put a smile on her face.

Teething biscuit. These hard, unsweetened, crackerlike biscuits are great for gnawing on when teeth are making their way through the gums.

Teething Ring. Water-filled teething rings, which can be frozen, are a safe way to keep the area cold.

LIFESTYLE REMEDIES

Avoid topical teething meds. Teething gels or other medicines that are rubbed directly onto baby's gums can give baby a bit of relief, but they get washed away too quickly to bring any real comfort.

Ease the pain with medicine. Over-the-counter pain relievers such as acetaminophen or ibuprofen, formulated for babies, are perfectly fine to relieve your little sweetie's teething pain. Ibuprofen lasts six to eight hours compared to the four-hour duration of acetaminophen. So for nighttime relief, you might want to use something that lasts a bit longer. The amount you give your baby is based on weight, so check with your pediatrician about how much to administer.

Warning! Never give aspirin to a baby. It may cause a life-threatening condition called Reye's Syndrome.

WHEN TO CALL THE DOCTOR
• If your baby has any of these symptoms: diarrhea, a mild temperature, trouble sleeping, pulling at the ears, spitting up, or little interest in eating. These symptoms are sometimes associated with teething but could indicate something more serious and should be double-checked with your pediatrician.

WHERE HAVE ALL THE TEETH GONE?

You start out with 20 teeth. You lose all those and get permanent teeth, plus some. By the time you get all your choppers, including your wisdom teeth, you should have 32 teeth. But how many teeth does the average American adult have? 24.

Rub down that gum. Massaging your baby's gums with a clean finger will make him feel so much better. Of course, if baby already has a few teeth you might want to watch where you put that finger.

Keep the mouth clean. The American Dental Association says it's never too early to keep your baby's teeth and gums clean. Rub those gums with some gauze or a fresh cloth to clean the area and soothe teething pain. If your baby has already sprouted some teeth, try brushing them with a soft, child-size toothbrush.

THE PATTERN OF LITTLE TEETH

Though there are deviations in the typical pattern of teeth eruption, most babies will debut their teeth in a fairly consistent style. The first teeth usually peek through the gum between four and eight months, but there have been variations as wide as two months to twelve months. When your baby gets her teeth depends on you. If you got your teeth late, chances are your baby will go toothless as long as you did. However, if your baby is still sporting a gummy grin after 12 months, you might want to check with your doctor. Here are the ages at which your baby's teeth will typically erupt.

Lower Teeth
Central incisor 6 to 10 months
Lateral incisor 10 to 16 months
First molar 14 to 18 months
Canine (cuspid) 17 to 23 months
Second molar 23 to 31 months

Upper Teeth
Central incisor 8 to 12 months
Lateral incisor 9 to 13 months
First molar 13 to 19 months
Canine (cuspid) 16 to 22 months
Second molar 25 to 33 months

Ulcers
HEALING THE HOLE

It's only in the last decade that scientific evidence conclusively proved that ulcers are most often caused by a bacterial infection, not by the pressure-cooker type-A personality that was the subject of countless jokes. Misconceptions and myths die hard, though, so there are some people who haven't gotten the word yet and still believe that the demanding boss or the overachiever are more likely to work themselves into an ulcer. Although these personality characteristics may aggravate or slow down the healing of an existing ulcer, they don't cause them.

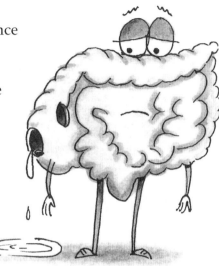

There's a Hole in the Bucket

An ulcer is a sore or hole in the protective mucosal lining of the gastrointestinal tract. Ulcers appear in the area of the stomach or the duodenum, the upper part of the small intestine, where caustic digestive juices, pepsin, and hydrochloric acid are present. Today we know that the majority of ulcers are the result of an infection with a bacteria called *Helicobacter pylori* (*H. pylori*). These bacteria makes the stomach and small intestine more susceptible to the erosive effects of the digestive juices. The bacteria may also cause the stomach to produce more acid.

There are some lifestyle factors that can contribute to the development of an ulcer. These include alcohol consumption, eating and drinking

FASCINATING FACT
Approximately 25 million Americans are expected to develop at least one ulcer during their lifetime, according to the University of Maryland Medical Center. Each year more than 40,000 people have surgery because of persistent symptoms or problems from ulcers, and about 6,000 die of ulcer-related complications.

DOWN WITH DECAF
Just when you thought you were being good by ordering decaf, along comes this discouraging news: Decaffeinated coffee may do as much harm to ulcers as the full-strength brew.

The effects of decaffeinated coffee were compared to those of peptone, a strong stimulant of acid secretion in the stomach. Researchers found that drinking unleaded brew produced more gastric acids than were produced by peptone. Who said decaf wasn't a stimulant?

foods that contain caffeine, significant physical (not emotional) stress such as severe burns and major surgery, and excessive use of certain over-the-counter pain medications such as aspirin or ibuprofen. Studies have shown that smoking also tends to increase the chances of developing an ulcer, slows the healing of existing ulcers, and makes a recurrence more likely. Family history of ulcers also appears to play a role in susceptibility.

Who Gets Ulcers?

If Type-A folks don't automatically get ulcers, then who does? The cause lies less in personality and more in stomach makeup. Researchers believe some people just produce more stomach acid than others. If stomach acid production isn't the problem, then a weak stomach may be. The stomach lining in certain individuals may be less able to withstand the onslaught of gastric acids. Lifestyle factors mentioned above can also weaken the stomach's lining.

Signs and Symptoms

You're probably familiar with the most typical symptom of a brewing ulcer: a burning or gnawing pain between the breastbone and navel. This pain is more common between meals (it improves with eating but returns a few hours later) and in the middle of the night or toward dawn.

Less typical symptoms include nausea or vomiting, weight loss and loss of appetite, and frequent burping or bloating.

If you have an ulcer or suspect you may have one, you should be under the care of a physician. Between visits to the doctor, there are ways to care for your digestive tract.

DIETARY REMEDIES

Bananas. These fruits contain an antibacterial substance that may inhibit the growth of ulcer-causing *H. pylori.* And studies show that animals fed bananas have a thicker stomach wall and greater mucus production in the stomach, which helps build a better barrier between digestive acids and the lining of the stomach. Eating plantains is also helpful.

Cabbage. Researchers have found that ulcer patients who drink 1 quart of raw cabbage juice per day can often heal their ulcers in five days. If chugging a quart of cabbage juice turns your stomach inside out, researchers also found that those who eat plain cabbage have quicker healing times as well. Time for some coleslaw! Just skip the mayonnaise because fat can aggravate an ulcer.

 Garlic. Garlic's antibacterial properties include fighting *H. pylori.* Take two small crushed cloves per day.

Plums. Red- and purple-colored foods inhibit the growth of *H. pylori.* Like plums, berries can help you fight the good fight, too.

HERBAL REMEDIES

Cayenne pepper. Used moderately, a little cayenne pepper can go a long way in helping ulcers. The pepper stimulates blood flow to bring nutrients to the 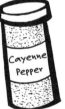 stomach. To make a cup of peppered tea, mix ¼ teaspoon cayenne pepper in 1 cup hot water. Drink a cup per day. A dash of cayenne pepper can also be added to soups, meats, and other savory dishes. Avoid this remedy if spices bother your stomach.

HERBAL RELIEF

By decreasing inflammation, chamomile helps speed up the healing process for ulcers. As an added bonus, chamomile contains a flavonoid called apigenin that can fight bacteria known to cause ulcers. To make chamomile tea, mix 1 teaspoon dried chamomile into 1 cup boiling water. Steep for 5 minutes and drink. Several cups per day may be helpful.

The medicine cabinet holds what many think is a cure-all for ulcers: antacids. When taken as directed, antacids are your stomach's ally and can relieve the discomfort of an ulcer attack. However, like all medications, antacids come with a dark side. Here's what you need to know to use antacids appropriately:

• Never self-medicate with antacids. Use them as directed by a physician.

• Aluminum-based antacids may cause constipation and may also interfere with absorption of phosphorus from the diet, resulting in weakness and bone damage over a long period.

• Magnesium-based antacids can act as a laxative and cause diarrhea.

• Consistent use of antacids may mask the symptoms of more serious disorders.

Licorice. Several modern studies have demonstrated the ulcer-healing abilities of licorice. Licorice does its part not by reducing stomach acid but rather by reducing the ability of stomach acid to damage the stomach lining. Properties in licorice encourage digestive mucosal tissues to protect themselves from acid. Licorice can be used in encapsulated form, but for a quick cup of licorice tea, cut 1 ounce licorice root into slices and cover with 1 quart boiling water. Steep, cool, and strain. (If licorice root is unavailable, cut 1 ounce licorice sticks into slices.) You can also try licorice candy if it's made with real licorice (the label will say "licorice mass") and not just flavored with anise.

Warning! Licorice can alter the action of a number of medications, including insulin, aspirin, ace inhibitors, and oral contraceptives. Large amounts can also contribute to water retention, headache, swelling, and heart attack. Follow package directions carefully and eat no more than recommended. Do not take licorice if you are pregnant or nursing.

LIFESTYLE REMEDIES

Control your stress. All that frustration and anxiety you carry around can aggravate ulcers or make the conditions ripe for one to appear. Work on ways to effectively control (and eliminate) stress. Take a stress management course, learn to meditate, do yoga, or exercise regularly! Do whatever it takes to let go of stress.

Don't smoke. Smokers have double the risk of developing ulcers. If that's not bad enough, ulcers heal more slowly in smokers, and their relapse rate is higher than average.

Limit alcohol intake. The question of alcohol's impact on ulcer formation remains unanswered, but many medical experts believe individuals who drink heavily are at higher risk for ulcer development compared to light drinkers or abstainers.

Nibble throughout the day. The key to keeping gastric juices from attacking the digestive tract lining is to keep them busy with food. Snacking on healthy treats, such as carrot sticks and whole-wheat crackers, should do the trick. Also, consider becoming a six-small-meals-per-day type person rather than a three-meals-per-day type.

WHEN TO CALL THE DOCTOR

- If you experience severe and sudden abdominal pain
- If your bowel movements are black or bloody
- If you vomit blood
- If you feel cold or clammy with no other explanation
- If you develop persistent nausea or vomiting
- If you lose weight for no reason
- If you have pain that radiates to your back

FOOD SURPRISES

Milk was an early treatment for ulcer flare-ups, but it is no longer considered a good drink if you have ulcers. Foods high in calcium, such as milk, stimulate stomach acid. And the fat in whole-milk can aggravate ulcer pain. Limit your milk intake according to your doctor's advice.

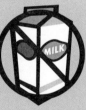

Highly spiced and fried foods, on the other hand, once were thought to be prime culprits in starting ulcers. However, research has shown that they have little or no bearing either on the development or the course of an ulcer. This is not to say that such food won't cause irritation. Watch what you pull from the refrigerator and note your gut reaction to each. If you experience discomfort, ban the food from the fridge. If nothing happens after popping that pizza slice into your pouch—rejoice and enjoy!

Urinary Tract Infection
BLASTING BACTERIA

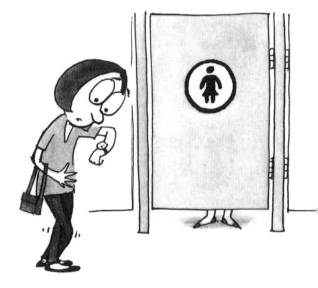

You stand in front of the bathroom door for the twentieth time in the last hour. You've got to go, but every time you do, you end up with only a painful trickle. You recognize the burning sensation that makes every trip to the toilet an ordeal. You've got a urinary tract infection.

Urinary tract infections (UTIs) are the second most common type of infection in the body. Men get UTIs, but they are much more common in women—one in five women will get a UTI in her lifetime.

If you've ever had a UTI, you'll probably never forget the symptoms. It usually starts with a sudden and frequent need to visit the potty. When you get there, you can squeeze out only a little bit of urine, and that's usually accompanied by a burning sensation in your bladder and/or urethra. In more extreme cases, you may end up with fever, chills, back pain, and even blood in your urine.

Bladder Control
UTIs are a result of bacteria, particularly *Escherichia coli* (*E. coli*) bacteria, taking temporary control of your bladder and your urethra (the tube that allows urine to flow from your bladder to the toilet). Women tend to get more UTIs for two reasons: They have a shorter urethra than men, and their urethral opening is precariously close to the vagina and the bacteria-loving anus, where *E. coli* and other bacteria normally hang out without causing harm. That means everyday body functions and sex are more likely to push bacteria into your urethra. Being pregnant also ups your risk of a UTI because your bladder is under a lot of pressure from your uterus and is more apt to entertain an infection. And if you use a diaphragm to protect against pregnancy, you put more

pressure on your urethra and are more likely to end up with a UTI.

Men get UTIs but not for the same reasons. If a man suspects he has a UTI, he should call his doctor; the UTI may be due to a bladder stone, an enlarged prostate, or a sexually transmitted disease such as gonorrhea. A prostate infection may also make its way to the bladder, causing a bladder infection.

When you have an infection in your lower urinary tract, the medically correct term for the condition is cystitis. If the infection is in your urethra, you've got urethritis. UTIs typically combine both cystitis and urethritis. Sometimes the infection is at the top of your urinary tract, closer to your kidneys. If you end up with this type of infection, it can easily spread to your kidneys, causing a condition called pyelonephritis. Pyelonephritis can cause more severe symptoms, including back pain, fever, nausea, and vomiting.

UTIs that last longer than two days require medical intervention. Untreated UTIs can infect the kidneys and turn into a much more serious problem. To help prevent a UTI from developing or nip one in the bud, try some of the remedies available in your own home.

DIETARY REMEDIES

Baking soda. Adding 1 teaspoon baking soda to your glass of water may help ease your infection. The soda neutralizes the acidity in your urine, speeding along your recovery. Don't do this if your doctor has told you to reduce your sodium intake.

A MATTER OF INCHES

The urethra in your average woman is about 1.5 inches long. The urethra in your average man: 8 inches.

HERBS FOR A BETTER BLADDER

In Germany, where herbs are treated as traditional drugs, asparagus, birch, couch grass, goldenrod, juniper, lovage, parsley, spiny restharrow, and nettle are often prescribed for UTIs.

TESTING FOR
BLADDER INFECTIONS
AT HOME

Do you get frequent bladder infections and don't want to leave a sample at the doctor every couple of months? Now you can test for bladder infections at home. The tests are FDA approved and cost about $12. Similar to a pregnancy test, you urinate in a cup and then check your urine with the dipstick. If the test shows infection, you can put a call in to your doctor and avoid having to spend time in a waiting room. If this is your first infection, though, you should see a doctor to get an accurate diagnosis and make sure nothing more serious, such as a kidney infection, is going on.

Blueberries. Blueberries and cranberries are from the same plant family and seem to have the same bacteria-inhibiting properties. In one study, blueberry juice was found to prevent UTIs. Since you're not likely to find a gallon of blueberry juice at your local store, try sprinkling a handful of these flavorful, good-for-you berries over your morning cereal.

Cranberry juice. Many studies have found that drinking cranberry juice may help you avoid urinary tract infections. It appears that cranberry juice prevents infection-causing bacteria from bedding down in your bladder because it makes your urine more acidic, and it also has a very mild antibiotic affect. Drinking as little as 4 ounces of cranberry juice per day can help keep your bladder infection-free. If you tend to get UTIs or are dealing with one right now, try to drink at least 2 to 4 glasses of cranberry juice per day. If pure cranberry juice is just too bitter for your taste buds, you can substitute cranberry juice cocktail. It seems to have the same effect as the pure stuff. Or purchase over-the-counter cranberry supplements designed for urinary tract health. Take note: If you have a UTI, cranberry juice is not a replacement for doctor-prescribed antibiotics in treating your infection.

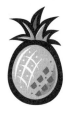 **Pineapple.** Bromelain is an enzyme found in pineapples. In one study, people with a UTI who were given bromelain along with their usual round of antibiotics got rid of their infection. Only half the people who were given a placebo plus an antibiotic showed no signs of lingering infection. Eating a cup of

pineapple tastes good and may just help rid you of your infection.

Water. If you tend to get urinary tract infections, be sure to drink plenty of water—about eight 8-ounce glasses per day. You should be urinating at least every four to five hours. If you are currently dealing with an infection, drink buckets of water to fight it off. Drink a full 8 ounces of water every hour. The river of water in your system will help flush out bacteria by making you urinate more frequently.

DIETARY SUPPLEMENT REMEDIES

Vitamin C. Some doctors are prescribing vitamin C for patients who develop recurrent urinary tract infections. Preliminary studies suggest that vitamin C may help pregnant women who are plagued with urinary tract infections. It keeps the bladder healthy by acidifying the urine, essentially putting up a no-trespassing sign for potentially harmful bacteria. Talk to your doctor before taking supplements if you are pregnant.

HERBAL REMEDIES

Goldenseal. This herb is a well-known infection fighter. It has a component called berberine that works much like cranberry juice in keeping harmful bacteria from camping out in your bladder. The typical recommended dose is 250 to 400 mg of goldenseal root extract containing 10 percent berberine, three times per day. Talk with your doctor before taking goldenseal if you have high blood pressure, are pregnant, or have diabetes.

Uva ursi. European doctors prescribe this herb for urinary tract infections. This herb has a chemical

WHY'S THAT LINE SO LONG?

You've been slurping sodas through the entire circus performance. But like everyone else under the big top, you don't want to miss the human cannonball, so you hold it until intermission. As soon as the lights come up, you run to the restroom, only to discover there's already a line around the corner. As your eyeballs begin to float, you glance over at the guy's restroom, where there's nary a man standing around waiting for a chance at the porcelain throne.

A group of researchers at Cornell University wanted to know if girls indeed spent more time in the restroom than guys. They set up shop at highway rest stops and counted the seconds each sex spent doing their duty. Men spent an average of 45 seconds using the toilet. Women spent almost twice as much time, an average of 79 seconds.

WHEN TO CALL THE DOCTOR

- If you have symptoms and also have shaking spells or have vomited in the last 12 hours
- If you have symptoms and a fever that get worse after a couple of days of home treatment
- If you have blood in your urine or pink-tinted urine
- If you have symptoms of a urinary tract infection and you have a history of kidney disease
- If you have symptoms of a urinary tract infection and have diabetes or are pregnant
- If you experienced a stomach or back injury during the two weeks before your symptoms started. This may indicate a kidney injury.
- If you have symptoms and high blood pressure
- If you have symptoms and are a man older than 50
- If you suspect you may have a sexually transmitted disease

that is converted by your urine to a bacteria-killing machine. If you have a urinary tract infection, the recommended amount of this herb is 3 to 5 mL of an uva ursi tincture three times per day.

TOPICAL REMEDIES

Hot water. Heat up some water on the stove, and pour it into a hot water bottle. Place the water bottle on your lower abdomen to help ease any pain caused by the infection.

LIFESTYLE REMEDIES

Consider cotton. Anything that comes into close contact with any of those ultra-personal areas should be cotton. Wearing cotton underwear or cotton-lined panty hose will help you stay fresher and dryer. Guys should go for boxer shorts.

Cut the caffeine. Also avoid caffeine-loaded drinks. Caffeine can irritate the bladder, which is the last thing you need when a UTI has taken hold.

Don't drink alcohol. Alcohol is an irritant to your bladder, just what you don't need when you're dealing with an infection.

Follow the rules for making love. If you're prone to getting UTIs, be sure you and your partner clean up before making love. After you make love, head to the bathroom to urinate and get rid of any potentially harmful bacteria. And try using a condom instead of a diaphragm. Diaphragms may promote UTIs.

Go with the flow. After urinating, be sure to wipe from front to back to keep bacteria from getting close to the urethra.

When you've got to go, go. If you hold your urine, you're more likely to get a backup of bacteria and end up with an infection.

Warts

BANISHING BUMPS

Old wives' tales abound about how people get warts. You've surely heard the one about catching them by touching a frog or toad. However, that's not how you get them.

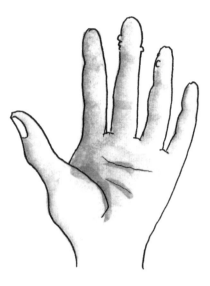

Warts are caused by the human papillomavirus (HPV), and there are more than 60 varieties of it. You get a wart from coming into contact with the virus through skin-to-skin contact. You can get the virus from another person, via a handshake for example, or you can actually give one to yourself if you already have a wart. You can spread the wart virus to other parts of your body by scratching, touching, shaving, or even biting your nails. All it takes is a little break in the skin for the virus to enter the system.

Culprit Categories

Before you can attempt to get rid of your wart, you have to be sure that little bump actually is one. There are three common varieties—common, plantar, and flat—according to the American Academy of Dermatology.

Common warts are found in areas where the skin has been broken: where fingernails are bitten down to the quick or hangnails are picked until they bleed. Often, they look like they have little dots or seeds in them, which is why they're frequently called "seed warts." But what you see aren't seeds; they're merely dots produced by the blood vessel supplying the infected area.

Common warts are:
- Small
- Flesh-colored
- Hard
- "Seedy" and rough to the touch
- Raised
- Often found on kids, because they always have some kind of sore on their fingers, and people with immune system deficiencies, since they are more susceptible to all types of viral infections.

WART STATS
- 10 percent of us get warts
- 50 percent of all warts disappear without treatment within 6 to 12 months

THOSE EMBARRASSING STRINGY THINGIES

You know those fat little strings of flesh that pop up on your face, neck, or eyelids? They're called filiforms, and yes, they're warts, too. You may be tempted to clip them right off, but don't! Clipping off any wart can cause the virus to spread and reinfect the area.

Plantar warts do not stick above the surface the way common warts do. That's because the pressure from walking pushes them back into the skin.

Plantar warts are:
- Usually found on the weight-bearing areas of the foot (*plantar* means bottom of the foot)
- Usually gray or brown
- "Seedy" and rough to the touch
- Hard
- Flat
- Painful. At the very least, a plantar wart can feel like a stone in the shoe. It can also cause a sharp, burning pain. At worst, the repetitive pounding of simple footsteps can irritate these nuisances, sometimes so badly they bleed.
- Able to grow to an inch in circumference or more and spread out into clusters called mosaic warts.

Flat warts are the smallest of the warts.

Flat warts are:
- Found in clumps of 20 to 100, usually on the face and neck, but also on the chest, knees, hands, wrists, and forearms. In men, they're common in the bearded area, most likely picked up from shaving irritations and nicks. In women, they're common on shaved legs.
- Tiny
- Flat
- Smooth
- Flesh-colored, gray, or brown

There are dozens of other kinds of warts, as well as other problems that may look like warts. If you have any concerns, consult your physician. What looks warty to you could be something much more serious, such as a skin cancer.

Waiting Them Out?

Warts can take a long time to go away, but most will if you wait long enough. Unfortunately, they also have a tendency to recur. Doctors aren't sure why, but some speculate that the "mother" wart sheds "babies" into the surrounding skin. And some people seem to have a susceptibility to warts. Adults get warts less frequently than children do, but warts in adults take longer to go away.

Wart Be Gone

There are many ways to rid yourself of a wart. Doctors can zap them with a laser, burn or freeze them, or give you topical medications that might do the trick. You can pay a pretty penny for these medical treatments, but if your warts are painful or multiplying rapidly, you may want to go the medical route. If not, and you have some time, there might just be a home remedy that will send your unsightly little nuisance into wart oblivion.

DIETARY REMEDIES

Foods. Eat foods that strengthen the immune system, such as broccoli, garlic, oranges, onions, red meats, rice, scallions, sunflower seeds, sweet potatoes, and whole-grain breads.

DIETARY SUPPLEMENT REMEDIES

Vitamin C. Crush 1 vitamin C tablet, and add water to make a thick paste. Apply it to the wart, then cover. The acid in the vitamin C may irritate the wart away.

Vitamin E. Break a vitamin E or A capsule, rub a little of the oil on the wart, and cover it with an adhesive

THE DANDELION CURE

If you've scorned the lowly dandelion growing in your lawn, you may change your mind if you've got recalcitrant warts. Pick a dandelion, break the stem, and rub the white milky juice on your wart two or three times per day until the wart is cured.

FASCINATING FACT

Some types of HPV cause common and plantar warts. These types of HPV do not cause genital warts.

GENITAL WARTS

Genital warts are also caused by the human papillomavirus, and they are one of the most common sexually transmitted diseases (STDs) in the world and the leading STD in the United States. Twenty million Americans are already infected, and 6.5 million cases are reported every year. Half of all sexually active people will contract genital warts in their lifetime.

Don't confuse genital warts with genital herpes (see page 211); they are not the same.

Curing genital warts is harder than preventing them, so protect yourself! Avoid sexual contact if you or your partner is infected. Latex condoms may reduce the risk of developing diseases that are linked to HPV, such as genital and anal cancers, but they cannot completely prevent the transmission of HPV. The only sure way to prevent HPV infection is to avoid all sexual activity.

A vaccine is now available that can protect girls and women from the four types of HPV that cause genital warts and most kinds of cervical cancer. The Centers for Disease Control recommends that girls receive the vaccine at age 11 or 12. It is also recommended for females ages 13–26 who have not already received the vaccine. There is no vaccine to prevent HPV diseases in men. Genital warts can cause serious complications during pregnancy and delivery and occasionally life-threatening problems in the newborn.

Go to the doctor if you suspect you have genital warts! There are treatments available. If the HPV infection is not cleared up, it can cause changes that lead to cancer in the cervix, vagina, and other areas.

bandage. Repeat three times per day. Remove the bandage at night to let it breathe, then start over with the oil in the morning.

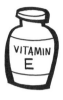

TOPICAL REMEDIES

Adhesive tape. Wrap a finger wart with four layers of adhesive tape. Wrap the first strip over the top of the finger and the second strip around the finger. Repeat both wrappings. Leave the adhesive in place 6½ days, then remove and let the wart breathe for half a day. Repeat the process until the wart is gone.

Baking powder. Mix baking powder and castor oil into a paste, then apply it to the wart at night, covering it with a bandage. Remove the bandage the next morning. Repeat as necessary.

Baking soda. Dissolve baking soda in water, then wash your wart-plagued hand or foot in it. Let your

hand dry naturally, with the baking soda still on it. Repeat often, until the wart is gone.

Figs. Mash up a fresh fig and place some on your wart for 30 minutes. Do this daily for two to three weeks.

Lemon juice. Squeeze a little lemon juice on your wart, then cover it with fresh, chopped onions for 30 minutes once per day for two to three weeks.

Pineapple juice. Soak your wart in pineapple juice. It has a dissolving enzyme.

HERBAL REMEDIES

Aloe. Break open an aloe leaf, and soak up the clear juice from the inner leaf on a cotton ball. Apply the cotton ball to the wart, and cover with a bandage. Repeat daily until the wart is gone.

Garlic. Rub crushed garlic or onion on your wart. Or eat fresh garlic. If you don't want to smell like an Italian cookery, try swallowing three garlic capsules three times per day—or munch on some breath-freshening parsley afterward.

MORE DO'S & DON'TS

- Don't scratch existing warts.
- Don't shake hands or share towels with someone who has an obvious wart.
- Use an electric razor if the area you shave has a wart. This helps to avoid the tiny nicks that will allow the virus to gain entry.
- Wash your hands with soap and hot water if you've touched a wart.
- Wear shoes or sandals in public places, including showers.
- Keep it dry. Warts love to multiply in moist areas.

WHEN TO SEE THE DOCTOR

- If the wart is causing problems: If it's unsightly or sore or it's in a place where it's constantly irritated, which increases the likelihood of spreading it.
- If the wart changes colors or bleeds
- If you're more than 45 years old and a new wart pops up. The doctor may want to look to make sure it's not skin cancer.
- If you have a plantar wart and also have diabetes or poor circulation in your feet

YOU'RE GETTING SLEEPY...AND WART-FREE

Hypnosis has helped rid many wart sufferers of their bumps. Some experts also suggest the power of positive thinking can do the trick, too. So keep a positive thought while you wish that wart away!

Water Retention
BEATING THE BLOAT

If you feel like the Goodyear blimp around "that time of the month," join the millions of other women who feel likewise. Water retention is part of the premenstrual syndrome (PMS) package. During this time, hormonal fluctuations can cause havoc in a woman's body. In some women, the monthly rise in estrogen turns on the faucet for the hormone aldosterone. Aldosterone, in turn, causes the kidneys to retain fluids and the woman to suddenly gain a few water-filled pounds.

Although PMS is the major cause of water retention in women, water retention for both men and women can also be related to kidney problems, both serious (kidney disease) and commonplace (not drinking enough water). Heart, liver, or thyroid malfunctions can also play a role in water retention. And, of course, eating too many salty foods can turn your body into a water-storage tank.

Thanks to the effects of gravity, retained water tends to flow southward and pool in the feet, ankles, and legs, although no area of the body is immune. Try to elevate your legs frequently. If you suffer from the occasional bloated-cow feeling due to PMS, eating too much, or not drinking enough water, there are ways to deflate yourself at home.

FASCINATING FACT
In an odd tribute to dandelion's diuretic effect, the French call it *pissenlit*, meaning to urinate in bed.

DIETARY REMEDIES

Bananas. Go ape and grab a few bananas. Slice them on your cereal, make a smoothie, or just peel and eat them plain. Bananas 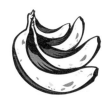 contain high amounts of potassium, which helps eliminate fluid retention. Not a banana fan? Munch on a handful of raisins instead.

Cabbage. A natural diuretic, cabbage can be added to salads or sandwiches. Enjoy a side of coleslaw for lunch.

Cranberry juice. Another natural diuretic. Drink it straight from the bottle.

 Salt. Around the time you expect your period, try to drastically reduce your salt intake. Sodium increases fluid retention, so don't use the salt shaker. If recipes call for salt, try adding more pepper or another spice instead. Most importantly, cut down on processed foods and fast foods, all of which are overflowing with salt.

Water. When you feel waterlogged, guzzling a glass of H_2O might be the last thing on your mind, but it may be the best thing for you. Water flushes out the system better than anything else and can reduce premenstrual bloating. Drink 8 to 10 glasses per day; more when you exercise.

 Yogurt. Too many rich treats will cause the stomach to bloat. If you've overindulged and are feeling the effects, treat your stomach to a cup of plain, low-fat yogurt that contains active cultures. The active cultures aid in digestion and increase the good bacteria in the gut.

BE KIND TO YOUR KIDNEYS

Kidneys, the two small bean-shaped organs located at the back of the abdominal cavity on either side of the spine, are the filters of the human body. Whatever enters the body, the kidneys sort like two efficient secretaries into a "Keep and Use" pile and a "Throw Out" pile. The "in" items are sent into the bloodstream, while the "out" items leave with body waste.

Unlike administrative assistants today, the kidneys are on duty 24–7 and hold down the extra job of making sure every office in the body is getting its share of water. When the water supply is diminished (for various reasons, including not drinking enough), the kidneys become sluggish and the entire body goes into panic mode. Every single cell and tissue holds on dearly to the water it already has, waiting for more.

Managing the kidneys is relatively easy. Keep them happy and functioning efficiently by drinking eight 8-ounce glasses of water per day, more if you exercise or it's hot or humid outside.

BLOAT BUSTER

It's the bane of the lawn, but it's the right plant for bloated people! The root of the lowly dandelion, especially when harvested after spring's first warm spell, is the best natural diuretic the garden delivers. In fact, dandelion's diuretic effect is comparable to prescription diuretics. But, unlike prescription drugs, this natural diuretic also delivers a wagon full of vitamins and minerals, including high amounts of vitamin A and moderate amounts of vitamins C and D, some B vitamins, iron, magnesium, manganese, and zinc. If you use your own dandelions for the following recipes, don't use any chemical sprays or fertilizers on your lawn. Also, don't pick dandelions from other people's lawns. Although the neighbors wouldn't mind, you can never be sure what chemicals have been used on their lawn.

Warning! Avoid dandelions if you have too much stomach acid, ulcers, diarrhea, irritable bowel syndrome, or ulcerative colitis. It is best to consult your doctor before using dandelions, especially if you are pregnant.

DIETARY SUPPLEMENT REMEDIES

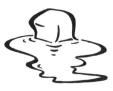

Vitamins A and C. When you feel like a balloon, try to increase your intake of vitamins A and C, both of which help diminish the fragility of capillaries and decrease water retention.

TOPICAL REMEDIES

Ice. When ankles puff up, applying an ice pack can help bring them back to normal size. Place ice cubes in a plastic bag with a zipper seal, wrap a light towel around the bag, and apply for five to ten minutes. A bag of frozen veggies also works well. In summertime, dip legs (ankle-deep) into a bath of ice water. People who have diabetes or poor circulation in their feet should skip the ice bath, however, unless directed to use it by their physician.

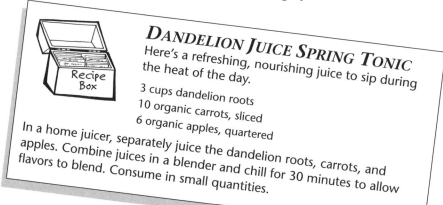

DANDELION JUICE SPRING TONIC

Here's a refreshing, nourishing juice to sip during the heat of the day.

3 cups dandelion roots
10 organic carrots, sliced
6 organic apples, quartered

In a home juicer, separately juice the dandelion roots, carrots, and apples. Combine juices in a blender and chill for 30 minutes to allow flavors to blend. Consume in small quantities.

Recipe Box

LIFESTYLE REMEDIES

Don't smoke.

Eat six small meals per day rather than three big ones.

Exercise. Ankles can swell like sour-
dough bread thanks to water retention. Luckily, avoiding la baguette
look just takes a little movement.
Exercises that work the calf muscles
help move blood and excess fluid out of the ankle
area. Regular walking, running, bicycling, and
aerobic dancing can work wonders. If ankles swell
while seated at work, try lifting your legs up
parallel to the floor every few minutes. During
breaks, walk around the office or up the stairs.
Spend a portion of the lunch hour on your feet,
exercising.

Junk the junk food. Not only is junk food bad for
you, but the excess salt tips the scales.

Keep your feet up. While resting, reading, or
watching television, prop a pillow under those
tootsies. A little help from gravity can go a long
way in draining fluid from swollen limbs.

Limit alcohol intake.

Stay loose. If you have to squeeze into your
pants, you can be guaranteed that pressure is
being placed on your upper thighs and waist, in
turn restricting the removal of fluids from the
lower legs.

Uncross your legs. Forget sitting ladylike! Doing
so limits the blood flow through the thigh veins,
in turn aggravating the swelling in the lower legs.

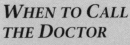

WHEN TO CALL THE DOCTOR

- If you are older than 45 and suddenly experience bloating and swelling, especially of the ankles
- If you are pregnant and experience water retention
- If water retention is disrupting your daily life
- If you're taking blood pressure medications or birth control pills and are retaining water. These can cause fluid retention.

NATURAL DIURETICS

A diuretic is a substance that tells the kidneys to increase the urine output above the normal call of duty. Diuretics help flush excess fluids from the body and, in doing so, make you feel less bloated. Unfortunately, many store-bought diuretics and caffeinated diuretics (coffee, tea) can also dehydrate you, deplete potassium reserves, unbalance electrolyte counts, and interfere with glucose production. In addition to the foods discussed in this profile, the following natural diuretics assist in ridding your body of excess H_2O without such side effects:

- Corn silk. The stringy stuff in corn makes an excellent diuretic. Fill a 1-quart jar ⅓ full of fresh corn silk. Pour boiling water to cover and let cool to room temperature. Strain and drink the quart in 4 doses each day for seven to ten days.

- Juniper berries. It seems everyone from the ancient Egyptians to various Native American nations has used these berries as a diuretic. Place 1 to 2 tablespoons juniper berries in the bottom of a 1-pint jar. Fill with boiling water and cover. Strain and drink the pint during the day. Do not use this remedy if you have kidney problems. Do not consume the tea for more than three weeks.

Warning! Diuretics are not advisable as a weight-loss method.

Yeast Infection
ACHIEVING A BALANCE

Normally, it's not a topic that comes up in polite conversation, and on the odd occasion that it does, it's approached in a whisper. No one wants to talk about a yeast infection, and no one wants to admit they have one. That's probably because it's known as one of those "personal" things that only affects women.

Well, in most cases that's true, but yeast infections are not restricted to women only. You know that diaper rash covering the cutest little bottom you've ever seen? Guess what? Yeast. And that condition called thrush that babies often develop in the mouth? Yeast again. So you see, yeast is not just about an unpleasant vaginal infection that no one wants to talk about. It's a fungus that can proliferate anywhere the breeding ground is right. And the breeding ground is right in the genital and oral areas because that's where *Candida albicans,* the fungus that causes a yeast infection, lives.

Yeast happens when the acidity of normal fluids is altered. Usually they're acidic enough to keep the yeast from flourishing. But when something goes

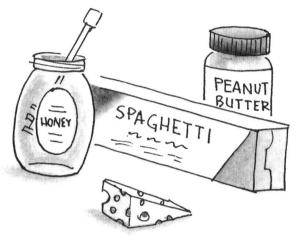

wrong, the balance is tipped and the yeast have a party, multiplying over and over. What causes the imbalance? Here are common factors:

- Weakened immune system
- Diabetes
- Overuse of antibiotics
- Steroids
- Certain medications used to treat cancer or suppress the immune system

In vaginal yeast infections, there may be additional factors:

- Hormonal changes, such as those that occur at puberty, pregnancy, or menopause
- Inadequate vaginal lubrication during intercourse

THE NO-NO FOOD LIST

Certain foods can contribute to conditions that give rise to a yeast infection. If you are prone to getting the infection or already have one, try avoiding these foods to see if that helps:

- Sugars, including white and brown sugar, honey, and molasses. Yeast feeds on sugar, so if you're prone to getting an infection, reduce the amount you eat. And during an infection, cut down further.
- Refined starches, such as refined pasta and white bread. Cut back if you're prone to getting yeast infections, and cut them out entirely when you have one. During the digestive process, refined starches break down into simple sugar.
- Alcohol. Those little *Candida albicans* really love the booze. It breaks down easily into sugar.
- Yeast and fermented foods, including breads and beer.
- Molds, including aged cheeses, mushrooms, dried fruits, fruit juice (unless it's fresh), peanuts, and peanut butter.

- Soap sensitivity
- Feminine hygiene deodorants and douches
- Spermicides

Yeast infections also can be transmitted between sexual partners. Using condoms or abstaining from sex during the infection are the best ways to prevent spreading it.

Typical symptoms of a vaginal yeast infection include intense itching and soreness accompanied by a thick white discharge. Symptoms of a genital yeast infection in men include irritation and itching in the genital area, sometimes accompanied by white discharge under the foreskin and/or swelling at the end of the penis. In the throat, yeast looks like creamy white patches (see "All About Thrush," page 441).

Most yeast infections can be cured with remedies found on the pharmacy shelf either in cream or suppository form. In addition, prescription medications are available that will stop the problem in as little as three days. There are also simple home panaceas that can bring relief or cure and even stop the disease from recurring.

DIETARY REMEDIES

Cranberry juice. Drink this one. Unsweetened, it may acidify vaginal secretions and equip them to fight off the yeast.

Yogurt. The live culture in plain yogurt is a great remedy for a yeast infection, helping to restore the acid-bacteria balance in more ways than one. Of course, you can eat yogurt. You can also insert 1 to 2 tablespoons into your vagina, apply it externally to the affected area (anal or vaginal), or use it as a douche by diluting it with warm water.

Salt. If mouth sores develop with thrush, gargle with a mixture of ½ cup lukewarm water and ½ teaspoon salt to promote healing.

Water. For a baby with thrush, give ½ ounce boiled, cooled water after a feeding to wash away milk remnants that contain milk sugars, which yeast love to feed on.

HERBAL REMEDIES

Basil. For thrush, make a basil tea and use it as a gargle. Boil 3½ cups water, remove from heat, and add 1¼ teaspoons ground basil. Cover and steep for 30 minutes. Cool and gargle. Or sweeten to taste with maple syrup and drink 1 cup twice per day.

Garlic. Eating 2 fresh garlic cloves per day, either plain or minced and tossed in a salad or sauce, may prevent yeast infections or help clear up a case of thrush. Garlic has antifungal properties.

Rosemary. To relieve itching and burning, make a tea of rosemary, and use it as a douche or dab it onto the external area.

Thyme. Make a thyme tea using 1 teaspoon dried thyme per 1 cup boiling water. Steep and drink 1 to 4 cups per day if you have a yeast infection.

TOPICAL REMEDIES

Baking soda. For thrush, brush your teeth after every meal with a mild toothpaste of baking soda and water. Commercial toothpaste may be too harsh if sores develop. Pour a little baking soda in your hand and add just enough water to make a paste. Then, rinse with ½ cup

---

THE THUMBS-UP FOOD LIST FOR YEAST INFECTIONS

It's important to keep the immune system strong when fighting off a yeast infection. Here are some immune-boosting foods to add to your grocery list:

- Raw vegetables and juice
- Green leafy vegetables
- Winter squash
- Whole grains

VAGINAL YEAST STATS

- 7 out of 10 women will have a yeast infection at some time in their lives
- 4 out of 10 women will have recurring yeast infections

WHEN TO CALL THE DOCTOR

- If you have abdominal pain
- If you have bloody discharge between menstrual periods
- If discharge gets worse or lasts longer than two weeks
- If you think you've been exposed to a sexually transmitted disease
- If you have recurrent yeast infections. This could be a sign of diabetes.
- If you have chills or fever
- If you have back pain
- If your symptoms resemble those for *Trichomonas* or *Gardnerella*.

warm water and 1 tablespoon of three percent hydrogen peroxide. Replace your toothbrush when the infection is cured.

Licorice powder. Boil 1 pint water and add 1 teaspoon licorice powder. Steep it, strain, but don't drink. Use the liquid as a vaginal douche.

Vinegar. Make a mild vinegar douche and use at the first sign of problems. Mix 1 to 3 tablespoons white vinegar with 1 quart of water.

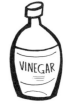

LIFESTYLE REMEDIES

Avoid stressful situations. They can bring on infection.

Be selfish. Don't share towels, and don't bathe with anyone. Yeast is contagious.

Choose contraceptives with care. Some people who take birth control pills or use the contraceptive sponge are more prone to getting yeast infections, so talk to your doctor about the best choices for you.

Don't use feminine hygiene products. That includes sprays, soaps, and perfumes. The chemicals in them cause irritation.

Dry yourself thoroughly after a shower.

Remove a wet bathing suit as soon as possible.

Skip the nylon undies. Nylon holds in moisture and heat. Instead use breathable cotton.

Trade in the tight jeans for baggies. Tight clothes can be responsible for creating the perfect breeding ground for yeast: moist and hot.

Try an over-the-counter antifungal cure.

THE PROPER DOUCHE

Regular douching isn't advised when you're not experiencing vaginal symptoms because it can disturb the natural pH balance and contribute to pelvic inflammatory disease. Certain studies have even linked regular, unnecessary douching to cervical cancer. So cancel the regular routine. If you're experiencing a yeast infection, a mild vinegar douche can return vaginal secretions to their proper acidic level. And douching with a yogurt solution may restore some of the vital yeast-fighting organisms that are reduced during an infection. For the best douche results, here are some easy steps:

1. Prepare the vinegar or yogurt solution.
2. Use a clean container, tube, and nozzle.
3. Lie in the tub with your legs parted and a folded towel under your buttocks.
4. Suspend the container 12 to 18 inches above the hips.
5. Insert the nozzle into the vagina with a gentle rotating motion until it encounters resistance, about two to four inches.
6. Use your fingers to close the vaginal lips until a little internal pressure builds up. This allows the solution to reach the entire internal surface.

   An effective douche takes about ten minutes.

ALL ABOUT THRUSH

This oral yeast infection shows itself as a heavy, whitish coat on the tongue and as patches that resemble cottage cheese curds on the mucous membranes in the mouth. It can spread to the gums, lips, and throat, and in rare cases, to the skin around the mouth or into the esophagus. Thrush is most common in newborns, who pick up a yeast infection from an infected mother during a vaginal birth; in people who practice oral-genital sex; in people who take certain medications such as antibiotics and corticosteroids; and in people with suppressed immune systems, especially AIDS.

Thrush must be treated by a physician, and there are several medications that will clear it up. For home helpers that relieve symptoms or prevent further outbreaks, see the cures in this profile.

In the meantime, if you or a household member has thrush, take the following precautions:

• Sterilize shared household items and boil eating utensils.
• Keep cups and glasses separate, or use disposables and dispose after one use.
• Rest, exercise, and eat a balanced diet to keep the body's resistance up.
• Until your infection clears up, run your toothbrush through the dishwasher or sterilize it daily in boiling water to prevent reinfection.

Index